Protein Purification
Second Edition

The Basics
Published Titles

Buffer Solutions, *by R. J. Beynon and J. S. Easterby*
Plant Cell Culture, *by D. E. Evans, J. Coleman, and A. Kearns*
Animal Cell Culture and Technology, *by Michael Butler*
PCR, Second Edition, *by Michael J. McPherson and Simon Geir Møller*
Measuring Gene Expression, *by Matthew Avison*
Protein Purification, *by Philip L. R. Bonner*
Working with DNA, *by Stan Metzenberg*
Protein Purification, Second Edition, *by Philip L. R. Bonner*

For more information about this series, please visit:
https://www.crcpress.com/THE-BASICS-Garland-Science/book-series/BS

Protein Purification
Second Edition

Philip L. R. Bonner

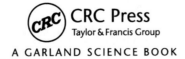

CRC Press
Taylor & Francis Group

A GARLAND SCIENCE BOOK

CRC Press
Taylor & Francis Group
6000 Broken Sound Parkway NW, Suite 300
Boca Raton, FL 33487-2742

© 2019 by Taylor & Francis Group, LLC
CRC Press is an imprint of Taylor & Francis Group, an Informa business

No claim to original U.S. Government works

Printed on acid-free paper

International Standard Book Number-13: 978-0-8153-4488-9 (Paperback)
International Standard Book Number-13: 978-1-138-31247-0 (Hardback)

Library of Congress Cataloging-in-Publication Data

Names: Bonner, Philip L. R., author.
Title: Protein purification / Philip L.R. Bonner.
Other titles: Basics (Taylor & Francis)
Description: Second edition. | Boca Raton : Taylor & Francis, 2018. | Series: Basics | Includes bibliographical references and index.
Identifiers: LCCN 2018013444| ISBN 9781138312470 (hbk. : alk. paper) | ISBN 9780815344889 (pbk. : alk. paper)
Subjects: | MESH: Proteins--isolation & purification
Classification: LCC QP551 | NLM QU 55 | DDC 612/.01575--dc23
LC record available at https://lccn.loc.gov/2018013444

**Visit the Taylor & Francis Web site at
http://www.taylorandfrancis.com**

**and the CRC Press Web site at
http://www.crcpress.com**

CONTENTS

DETAILED CONTENTS

Chapter 5   Non-Affinity Absorption Techniques Used to Purify Proteins   119

PREFACE

This book *Protein Purification* (Second Edition) remains a basic guide to the various protein purification techniques currently available, which enable scientists to enrich a protein of interest from extracts of prokaryotic and eukaryotic cells. It is designed for use in the laboratory and for self-study on the properties of proteins. The book has been expanded from the first edition with a starting chapter on the properties of water, pH and buffers. I have added a chapter on the structure and properties of proteins, which prior to a short description of chromatography. These introductory sections precede chapters on ion exchange, hydrophobic interaction, affinity and size exclusion chromatography, finishing with the techniques required to assess the purity of the prepared sample. I hope that the new organisation allows the reader to acquire progressively the information required for the successful chromatography of proteins. There are the usual flowcharts, diagrams, additional exercises and protocols to help in the analysis of any protein purification results obtained. The list of abbreviations and extensive glossary have been included to help the reader with the nomenclature. Throughout the book, there are comparisons drawn between the use of techniques in a laboratory with those in a larger-scale setting. The book is aimed at those who are relatively new to purifying proteins as well as providing a useful resource for more experienced scientists.

I would like to acknowledge the support of Liz (my wife), Francesca (my daughter) and my family, including Mark, Sarah, Erin, Harry, Neil, Clare, Ewan, Keira and James. I would also like to thank my work colleagues/friends Alan and David (Taylor & Francis) for their help and support throughout the preparation of this book.

ABBREVIATIONS

A_{280nm}	Absorbance at 280nm
ΔA_{440nm}	change in absorbance at 440nm
ADP	Adenosine 5′-diphosphate
AMP	Adenosine 5′-monophosphate
ATP	Adenosine 5′-triphosphate
BCA	Bicinchoninic acid
BCIP	5-bromo-4-chloro-3-indolyl phosphate
BICINE	N,N-bis-(2-Hydroxyethyl)glycine
bis-Tris propane	1,3-bis[Tris(hydroxymethyl)methylamino]propane
BSA	Bovine serum albumin
CAPS	3-[(3-cholamidopropyl)dimethylammonio]-1-propanesulfonate
CE	Capillary electrophoresis
CHAPS	3-[3-(cholamidopropryl) dimethylammonia]-1-propane sulfonate
CHAPSO	3-[(3-cholamidopropyl)dimethylammonio]-2-hydroxypropanesulfonic acid
CHES	2-(N-cyclohexylamino)ethanesulfonic acid
CMC	Critical micelle concentration
CTAB	Cetyl trimethylammonium bromide
Da	Dalton
DEAE	Diethylaminoethyl (as in DEAE IEX)
DIECA	Diethyldithiocarbamate
DMF	Dimethyl formamide
DTT	Dithiothreitol
E64	Trans-epoxy succinyl-L-leuculamido-(4-guanidino) butane
E.C.	Enzyme classification
E. coli	*Escherichia coli*
ECL	Enhanced chemiluminescence
EDTA	Ethylenediaminetetraacetic acid
FITC	Fluorescein isothiocyanate
GPI	Glycosylphosphatidylinositol
HA	Hydroxyapatite

HCIC	Hydrophobic charge induction chromatography
HEPES	N-2-hydroxyethylpiperazine-N′-2-ethanesulphonic acid
HIC	Hydrophobic interaction chromatography
HPLC	High-pressure liquid chromatography
HRP	Horseradish peroxidase
IDA	Iminodiacetate
IEF	Isoelectric focusing
IEX	Ion exchange chromatography
IgA	Class A immunoglobulin
IgG	Class G immunoglobulin
IgM	Class M immunoglobulin
IMAC	Immobilised metal ion affinity chromatography
I.U.	International units of enzyme activity
KSCN	Potassium thiocyanate
LDH	Lactate dehydrogenase
Lubrol (PX;12A9)	2-dodecoxyethanol
2-ME	2-mercaptoethanol
MBI	Mercapto-benzimidazole sulfonic acid
MEP	4-mercapto-ethyl-pyridine
MES	2(N-morpholine)ethane sulphonic acid
MMC	Mixed mode chromatography
MOPSO	3-(N-morpholino)-2-hydroxypropanesulfonic acid
M_r	Relative molecular mass
MWCO	Molecular weight cutoff (used in ultrafiltration membrane selection)
NAD^+	Nicotinamide adenine dinucleotide (oxidised)
$NADP^+$	Nicotinamide adenine dinucleotide phosphate (oxidised)
NaSCN	Sodium thiocyanate
NBT	Nitroblue tetrazolium
Nonindet (P40)	Ethylphenolpoly(ethylenglycolether)$_{11}$
NTA	Nitrilotriacetate
PAGE	Polyacrylamide gel electrophoresis
2D PAGE	2-dimensional polyacrylamide gel electrophoresis
PBS	Phosphate buffered saline
PEEK	Polyetheretherketones
PEG	Polyethylene glycol

PIPES	1,4-piperazinebis(ethanesulphonic acid)
PMSF	Phenylmethylsulphonyl flouride
psi	Pounds per square inch (a unit of pressure)
PVPP	Polyvinylpolypyrrolidone
RCF	Relative centrifugal force
R$_f$	Relative mobility (retention factor or relative to the front)
RPC	Reversed-phase chromatography
r.p.m.	Revolutions per minute
SDS	Sodium dodecyl sulphate
SEC	Size exclusion chromatography
S.I.	Système International
TBS	Tris buffered saline
TCA	Trichloroacetic acid
TCE	Trichloroethanol
TCEP	Tris(2-carboxylethyl)phosphine/HCl
TEMED	N,N,N′,N′,-tetramethylethylenediamine
Tricine	N-[Tris(Hydroxymethyl)methyl]glycine
Tris	2-amino-2-hydroxymethylpropane-1,3-diol
Triton	t-Octylphenoxypolyethoxyethanol
Tween	Polyoxyethylene sorbitan monolaurate polysorbate
UV	Ultraviolet
V$_e$	SEC elution volume
V$_o$	The void volume of an SEC column
V$_t$	The total volume of an SEC column
v/v	Volume/volume
w/v	Weight/volume

Water, pH and Buffers

1.1 INTRODUCTION

The surface of the Earth is covered in 70% water and approximately 98% of the total water is contained within the oceans, inaccessible as **potable** water. Fresh water comprises the remaining 2% of global water, which is predominantly locked up in the polar ice caps (1.6%), aquifers (0.36%) and lakes/rivers (0.036%). The small percentage of the total water that remains is contained within the atmosphere as clouds and living matter.

The composition of cells that make up living matter is dominated by water, which accounts for between 60–70% of the cell's weight. The solubilising properties of water help to keep **polar** molecules in solution and the non-polar molecules (e.g., lipids) are driven to adopt structures that avoid contact with water. The contents of every cell, from small metabolites to large macromolecular structures like proteins, have an intimate association with water, such that proteins lack biological activity when hydrating water is not present. The movements (**conformational** changes) that proteins undergo during biological activity are also linked to the protein's hydration level, with the water molecules acting as a lubricant to facilitate conformational changes. Water is also involved in an **enzyme's substrate** specificity and catalytic mechanism.

Within the cell, proteins are required for a variety of tasks, including structural support, catabolic and anabolic processes, replication and cell division. To achieve these tasks proteins must fold into their structurally active conformations, with approximately 80% of the protein's peptide groups and non-polar side chains of amino acids tightly embedded in the centre of the protein's structure. The amino acids with polar side chains are presented on the surface of the protein, interacting with water molecules (see Chapter 2) helping to maintain the protein in solution. The water molecules associated with the surface of a protein make up the protein's solvation (hydration) shell. This dynamic coating of the protein's surface is approximately two layers deep, and the water molecules are constantly exchanging places with water molecules in the surrounding cell medium (bulk phase). The depth of the solvation shell can vary, because the surface topography of a protein is not smooth like a snooker ball; it contains a variety of ridges and valleys where water molecules may form a closer association with the protein's surface polar groups or an enzyme's active site. The solubility of a protein is not solely dependent on its association with water; the presence and concentration of **anions**, **cations** (see Chapter 2) and the **pH** of the surrounding medium are critical to maintaining a protein in solution. An appreciation of the structure and properties of water, the basis of pH and the concept of buffering are invaluable in experimental biochemistry and designing a protein purification protocol.

1.2   THE STRUCTURE OF WATER

Water comprises two molecules of hydrogen covalently bonded to a molecule of oxygen (H_2O). This structure provides the molecule of water with an uneven distribution of electrons (see Figure 1.1A) described as a **dipole** moment. The presence of this dipole moment in water is fundamental to many of the unique properties of water. The electron-depleted area in one water molecule (Δ+ve) can form an attractive interaction called a **hydrogen bond** (H-bond; see Figure 1.1B) with the electron-enriched areas (Δ-ve) of other water molecules. The hydrogen bond donor is the atom attached to the hydrogen atom which is characterised by electron withdrawing negativity (e.g., oxygen or nitrogen). This results in the hydrogen atom showing the dipole positivity (Δ+ve). The hydrogen bond acceptor is an adjoining molecule with a lone pair of electrons (Δ-ve), providing the attractive interaction in the hydrogen bond between the positively charged donor atom and the negatively charged acceptor atom. Table 1.1 indicates the common hydrogen bond donor and acceptor interactions in biology.

In water, most of the molecules are engaged in hydrogen bonding with neighbouring water molecules, each bond lasting between 1–20 picoseconds (1 picosecond = 10^{-12} seconds) before a new H-bond is reformed or another H-bond formed with another neighbouring water molecule.

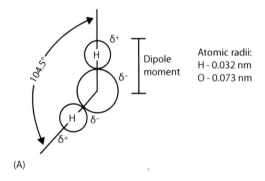

Dipole moment

Atomic radii:
H - 0.032 nm
O - 0.073 nm

104.5°

(A)

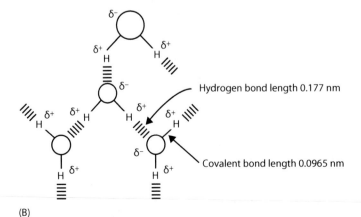

Hydrogen bond length 0.177 nm

Covalent bond length 0.0965 nm

(B)

Figure 1.1 (A) Shows the dimensions and structure of water. In (B) the hydrogen bonding network in water indicates that the covalent bond length is shorter and stronger than the hydrogen bond length. Small increases in heat will be sufficient to break the hydrogen but not the covalent bonds.

Table 1.1 Hydrogen bonding found in the interactions between other biological molecules.		
Hydrogen bond donor	Hydrogen bond acceptor	Comments
-O-H	O< H O=C<	Water and H-bonding to other biological molecules in solution
>N-H	O< H	

The amount of H-bonding in water decreases as the temperature rises because the H-bond dissociation energy is relatively low (23 kJ mol^{-1}) compared to the energy required to break an O-H covalent bond (470 kJ mol^{-1}) or a C-C covalent bond (348 kJ mol^{-1}). The increase in thermal energy on heating is sufficient to disrupt the H-bond network in water.

Many of the anomalous properties of water can be attributed to the dipole moment within the structure of the water molecule. For example, most solids are denser than their liquid or gaseous forms (with density defined as the mass of a substance divided by its volume). Pure water is the only substance that has its maximum density in its liquid form at 4°C, which is why ice floats on cold water. In addition, the surface tension of water results from the attractive dipole forces. Below the air-liquid interface (bulk phase) water molecules are attracted equally in all directions, whereas at the interface between air and water the top layer of water molecules does not have neighbouring water molecules on all sides. This means the water molecules at the surface are pulled together into a smaller space, creating internal pressure. This internal pressure or surface tension allows some insects to walk across the surface of water.

1.3 WATER AS A SOLVENT

Polar molecules with separate regions of positive and negative charge (dipole moment) will align themselves when an electrical field is applied. This is called the **dielectric constant (permittivity)**. Water has an extensive network of H-bonded molecules that opposes alignment, dispersing the applied electric field. The high dielectric constant of water (80.1 at 20°C) means that water has the ability to overcome the attractive ionic forces between two oppositely charged ions. For example, when sodium chloride (NaCl) crystals are placed in a solution of water, the positive end of the water molecules' dipole moment will surround the negative chloride ions in the crystal lattice, drawing the chloride ion into solution. The same process is repeated for the positive sodium ions (see Figure 1.2) until all the ions are held in solution. There is a limit to the amount of any salt that can be dissolved in a given volume of water at a given temperature (e.g., NaCl 359 mg ml^{-1} at 20°C; $(NH_4)_2SO_4$ 754 mg ml^{-1} at 20°C). When the solubility limit has been exceeded, the salt will remain solid in the liquid environment and over time will gather at the bottom of the vessel, resulting in a saturated solution.

Compounds in nature exhibit a range of solubility in water. Polar and ionic compounds readily dissolve in water and are described as **hydrophilic**. Compounds that have few or no polar elements to their structure are described as **hydrophobic** because they cannot interact with water. Water molecules near these hydrophobic elements form ordered **clathrate** structures around the hydrophobic element (see Figure 1.3).

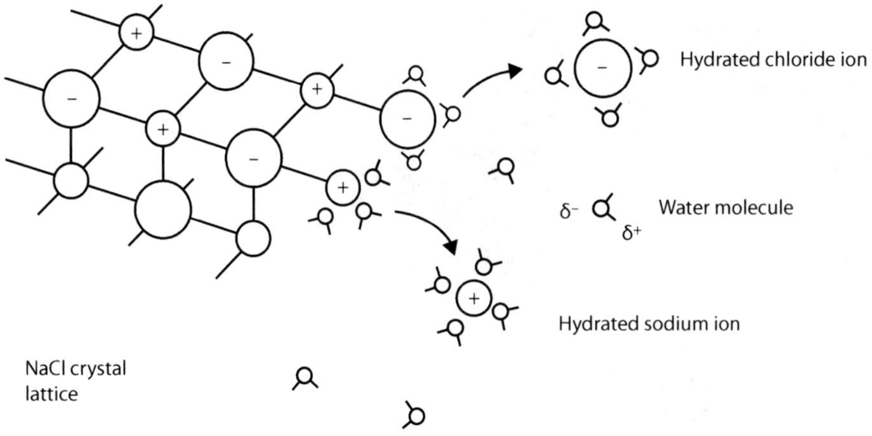

Hydrated chloride ion

Water molecule

Hydrated sodium ion

NaCl crystal lattice

Figure 1.2 Water as a solvent solubilising ionic crystals.

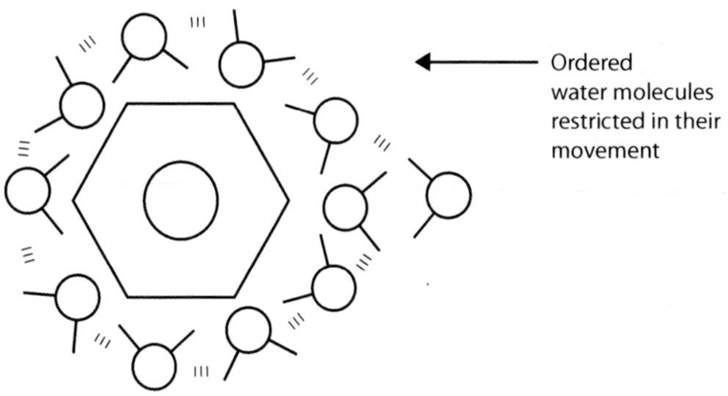

Ordered water molecules restricted in their movement

Figure 1.3 Clathrate water forms around hydrophobic molecules.

Interactions between water and non-polar compounds can be explained in terms of thermodynamics (see Appendix 1). An increase in clathrate water molecules with restricted movement is thermodynamically unfavourable because the entropy within the system decreases. Hydrophobic compounds in water will gather together, releasing water from the restricting clathrate structures thus presenting a smaller surface area of clathrate water ($-\Delta G$; therefore thermodynamically favourable). For example, when olive oil (composed of a variety of hydrophobic fatty acids) is introduced to a flask containing water, it does not mix with water but remains floating on the surface of the water, forming an interface between the two **immiscible** liquids (see Figure 1.4). If the vessel is agitated the oil will be dispersed into many small self-contained oil droplets, each with a coating of clathrate water. This is thermodynamically unfavourable because the entropy of the system has decreased due to the increase in clathrate water. The oil droplets will coalesce, releasing water from the restricting clathrate structures and presenting a smaller total of clathrate water molecules ($-\Delta G$; therefore thermodynamically favourable). Eventually the two immiscible phases will reform to produce the lowest number of clathrate water molecules in the system and the best possible thermodynamic state for the system. Please note that when oil floats on the surface of water, there are still water molecules with clathrate water structures at the interface between the water and oil (see Figure 1.4). This represents the lowest number of clathrate water molecules for this system and hence the most favourable thermodynamic level for this system.

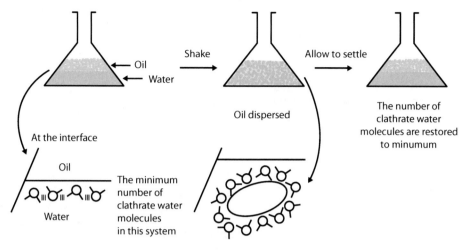

Shake

Allow to settle

Oil

Water

Oil dispersed

The number of
clathrate water
molecules are restored
to minumum

At the interface

Oil

Water

The minimum
number of
clathrate water
molecules
in this system

Oil droplets dispersed increasing
the number of clathrate water
molecules (thermodynamically
unfavourable)

**Figure 1.4 The interaction
between oil and water (two
immiscible liquids).**

1.4   THE IONISATION OF WATER

The dipole moment in the structure of water (see Figure 1.1B) allows adjacent water molecules to form H-bonds. In the dipole, the relatively large oxygen atom tends to hog the electrons, making the hydrogen protons loosely held in the structure and allowing protons to be exchanged between water molecules (and other molecules containing hydrogen). This exchange of protons does not alter the charge on the molecule, but at a relatively low level (two molecules in every billion) water molecules can ionise into a negatively charged hydroxyl group (OH$^-$) and a positively charged **hydronium ion** (H$_3$O$^+$). This represents another very important property of water.

$$H_2O \rightleftharpoons H^+ + OH^-$$

$$H_2O + H^+ \rightleftharpoons H_3O^+$$

Summary: $2H_2O \rightleftharpoons H_3O^+ + OH^-$

In a reaction at a given temperature, when the rate of dissociation is equalled by the rate of association, the reaction is at equilibrium. The equilibrium constant for water (K_{eq}) at 25°C is given by the equation:

$$K_{eq} \rightleftharpoons \frac{[H_3O^+][OH^-]}{[H_2O]^2}$$

$$K_{eq}[H_2O]^2 \rightleftharpoons [H_3O^+][OH^-]$$

The concentration of water [H$_2$O] (can be assumed to be constant and in excess to [H$_3$O$^+$][OH$^-$] (The square brackets [ ] signify a **molar** concentration). The equation can be simplified to give the ionisation constant or ion product of water (K_w):

$$K_w = [H_3O^+][OH^-]$$

In pure water the molar concentration of water is 55.5 M (divide the weight of 1.0 litre of water (1000 g) by the relative molecular mass of water; M_r = 18) and the K_{eq} for water has been determined to be 1.8×10^{-16}.

$$K_w = [1.8 \times 10^{-16}][55.5] = [H_3O^+][OH^-]$$
$$K_w = 1 \times 10^{-14} \text{ M at } 25°C$$

(The ion product of water [K_w] varies with temperature from 0.114×10^{-14} at 0°C to 51.3×10^{-14} at 100°C.)

In pure water the ionisation of two water molecules produces equal amounts of hydronium ions and hydroxyl ions.

$$K_w = [H_3O^+][OH^-] = [H_3O^+]^2$$
$$K_w = \sqrt{1 \times 10^{-14}}$$
$$= 1 \times 10^{-7} \text{ M}$$

1.5   THE pH SCALE

The ion product of water is constant and this means that when the concentration of H_3O^+ increases, there is a corresponding decrease in the concentration of OH^-. This forms the basis of the pH scale, which signifies the molar concentration of H_3O^+ in solution (for simplicity [H^+] is often quoted). The various exponential (1×10^{-X}) values of the molar concentrations of H_3O^+ (see Table 1.2) can be converted to a linear scale by taking the negative logarithm (the symbol p denotes "negative $\log_{10}$ of").

$$pH = \log \frac{1}{[H_3O^+]}$$
$$= -\log[H_3O^+]$$

Table 1.2 The molar concentrations of hydronium ions in the pH scale.

[H_3O^+] (M)	pH	[OH^-] (M)
10^0	0.0	10^{-14}
10^{-1}	1.0	10^{-13}
10^{-3}	3.0	10^{-11}
10^{-5}	5.0	10^{-9}
10^{-7}	7.0	10^{-7}
10^{-9}	9.0	10^{-5}
10^{-11}	11.0	10^{-3}
10^{-14}	14.0	10^0

so pH is the negative $\log_{10}$ of the $[H_3O^+]$ (often seen as the negative $\log_{10}$ of the $[H^+]$).

At 25°C K_w and the $[H_3O^+] = 1 \times 10^{-7}$ M (see above).

$$\text{Conversion to pH} \qquad pH = \log\frac{1}{[H_3O^+]}$$
$$= \log 1/\log(1 \times 10^{-7})$$
$$= \log(1 \times 10^7)$$
$$= \log 1 + \log 10^7$$
$$= 0 + 7$$
$$= 7$$

At 25°C the pH of a neutral solution is pH 7.0.

1.6   ACIDS AND BASES

Brønsted proposed that acid-base reactions involve the transfer of an H^+ ion (proton). A Brønsted acid is a proton donor and a Brønsted base is a proton acceptor. Every Brønsted acid has a conjugate base and the same is true for the Brønsted base.

$$\text{e.g.,} \qquad HCl + H_2O \quad \rightleftharpoons \quad H_3O^+ + Cl^-$$
$$\text{acid} \quad \text{base} \qquad\qquad \text{acid} \quad \text{base}$$

Acids are often referred to as being "strong" or "weak" and a measure of the strength of an acid is the acid-dissociation equilibrium constant (K_a) for that acid. (The **pK_a** is the negative log of the K_a, converting the exponential values of K_a into a linear scale.)

$$HA + H_2O \quad \rightleftharpoons \quad H_3O^+ + A^-$$
$$\text{acid} \quad \text{base} \qquad\qquad \text{acid} \quad \text{base}$$

$$K_a = \frac{[H_3O^+][A^-]}{[HA]}$$

A strong acid (the proton donor) readily dissociates at all pH values and has a high K_a value (HCl: $K_a = 1 \times 10^6$). A strong acid will have a low pK_a.

For example, strong acid dissociation
$$HCl \rightarrow H^+ + Cl^-$$
(readily dissociates from pH 0–14)

The dissociation of a weak acid (the proton donor) is pH dependent and has a small K_a value (CH_3COOH $K_a = 1.8 \times 10^{-5}$; pK_a 4.75). At low pH values the proton concentration (in reality $[H_3O^+]$) is high which drops off exponentially as the pH increases (see above).

e.g., Weak acid dissociation
$$CH_3COOH \rightleftharpoons H^+ + CH_3COO^-$$
pK_a 4.75   (below pH 3.0) (Fully dissociated above pH 7.0)

1.7   BUFFERS

Proteins have pH optima for their designated roles within the cell or body and they may well have a different optimal pH for their storage. The **native** (biologically active) conformation of a protein can become unravelled (biologically inactive) by changes in pH, temperature and the presence of detergents (see Chapter 2). Therefore, in biology maintaining the pH within the cell (*in vivo*) and of any protein in solution (*in vitro*) is vitally important.

A buffer, comprised of a weak acid and one of its salts (conjugate base) or a weak base and one of its salts (conjugate acid), can maintain the pH of a solution.

$$HA + H_2O \quad \rightleftharpoons \quad H_3O^+ + A^-$$
$$\text{acid} \quad \text{base} \qquad \qquad \text{acid} \quad \text{base}$$

The dissociation contants $K_a = \dfrac{[H_3O^+][A^-]}{[HA]}$

The Henderson–Hasselbalch equation can be used to determine the quantitative aspects of buffers (see Exercise 1.1 and Appendix 8).

$$pH = pK_a + log_{10}\frac{[A^-]}{[HA]} \quad \text{or } pH = pK_a + log_{10}\frac{[\text{proton acceptor}]}{[\text{proton donor}]}$$

where $[A^-]$ is the concentration of base and $[HA]$ is the concentration of acid. (The square brackets [ ] signify a molar concentration; however, because $[A^-]/[HA]$ is a ratio any concentration unit will suffice.)

It is the $[A^-]/[HA]$ ratio that determines the pH of a solution. When the acid concentration is equal to the base concentration, pH = pK_a. Buffers are most effective at their pK_a because they can soak up or release protons upon the addition of an acid or an alkali (see Figure 1.5).

When [acid] > [base] the pH of the buffer is less than the pK_a, and when [base] > [acid] the pH is greater than the pK_a. For buffering, the $[A^-]/[HA]$

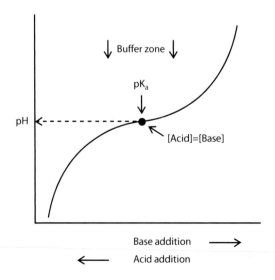

Figure 1.5 A buffer titration curve.

Table 1.3 A list of common buffers and their effective pH ranges.

Buffer	pK$_a$	Effective buffer range
Maleate	1.97	1.2–2.6
Glycine/HCl	2.35	2.2–3.6
Citric acid/ Na$_2$HPO$_4$	Citrate: 3.13, 4.76, 6.40 Phosphate: 7.20	2.6–7.6
Acetate/CH$_3$COOH	4.75	3.6–5.6
MES	6.10	5.5–6.7
bis-Tris propane	6.46	5.8–7.2
PIPES	6.76	6.1–7.5
MOPSO	6.87	6.2–7.6
NaH$_2$PO$_4$/Na$_2$HPO$_4$	7.20	5.8–8.0
HEPES	7.48	6.8–8.2
Triethanolamine	7.76	7.0–8.3
Tricine	8.05	7.4–8.8
Tris/HCl	8.06	7.5–9.0
BICINE	8.26	7.6–9.0
CHES	9.50	8.6–10.0
CAPS	10.40	9.7–11.1
Na$_2$CO$_3$/NaHCO$_3$	10.33	9.0–10.7

ratio can only be varied within certain limits—usually to 1.0 pH unit on either side of the pK$_a$ value. This means that there is little or no buffering at the extremes of the buffering range and it may be necessary to alter the molarity of the buffer to maintain good buffering capacity or switch to a different buffer (see Table 1.3). The components of some buffers (e.g., citrate/phosphate) have several pK$_a$ values, which allows this buffer to operate over a wide pH range.

1.7.1 Points to remember about buffers

- Components (e.g., EDTA) included in a buffer may alter the pH, so adjust the pH after all the additions have been dissolved in the highest grade of water available.
- Avoid the temptation to adjust the pH of a buffer with strong acids or bases (unless they are integral in the buffer) as this will mop up the available buffering capacity. Make minor adjustments to the pH with concentrated solutions of either the acid or base component of the buffer. This will slightly increase the concentration of one of the buffer components but the buffering capacity will be maintained.
- The pK$_a$ value for buffers can vary with temperature (e.g., pK$_a$ of Tris is 8.8 at 4°C and 8.3 at 20°C). Equilibrate the buffer to the temperature it is to be used at before adjusting the pH.

- For convenience make 10- to 100-fold stock solutions of the buffers. These can be autoclaved (or filtered through 0.2 μm membrane) and then stored at RT, 4°C or −25°C. When the buffer is required, warm the buffer to the desired working temperature and check the pH after dilution to the working concentration.
- Before using a buffer for chromatography always filter the buffer through a 0.2 μm membrane to remove **particulate** matter and trace bacterial contamination.
- Check that a buffer is compatible with the target protein by assaying the target enzyme in the chosen buffer. Also check that the target protein remains active in the buffer during storage.
- Phosphate will form insoluble complexes with some divalent metal ions at physiological pH values (e.g., Ca^{2+} and Zn^{2+}) and borate buffers will complex with hydroxyl groups, so borate buffers should be avoided when purifying glycoproteins.

1.8   SUMMARY

Water as a solvent has many unique properties, most of which can be attributed to its structure. The uneven arrangement of electrons in water imparts a transient uneven distribution of charge, with one end of the molecule becoming more electronegative than the other end. The oppositely charged areas within a cluster of water molecules briefly become attracted to each other in a process called hydrogen bonding. These fleeting interactions between water molecules result in properties such as surface tension and the migration of water up glass capillary tubing.

Water can also ionise to form negatively charged hydroxyl (OH^-) and positively charged hydronium (H_3O^+) ions. This property underpins the pH scale, the concept of acids/bases and the concept of buffers.

EXERCISE 1.1 PRACTICE CALCULATIONS USING THE HENDERSON–HASSELBALCH EQUATION

Calculate the pH of a sodium acetate buffer solution (see Table 1.3) containing 0.25 M acetic acid and 0.5 M sodium acetate.
The pK_a of acetic acid is 4.76.

$$CH_3COOH + H_2O \rightleftharpoons H_3O^+ + CH_3COO^-$$

$$\quad\ \text{acid} \qquad\quad \text{base} \qquad \text{acid} \qquad \text{base}$$

The Henderson–Hasselbalch equation

$$pH = pK_a + \log_{10}\frac{[A^-]}{[HA^+]} \quad \text{or} \quad pH = pK_a + \log_{10}\frac{[\text{proton acceptor}]}{[\text{proton donor}]}$$

$$pH = pK_a + \log_{10}\frac{[\text{acetate}]}{[\text{acetic acid}]}$$

$$pH = 4.76 + \log_{10} \frac{[0.5]}{[0.25]}$$

$$pH = 4.76 + 0.30$$

$$pH = 5.06$$

RECOMMENDED READING

Research papers

Brovchenko, I. and Oleinikova, A. (2008) Multiple phases of liquid water. *Chem Phys Chem* 9:2660-2675.

Ebbinghaus, S., Kim, S.J., Heyden, M., Yu, X., Heugen, U., Gruebele, M., Leitner, D.M. and Havenith, M. (2007) An extended dynamical hydration shell around proteins. *Proc Nat Acad Sci USA* 104:20749-20752.

Lewicki, P.P. (2004) Water as the determinant of food engineering properties. A review. *J Food Eng* 61:483-495.

MacCallum, J.L. and Tieleman, D.P. (2011) Hydrophobicity scales: a thermodynamic looking glass into lipid–protein interactions. *Trends Biochem Sci* 36:653-662.

Pace, C.N., Trevino, S., Prabhakaran, E. and Scholtz, J.M. (2004) Protein structure, stability and solubility in water and other solvents. *Philos Trans R Soc Lond B Biol Sci* 359:1225-1235.

Books

Berg, J.M., Tymoczko, J.L. and Stryer, L. (2015) *Biochemistry.* 8th ed. W.H. Freeman, New York, USA.

Beynon, R.J. and Easterby, J.S. (1996) *Buffer Solutions.* Biosis Sci Publishing Ltd, Oxford, UK.

Eisenberg, D. (1997) *The Structure and Properties of Water.* Oxford University Press, New York, USA.

Nelson, D.L. and Cox, M.M. (2013) *Lehninger: Principles of Biochemistry.* 7th ed. W.H. Freeman, New York, USA.

Protein Structure and Properties

2.1 INTRODUCTION

There are a limited number of physical properties that proteins possess which can be utilised to aid protein purification; some are linked to the functional groups contained within the structure of amino acids (see Section 2.2 below). These properties include a protein's solubility (see Section 4.11.2), surface charge (see Section 5.2) and hydrophobicity (see Section 5.5). The total content of amino acids within a protein's structure dictates the final size and shape of the protein (see Section 7.1) and its functionality (see Section 6.1), both of which can also be exploited to aid purification. Finally, many proteins are modified, either as they are synthesised (**co-translational modifications**, e.g., *N*-glycosylation; see Section 6.10) or after they are synthesised (**post-translational modifications**, e.g., phosphorylation; see Section 6.9), and some of these modifications can also be exploited in order to purify proteins.

2.2 AMINO ACIDS

Amino acids are organic acids that form the basic building blocks of a protein's structure (see Appendix 2). As their name implies, contained within their structure are both a basic amino group ($-NH_2$) and an acidic carboxyl group ($-COOH$) (see Figure 2.1A). They are described as **zwitterions** (see Figure 2.1B) because they have the properties of both an acid and a base. The amino group and the carboxyl group are both described as weak acid charges (see Section 1.6), which means that the overall charge on the amino acid depends on the pH of the medium in which it is dissolved. At acidic pH values (see Section 1.5; a low pH and elevated $[H^+]$) the amino group is protonated ($-NH_3^+$) and the carboxyl group is non-dissociated ($-COOH$). When the pH increases, the proton on the carboxyl group starts to dissociate ($-COO^-$), resulting in an amino acid with both a positive and negative charge, which remains until the pH reaches 9.0. Around pH 9.0 the amino group loses its proton ($-NH_2$), leaving only the negative charge on the carboxyl group ($-COO^-$). Thus, as the pH increases and the $[H^+]$ exponentially decreases, the overall charge on the amino acid changes from predominantly positive to predominantly negative.

In general, all the amino acids found in proteins are alpha (α) amino acids, comprising a central α-carbon atom attached to an amino group ($-NH_2$), a carboxyl group ($-COOH$), a hydrogen atom ($-H$) and characteristic functional group ($-R$). The exception is proline, which is not an amino acid but an imino acid (containing an imino group $>C = NH$ and a carboxyl group $-COOH$). However, for simplicity, proline is always included with the other 19 amino acids. The vast majority of proteins in nature

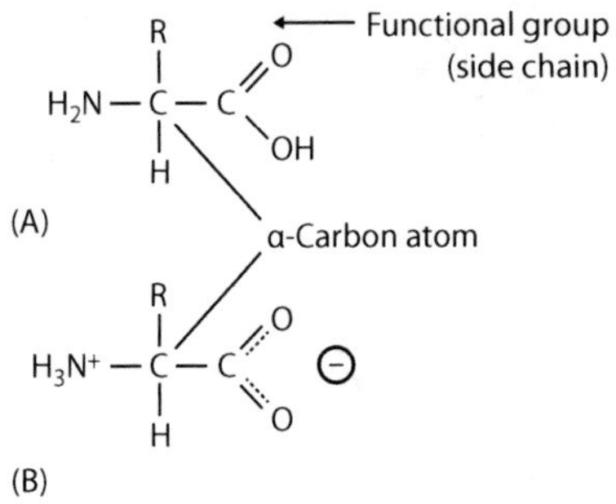

Figure 2.1 The basic structure of an amino acid (A) non-ionised and (B) zwitterionic form.

are constructed from amino acids containing twenty different functional groups (see Table 2.1). These different functional groups impart hydrophobicity, hydrogen bonding and charge properties to a protein. They provide sites for interactions with other proteins and the attachment of additional functional groups (e.g., co-translational and post-translational modifications; see Table 2.2), and collectively the different amino acids in a protein establishes a protein's three-dimensional shape and size.

A property that amino acids share with a lot of other organic molecules is the presence of an asymmetric carbon atom. When a carbon atom in a molecule has four different groups attached, it is described as asymmetric and as such can exist in different structural forms. A molecule containing one asymmetric carbon atom will have two stereoisomers; a larger molecule containing more than one asymmetric carbon atom will not exceed 2^n stereoisomers (where n = the number of asymmetric carbon atoms in the structure).

The basic structure of an amino acid (see Figure 2.1) has a tetrahedral α-carbon atom attached to four different groups. The exception is glycine, which has two hydrogen atoms attached to the α-carbon atom (see Table 2.1) and does not have an asymmetric carbon atom. Also exceptional are threonine and isoleucine, which have two asymmetric carbon atoms in their structure and exist in four different structural forms.

Identification of the isomeric forms of any organic compound is difficult because the properties of isomers are essentially the same. French physicist Jean-Baptiste Biot (1815) demonstrated that polarised light could be rotated clockwise (dextrorotary to the right) or anticlockwise (laevorotary to the left) when passed through a solution of organic material. Emil Fisher, a German chemist working on carbohydrates at the turn of the last century, devised the D- and L- labels for enantiomeric isomers. The three-carbon sugar glyceraldehyde with one asymmetric carbon atom was used as the blueprint to assign labels to particular isomeric configurations. The enantiomeric isomer of glyceraldehyde that rotated the plane of light to the right (clockwise; positive) was designated the D-isomer (derived from the Latin *dexter*, meaning "on the right"). The isomer that rotated the plane of polarised light to the left (anticlockwise; negative) was designated the L-isomer (derived from the Latin *laevus*, meaning "on the left") (see Figure 2.2A). Amino acids were designated as either L- (Laevo) or D- (Dextro) with reference to the L- and D-optical isomers of glyceraldehyde (see Figure 2.2B). This label refers to the spatial arrangement of the groups attached to the α-carbon atom (see Figures 2.2A and 2.2B). However, to complicate matters, the L- and D- labels do not indicate that all the L-isomers of amino acids will rotate the plane of polarised light to the left, as this property differs for each amino acid. For example, L-alanine

Table 2.1 Some properties of the twenty amino acids found in proteins.

Negatively charged amino acids	Typical pK$_a$ values	One-letter abbreviation	Three-letter abbreviation	Notes
Aspartate	4.1	D	Asp	The side chain will be negatively charged at pH 7.0.
Glutamate	4.1	E	Glu	The side chain will be negatively charged at pH 7.0.
Positively charged amino acids				
Arginine	10.8	R	Arg	The side chain will be positively charged at pH 7.0.
Lysine	12.5	K	Lys	1. The side chain will be negatively charged at pH 7.0. 2. Can be post-translationally modified by hyroxylation
Histidine	6.0	H	His	1. The side chain will be neutral or slightly positively charged at pH 7.0, depending on the local environment. 2. Histidine at the active site of enzymes functions to bind and release protons.
Polar amino acids				
Cysteine	8.3	C	Cys	1. The sulphydryl group in cysteine may react with another to form cystine. This is a covalent disulphide bond (-S-S-), which helps to stabilise the final structure of some **eukaryotic** proteins exported from the cell. 2. Free cysteines can be post-translationally modified by nitric oxide to form S-nitrothiols.
Tyrosine	10.9	Y	Try	1. A phosphate group can be attached to the hydroxyl group. 2. Absorbs light at 280 nm (fluorescence emission at 310 nm). 3. Can be sulphated particularly in eukaryotic proteins exported from the cell.
Serine		S	Ser	1. A phosphate group can be attached to the hydroxyl group. 2. O-glycosylation can occur on the amide nitrogen of serine.
Threonine		T	Thr	1. The side chain of threonine has an additional chiral centre. 2. A phosphate group can be attached to the hydroxyl group. 3. O-glycosylation can occur on the amide nitrogen of threonine.
Asparagine		N	Asn	1. *N*-glycosylation can occur on the amide nitrogen of asparagine. 2. The carboxamide deamidates at all pH values converting uncharged asparagine to negatively charged aspartate.
Glutamine		Q	Gln	The carboxamide deamidates at all pH values converting uncharged glutamine to negatively charged glutamate.

(Continued)

Table 2.1 (Continued) Some properties of the twenty amino acids found in proteins.				
Negatively charged amino acids	**Typical pK$_a$ values**	**One-letter abbreviation**	**Three-letter abbreviation**	**Notes**
Simple hydrophobic amino acids				
Glycine		G	Gly	Glycine does not exist as optical isomers because the α-carbon in glycine does not have four different groups attached.
Alanine		A	Ala	
Proline		P	Pro	1. Proline is an imino acid containing an imino group (>C=NH) and a carboxylic acid group (–COOH). 2. Can be post-translationally modified by hydroxylation.
Aliphatic hydrophobic amino acids				
Valine		V	Val	
Leucine		L	Leu	
Isoleucine		I	Ile	The side chain of isoleucine has an additional chiral centre.
Aromatic Hydrophobic amino acids				
Phenylalanine		F	Phe	
Tryptophan		W	Trp	Absorbs light at 280 nm (fluorescence emission at 360 nm).

rotates the plane of polarised light to the left, whereas L-leucine rotates the plane of polarised light to the right. The direction that the plane of polarised light moves is also temperature-dependent and in some instances can switch from clockwise to anticlockwise with an increase in temperature. If amino acids are chemically synthesised in an uncatalysed reaction, an equal mixture of the two isomers (D- and L-) will form and this is described as a racemate mixture. This mixture will not rotate a plane of polarised light to the right or left, which helps to differentiate between racemate mixtures and pure solutions of the isomers. Additionally, optical isomers do not readily convert from one configuration to the other because a change would require the breaking of bonds and structural rearrangement.

In the 1960s, another system for labelling stereoisomers was proposed by the English chemists Robert Sidney Cahn and Christopher Ingold and the Swiss chemist Vladimir Prelog. They proposed labelling structural isomers with the prefixes R- (derived from the Latin *rectus*, meaning "right") and S- (derived from the Latin *sinister*, meaning "left"), according to a list of priority rules. The first priority rule assigns a number to each group attached to the asymmetric carbon atom, with the highest atomic number given the number 1 and the lowest atomic number

Table 2.2 Common enzymic and non-enzymic post-translational modifications of proteins.

Post-translational modification	Amino acid	Notes
Phosphorylation	Serine Threonine Tyrosine	See Section 2.6
Glycosylation	N-linked (Asparagine) O-linked (Serine, threonine, tyrosine, hydroxylysine or hydroxyproline see below). N-acetylglucosamine (O-linked serine, threonine)	See Section 2.6
Glycation		Non-enzymic additions of reducing sugars to proteins
Lipid (A) Prenylation	Cysteine The conserved motif (–CAAX-) near the C-terminus of the target protein, where X is any amino acid	Attachment of farensyl or gerenylgerenyl isoprenoid residues. The isoprenoid attachment allows for membrane association
(B) Acylation	Cysteine N-terminus glycine	Palmitoylation or Myristoylation Fatty acid attachment allows for membrane association
(C) **GPI**-anchor	Amide link to N-terminus amino acid	The glycosophospholipid attachment allows membrane association in the **endoplasmic reticulum**. The proteins are resident in the external leaflet of the plasma membrane in lipid rafts
Sulphation	Tyrosine	Mainly on proteins exported from the cell or those that span the plasma membrane
Acetylation	Amino terminus Lysine	Very common e.g., histones and tubulin
Methylation	Lysine and arginine	e.g., histones
Hydroxylation	Proline and lysine	e.g., collagen
Polyglutamylation	glutamate	e.g., α- and β-tubulin
Polyglycylation	Glutamate near carboxyl terminus	e.g., tubulin
Deamidation	Asparagine and glutamine	Conversion to aspartate or iso-aspartate and glutamate The surface charge on the protein becomes more negative
	Glutamine to glutamate	Transglutaminase mediates deamidation of protein/peptide bound glutamine. The surface charge on the protein becomes more negative
Polyamination	Glutamine	Transglutaminase mediates the covalent incorporation of polyamines into proteins. The surface charge on the protein becomes more positive
Ubiquitinylation	Lysine	The addition of ubiquitin to proteins targets them for recycling by the proteasome
Proteolytic cleavage	Enzymic removal of fragments of proteins	e.g., conversion of proinsulin to insulin
Nitrosylation	(a) Cysteine (b) Tyrosine	Nitrosylation to (a) nitrothiols and (b) 3-nitrotyrosine related to oxidative stress
Oxidation	Cysteine Methionine Tryptophan	Reactive oxygen species generated as a result of oxidative stress oxidising

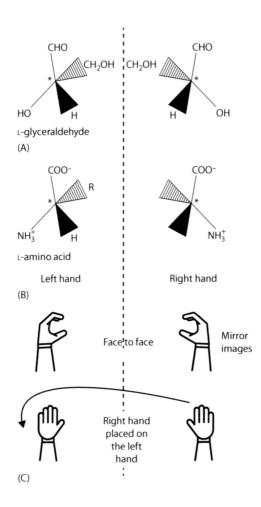

Figure 2.2 The three-dimensional arrangement of (A) glyceraldehyde (B) amino acids (C) human hands as examples of non- superimposable mirror images of each other (enantiomeric isomers). (*Is the assymetric carbon atom.)

assigned the number 4. The isomer is desigated R- if the numbers (1–4) move in a clockwise direction, and S- if the numbers move in an anti-clockwise direction. Other rules of priority are brought into play when the structures involved become more complex.

In the vast majority of biochemistry textbooks, the D- and·L- system of labelling amino acid stereoisomers is preferred, so an amino acid with one asymmetric carbon atom will have two enantiomeric stereoisomers (D- and L-). These amino acid isomers are described as being non-superimposable mirror images of each other (see Figure 2.2B). An immediate and straightforward example to illustrate the idea of enantiomeric stereoisomers are human hands. The left and right hands, if placed with the palms together, are mirror images of each other, but if the left hand is placed on top of the right hand the thumbs are positioned on opposite sides, indicating that the hands cannot be superimposed on each other (see Figure 2.2C).

The two isomeric forms of amino acids are chemically identical but proteins contain only the L-isoform of amino acids. The selection of the L-isomer for all twenty amino acids to form proteins may be a quirk of evolution or it may be that the L-isomers of amino acids are slightly more soluble. Either way, in nature the enzymes involved in protein synthesis have evolved to accommodate only the L-isoform of amino acids. In other words, the enzymes involved with amino acid metabolism have a three-dimensional **stereospecific** active site accommodating only the L-isomer of amino acids.

2.3   THE PEPTIDE BOND

Water is produced when the α-carboxyl group of one amino acid is joined to the α-amino group of another amino acid (see Figure 2.3A). The product of this condensation reaction is a dipeptide linked by a peptide bond (see Figure 2.3A). To form a polymer, additional amino acids can be added to the free carboxyl group of the dipeptide, elongating the peptide chain in a linear fashion (an oligopeptide has between 4–15 amino acids, whereas a polypeptide is >15 amino acids) and giving the polypeptide chain both polarity and direction. The first amino acid in a polypeptide chain has a free amino group (pK_a 8.0) and the last amino acid has a free carboxyl group (pK_a 3.1). Glutathione (M_r 307.32: Glu-Cys-Gly) is among the smallest functional tripeptides, while the muscle protein titin (comprising 34,000 amino acids with an M_r 3,800,000) is the largest known protein.

The polypeptide chain has a repeating core structure consisting of the linked α-carboxyl groups in each amino acid and a variable structure consisting of the different functional groups in each amino acid (see Table 2.1), which point away from the repeating core structure in the trans-configuration (see Figure 2.3B). A polypeptide may have elements of stabilising secondary structure but it is *not* a protein, whereas a protein does have a polypeptide chain.

There are several features of the peptide bond which dictate the spatial properties of a polypeptide chain. The carbonyl oxygen has a slight negative character and the amide nitrogen a slight positive character, establishing a dipole across the peptide bond. The electrons in the peptide bond resonate across the carbonyl carbon, oxygen and nitrogen in the peptide bond, resulting in a partial double bond character (see Figure 2.4). This is reflected in the carbon–nitrogen peptide bond length, which is typically 1.32 Angstroms (Å), a distance between the length of a carbon = nitrogen

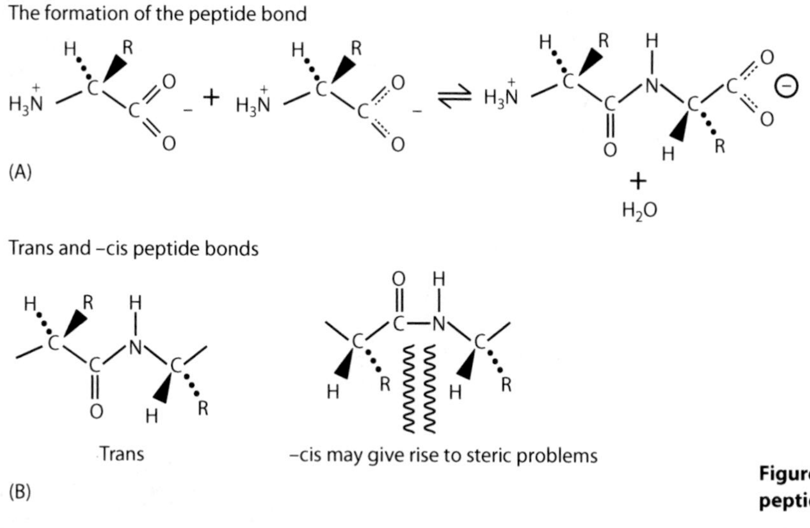

The formation of the peptide bond

(A)

$+$

H_2O

Trans and –cis peptide bonds

Trans   –cis may give rise to steric problems

(B)

Figure 2.3 The formation of the peptide bond.

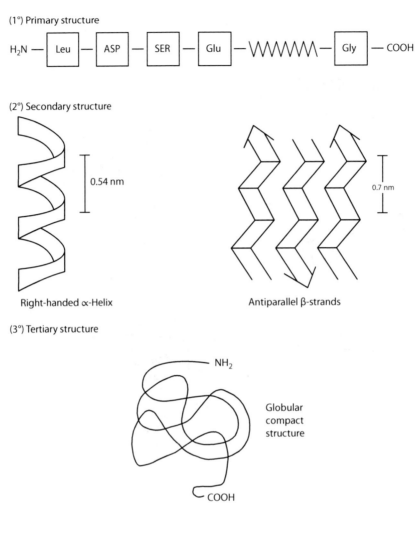

(1°) Primary structure

(2°) Secondary structure

0.54 nm

0.7 nm

Right-handed α-Helix

Antiparallel β-strands

(3°) Tertiary structure

Globular compact structure

(4°) Quarternary structure

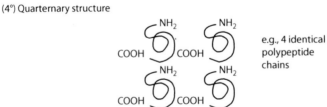

e.g., 4 identical polypeptide chains

Figure 2.4 The hierarchical nature of protein structure.

double bond (1.27 Å) and a carbon-nitrogen single bond (1.49 Å). This partial double bond character results in a planar configuration of electrons about the peptide bond (see Figure 2.4), restricting rotation. The peptide bond itself carries no net charge, which favours close interactions when proteins fold into the tightly packed tertiary structures.

The majority of peptide bonds in proteins are in present in a trans-configuration (see Figure 2.3B), wherein the functional groups of amino acids attached to the α-carbon atom are on opposite sides of the peptide chain. This prevents bulky amino acid functional groups from impinging on each other's space (steric exclusion means two atoms cannot occupy the same space). The imino acid proline is an exception (see Table 2.1), as the α-carbon atom is accommodated in an imino ring. If there is an amino acid (X) linked to proline (X-Pro), both cis- and trans-configurations can be accommodated without steric problems.

Embedded in a peptide chain is the repeating element of a planar double bond with restricted movement. However, the peptide chain is not a linear rigid polymer because there is rotation about the α-carbon atoms to which are attached the various amino acid functional groups (see Figure 2.4). The angle of rotation about the α-carbon–nitrogen bond is called phi (φ) and the angle of rotation about the α-carbon–carbonyl carbon bond is called psi (Ψ). The Indian scientist Gopalasamudram Ramachandran (1963) plotted all the possible phi- and psi- angles and showed that unlimited movement is not possible due to steric interactions between the rotating amino acid functional groups. In fact, 75% of the potential angles are restricted.

The planar element and the restrictions in movement about the peptide bond (phi and psi angles) limits the number of secondary structures that a polypeptide chain can assume. On the face of it, the properties of the peptide bond may seem to impose many limitations. However, a polypeptide chain with freedom to fold in many different forms would give a polymer with a variety of shapes many without functionality. Cells would have to expend a lot of energy synthesising and recycling functionless amino acid polymers. The limitations in movement of the peptide bond favour non-random folding of polypeptide chains into proteins with consistent shape and functionality.

2.4   OVERVIEW OF PROTEIN STRUCTURE

2.4.1   Primary structure

Proteins are polymers made from twenty amino acids in the L-configuration, each with a different functional group (see Table 2.1). The content and sequence of the amino acids within a protein are determined by the gene sequence for that protein. The primary structure of a protein is the arrangement of the amino acids in a protein sequence, from the first amino acid at the amino terminus and to the final amino acid at the carboxyl terminus.

2.4.2   Secondary structure

During protein synthesis, as the length of the polypeptide chain increases, sequences of amino acids can fold into regular secondary structures stabilised by hydrogen bonding. Two American scientists (Linus Pauling and Robert Corey) in 1951 correctly predicted the alpha-helix (alpha because they proposed this structure first) and the beta-(pleated) sheet as two secondary structures for proteins. Most proteins have a mixture of both α-helix and β-sheet secondary structures. The distance between amino acids in the α-helix is 1.5 Å, whereas in the β-sheet the distance is 3.5 Å. Hence, the β-sheet can be described as extended polypeptide sequences called β-strands.

The α-helix is a right-handed cylindrical structure with 3.6 amino acid residues in each turn (see Figure 2.5). This means that amino acids in the polypeptide chain which are separated by three to four amino acids in the primary structure become close neighbours in the α-helix. The α-helix is stabilised by intra-chain hydrogen bonding and the amino acid functional

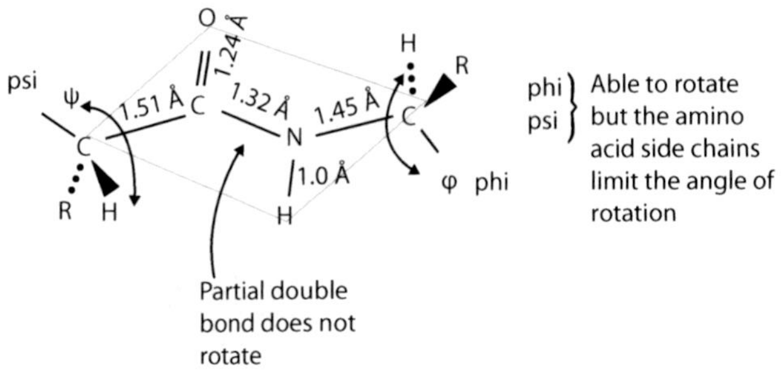

Figure 2.5 The planar nature of the peptide bond showing the rotation (phi and psi) about the peptide bond.

groups point away from the core of the structure. Some amino acids (valine, threonine and isoleucine) destabilise the formation of the helix due to steric problems and others (serine, aspartate and asparagine) due to conflicting hydrogen bond formation. The structure of proline (see Table 2.1) does not fit easily into the helical structure and consequently breaks the continuation of the α-helix. A chaperone protein, prolyl isomerase, ensures that proline exists in either the cis- or trans-conformation to ensure the correct location of β-hairpin turns in the secondary structure of proteins.

The β-sheet secondary structure (see Figure 2.5) is composed of two or more polypeptide sequences (β-strands) in close proximity to each other, stabilised by inter-chain hydrogen bonding. The β-strands can run parallel or anti-parallel to each other and β-sheets can be comprised of 4–10 β-strands (parallel, anti-parallel or mixed).

To ensure proteins assume a compact structure, strands and helices reverse direction by means of either a β-turn (can be referred to as a reverse or hairpin turn) or an omega (Ω) loop. These turns or loops are situated on the surface of the protein's structure and provide sites for interactions with other proteins and chromatographic media.

2.4.3 Tertiary structure

When the mRNA for a protein is translated in the cell on the ribosomes, peptide bonds are formed between sequentially added amino acids. The polypeptide chain emerging from the ribosome is subjected to the constraints about the peptide bond (see Section 2.3) and the emerging polypeptide chain rapidly twists and turns into folding intermediates (60ns). This process takes into account the size, shape and properties of the functional groups on the covalently linked amino acid chain. As the polypeptide chain starts to elongate, stabilising secondary structures will form, with an α-helix folding in 16ns and a β-turn taking 6μs. Overall, the formation of the final secondary and tertiary structures can take seconds to minutes to complete depending on the size of the protein.

The tertiary structure of a protein describes the final three-dimensional shape the folded protein finally assumes. This final folded structure takes into account the many properties of the amino acid functional groups contained within the protein's primary structure. The driving force that determines the tertiary structure of a protein is the accommodation of the amino acids with hydrophobic functional groups ("hydrophobic collapse"). In the cell's aqueous environment, the interaction between the amino acid hydrophobic functional groups and water is thermodynamically unfavourable, whereas their association with other amino acids with hydrophobic functional groups in the close vicinity is thermodynamically favourable.

The hydrophobic functional groups of amino acids very quickly adopt close associations with each other, allowing the rest of the polypeptide structure containing the hydrophilic functional groups to fold around this hydrophobic core. However, not all the hydrophobic residues in a protein's primary structure can be accommodated in the protein's core. If an amino acid with hydrophobic functional groups is close to the surface of the protein's structure, the hydrophobic functional groups will be shielded from the water by neighbouring polar amino acid functional groups. These pockets of hydrophobicity can play a key role in a protein's function by interacting with other proteins. They also can be exploited in the "salting out" of proteins (see Section 4.11.2) and hydrophobic interaction chromatography (HIC) (see Section 5.5).

Most proteins contain a variety of amino acids with hydrophobic functional groups, and these emerge from the ribosome as the messenger RNA sequence is translated. Non-functional interactions between hydrophobic amino acid functional groups can cause misfolding or aggregation. A group of proteins called chaperones (e.g., BIP) bind to the emerging polypeptide and folding intermediates, helping to prevent misfolding and aggregation before the whole protein has been synthesised. Many α-helices and β-strands have a polar and non-polar face. The non-polar face of the α-helix will point towards the core of the protein's structure and the polar face will point out towards the water phase of the cytoplasm.

Thus, in a protein's tertiary structure, the thermodynamic properties of the amino acid functional groups are satisfied, with the protein's hydrophobic functional groups as far away from water as possible and the hydrophilic amino acid functional groups on the protein's surface in contact with the water. This shell of water (approximately two to three water molecules deep) surrounding the protein enables the protein to remain in solution. Hydrophobic collapse directs the formation of the three-dimensional shape of the protein, but the final structure is held together by a variety of weak non-covalent forces, including:

a. Hydrophobic forces: maintenance of the hydrophobic interactions within the protein (see above)
b. Hydrogen bonding: between neighbouring dipoles (see Section 1.3)
c. Salt bridges: these are a combination of H-bonding (see Section 1.2) and electrostatic interactions between oppositely charged amino acid functional groups (positively charged functional groups of Lys, Arg or His and negatively charged functional groups of Asp and Glu). The functional groups participating in salt bridging must be in close proximity (<4.0 Å) and the interaction is influenced by the local pH environment (see Section 1.5). Depending on the local pH environment, other amino acids with ionisable functional groups may also participate in salt bridging (see Table 2.1).
d. van der Waal interactions: These are a summation of the weak non-covalent and non-ionic attractions between molecules (including London dispersion forces). They result from the constant fluctuations in the electron clouds surrounding atoms within a protein's structure, which mean that in any instant there is likely to be an uneven electron distribution within an atoms' electrons, resulting in a momentary dipole (see Section 1.3). This transient dipole results in an attractive force between surrounding atoms. However, the force is dependent on the distance between neighbouring atoms, because at close proximity (<4.0 Å) repulsion is greater than the induced attraction.

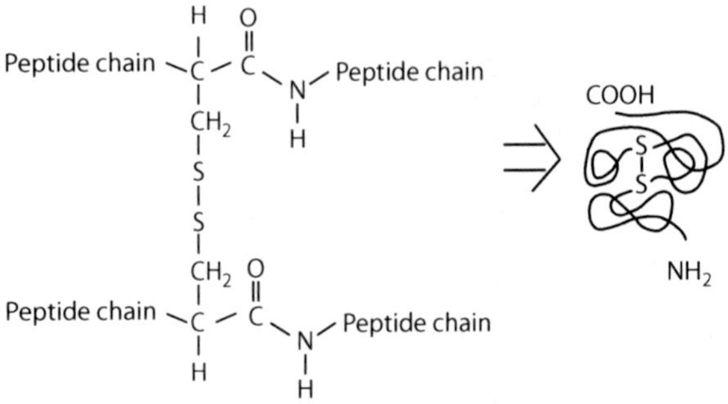

Figure 2.6 The structure of an intraprotein disulphide bonds between two cystein residues.

Individually these non-covalent forces present within a protein structure are weak but collectively they are strong enough to hold a protein in its three-dimensional shape. The thermal instability of proteins emphasises the weak nature of the forces that keep a protein's structure intact. Enzymes have stereospecific active sites (meaning they will only accommodate substrates with the correct three-dimensional shape) and most eukaryotic enzymes show maximal activity between 35–40°C. An increase in the surrounding temperature above 40°C provides sufficient thermal energy to overcome some of the weak interactions that hold a protein's structure together, partially unravelling the protein's tertiary structure. Non-specific interactions will then start to occur between neighbouring proteins, which may prevent the correct refolding of the enzyme (protein) if the temperature is again lowered below 40°C. Elevation to higher temperatures >50°C will result in protein aggregation and the subsequent loss of enzyme activity.

Proteins that are exported from the cell (e.g., insulin) and membrane proteins that have areas of their structure pointing away from the plasma membrane into the extracellular matrix can have an additional covalent bond to help maintain their tertiary structures. When two cysteine residues are in close proximity, an intra-chain disulphide bond can form between them (-S-S-) (see Figure 2.6). This covalent bond increases the stability of the protein's final tertiary structure. Protein disulphide isomerase, a chaperone protein present in the endoplasmic reticulum of eukaryotic cells, catalyses the formation of disulphide bonds within a protein as the protein folds. This helps prevent misfolding of proteins by correctly aligning the disulphide bonds.

The final three-dimensional shape of proteins can be roughly divided into two groups: the fibrous ("rope like") and the globular (compact) proteins. Fibrous proteins can be present inside (e.g., spectrin in erythrocytes) or outside (e.g., collagen) the cell to provide structure, strength, support and sites of adhesion. They are not normally required to move very far. The majority of proteins are described as globular, assuming compact shapes to help reduce frictional and drag forces as they diffuse within the cytoplasm and/or the extracellular fluid.

2.4.4   Quaternary structure

Some proteins are comprised of more than one folded polypeptide chain or a number of the same folded polypeptide chains gathered together in a superstructure. The individual folded polypeptide chains are called subunits of the whole protein and the arrangement of these subunits within the protein is described as the quaternary structure (see Figure 2.3).

Haemoglobin ($\alpha_2\beta_2$) (see Exercise 7.2) is functionally active as a tetrameric protein, comprising two α-subunits and two β-subunits. Proteins at key control points in metabolic pathways often have quaternary structure. For example, phosphofructokinase (PFK) in the glycolytic pathway is comprised of four identical subunits.

2.5   MOTIFS AND DOMAINS (SUPER SECONDARY STRUCTURE)

Frequently occurring folding patterns (motifs) can be found in many proteins. These can be relatively simple structures like the β-turn (two adjacent anti parallel β-strands), the omega loop (residues at the start and the end of the loop are close together) and a calcium-binding motif present in a number of proteins (e.g., calmodulin) called the EF hand (α-helix turn α-helix), or more complex structures like the Greek key (four adjacent anti-parallel β-strands) (see Figure 2.7).

Domains (30–400 amino acids) are stable, distinct folded areas in globular proteins sometimes comprising several motifs. A protein may consist of several domains joined by short polypeptide chains, with each domain having a distinct function. When a domain appears in a different protein it will retain its functionality. This could be catalytic or involve protein–nucleic acid, protein–protein or protein–membrane interactions (see Table 2.2).

2.6   POST-TRANSLATIONAL MODIFICATIONS

The human **genome** contains approximately three billion nucleotide base pairs, but only a small fraction of the total genomic DNA (1.5%) contains gene sequences for approximately 30,000 proteins. However, it has been estimated that there are approximately 400,000 different proteins. This is in part due to alternative gene splicing but predominantly due to post-translational modification of proteins. There are many examples of enzymic and non-enzymic (see Table 2.3) post-translational modifications of proteins, which can be temporary and cell-specific. They are used by the cell to alter a protein's functionality, location and ability to interact with other proteins.

For example, it has been estimated that 30% of the proteins present in a cell at any one time will have a phosphate residue ($-PO_4^{2-}$) attached to the functional group of serine, threonine or tyrosine (with a ratio of phosphorylation distribution 100:10:1) by kinase enzymes. The attachment of the negatively charged phosphate group will cause conformational changes in

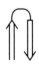

β-turn

α-Helix
turn
α-Helix
e.g., EF hand

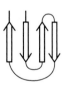

Greek key
4 antiparallel
β-Strands

Figure 2.7 Representations of three common motifs in the structure of globular proteins.

Table 2.3 Examples of domains that are found within globular proteins.		
Domain	**Interaction**	**Examples**
C1	Phospholipid binding	Protein kinase C, Diacylglycerol kinase and c-Raf kinase
CH	Cytoskeletal interactions	β-Spectrin and Dystrophin
CARD	Apoptosis signalling	Procaspase-2 and Apaf-1
MIU	Ubiquitin binding	Myosin VI and Rabex-5
SH3	Phosphotyrosine binding	Phospholipase C-γ and Src tyrosine kinase
WW	Proline-rich sequence binding	Nedd 4 ubiquitin ligase and Dystrophin

the protein structure by attracting or repelling any amino acid functional group with positive or negative charges in the near vicinity. This may activate a previously quiescent enzyme for a brief period of time before cellular phosphatases remove the phosphate group, restoring the enzyme to an inactive configuration. Monoclonal antibodies can be raised to both the phosphorylated and non-phosphorylated forms of a protein, providing a means to purify the non-phosphorylated from the phosphorylated protein by immunoaffinity chromatography (see Section 6.9).

Another common post-translational modification is the attachment of saccharide residues (**glycosylation**) to the asparagine (N-linked) or serine (O-linked) functional groups (see Table 2.2). These modifications occur within the endomembrane system of eukaryotic cells for proteins destined for cellular export or to reside in the plasma membrane. The attachment of a multi-branched chain of saccharide residues will alter the size, shape and surface charge of the original protein. In addition, cytoplasmic and nuclear enzymes may be temporarily glycosylated with N-acetyl glucosamine to moderate their function. Lectins are a group of proteins (originally identified in extracts from leguminous plants) that bind to saccharide residues and can be used in lectin affinity chromatography (see Section 6.10) to enable the purification of glycosylated proteins, including membrane proteins.

2.7   THE CHARACTERISTICS OF A PROTEIN WHICH CAN BE EXPLOITED TO PURIFY A TARGET PROTEIN

There are a limited number of physical properties of proteins which can be utilised to aid purification.

2.7.1   Surface charge

The surface of proteins is covered with a charge contributed by amino acids with functional groups that have weak acid properties (see Section 1.5–1.6). The charge on a weak acid depends upon the pH. The carboxyl groups on the amino acid functional groups of aspartic (D) and glutamic acid (Q) have little charge below pH 3.0 but are negatively charged at a physiological pH of around pH 7.0. The amino groups on the amino acid functional groups of lysine (K) and arginine (R) have little charge above pH 9.0 but are positively charged at a physiological pH of around pH 7.0. In addition, below pH 6.0 histidine (H) gains positive charge. If oppositely charged amino acid functional groups are in close proximity in the protein's structure, they may form a salt bridge to help stabilise the protein's tertiary structure.

When amino acids are incorporated into a protein's structure, the functional groups of the amino acids with weak acid charges (aspartate, glutamate, lysine and asparagine) point into the external medium. The charged groups make contact with water molecules and their overall charge is pH-dependent. This makes a protein a large zwitterionic structure and the overall charge on the protein's surface is pH-dependent. At a low pH the overall charge will be positive, and at a high pH the overall charge will be negative. There is a point on the pH scale where the positive charges on the protein's surface are balanced by the negative charges; at this point there is no net charge on the protein. There are still both positive and negative charges, but the summation of the charges contributed by all the positive and negative charges is zero. This point on the pH scale is called the **isoelectric point** (pI) of a protein.

Because proteins arise from different genes they have a variable number of amino acids with charged functional groups, resulting in different surface charges and a variety of isoelectric points. The differences in net charge on proteins can be exploited to resolve proteins in a complex mixture.

2.7.2 Hydrophobic nature

There are eight amino acids with functional groups that demonstrate varying degrees of hydrophobicity. The amino acids with aromatic functional groups are tyrosine (Y), tryptophan (W) and phenylalanine (F). The amino acids with aliphatic functional groups are leucine (L), isoleucine (I), valine (V), alanine (A) and methionine (M). If not situated in the core of a protein's structure, they are usually hidden in pockets at the surface of a protein by the functional groups (charged or polar) of neighbouring amino acids. These pockets of surface hydrophobic amino acids can be exploited to purify a protein from a complex mixture. Again, because proteins arise from different genes, they have varying combinations of the eight hydrophobic amino acids and thus possess different degrees of hydrophobicity. These differences in surface hydrophobicity can be exploited to resolve a protein from a complex mixture (see Chapters 4 and 5).

2.7.3 Solubility

Proteins are usually soluble in water because of the interaction between water molecules and the hydrophilic/polar amino acids functional groups in their structure (different proteins will have different hydrophilic/polar amino acid functional groups). The solubility of proteins in solution can be altered by temperature, pH and ionic strength. At low salt concentrations, proteins show increased solubility ("salting in"). As the concentration of salt increases, proteins show differential solubility ("salting out"), which can be used to fractionate complex protein mixtures or concentrate dilute solutions of proteins (see Section 4.11.2).

2.7.4   Biospecificity

Proteins have evolved to serve specific biological functions. For example, enzymes have stereospecific active sites, making them highly specific for their substrates. This biospecificity can be utilised in a protein purification protocol to isolate an individual protein from a complex mixture. For example, the tripeptide glutathione attached to an agarose/Sepharose resin can be used to purify the enzyme glutathione S-transferase. In addition, the relatively large bacterial protein G attached to agarose/Sepharose can be used to purify IgG from a sample of serum (see Chapter 6).

2.7.5   Molecular mass (M$_r$)

Different proteins have different numbers of amino acids and thus have different molecular masses. These differences in size and shape can be exploited to resolve a target protein from a complex mixture (see Chapter 7).

2.7.6   Post-translational modifications

For proteins destined for the endomembrane system, the plasma membrane or for export from the cell, sugar residues can be attached during the process of protein synthesis (co-translational modification). Other proteins in the cytoplasm or the nucleus can have additional groups added to the functional groups of specific amino acids. These additions alter the structure of the original amino acid functional group, which in turn alters the proximity of neighbouring amino acid functional groups, leading to a conformational change in the protein's structure. Protein phosphorylation is a common cellular post-translational protein modification temporarily attaching a big negative charge to an area of a protein's structure. In the vicinity of the phosphate group some amino acid side chains will be attracted to the phosphate group and others repelled. The net result will be a conformational change which can result in the protein becoming temporarily biologically active. The duration of the phosphorylation event is moderated by the action of phosphatases, which remove the attached phosphate groups from proteins.

Post-translational modifications alter the size and surface charge of the original protein and these changes can be utilised to isolate the protein from a complex mixture. The addition of sugar residues to a protein can be exploited in a purification protocol by using lectin affinity chromatography (see Section 6.10) and size exclusion chromatography (see Sections 7.1–7.5). The addition of phosphate groups to a protein can be exploited by the use of ion exchange chromatography (see Section 5.2), chromatofocusing (see Section 5.3), hydroxyapatite chromatography (see Section 5.4), immunoaffinity chromatography using monoclonal antibodies specific for functional groups (e.g., phosphoserine) (see Section 6.9), and preparative isoelectric focusing (see Section 7.12).

2.7.7   Engineering proteins to aid purification

If the gene for a protein is available (and there are many commercial companies that can provide genes at a modest price), it is possible to express the gene in another organism to overproduce the protein of interest. The increase in the total amount of the protein of interest in the initial extraction will aid purification. It is also possible to add additional components to the recombinant protein's structure to provide an affinity tag which will promote the purification process (see Sections 6.11–6.12).

2.8   A RANGE OF TECHNIQUES THAT CAN BE USED IN PROTEIN PURIFICATION

There are a wide variety of techniques that can be used in a purification procedure. The most popular of these techniques are covered in the later chapters of this book.

2.8.1   Surface charge

Techniques that exploit the differences in proteins' surface charge include: ion exchange chromatography (IEX), chromatofocusing, hydroxyapatite chromatography (HA) (see Chapter 5), non-denaturing polyacrylamide gel **electrophoresis** (PAGE) and preparative isoelectric focusing (IEF) (see Chapter 8).

2.8.2   Hydrophobicity

Techniques that exploit the hydrophobic character of a protein include: salting out of proteins (see Section 4.11.2), hydrophobic interaction chromatography (HIC) (see Section 5.5), and reversed-phase chromatography (see Section 8.8).

2.8.3   Biospecificity

Techniques that exploit some aspect of biospecificity, post-translational modification or engineering include: affinity chromatography, covalent chromatography, immunoaffinity chromatography and immobilised metal affinity chromatography (IMAC) (see Chapter 6).

2.8.4   Molecular mass

Techniques that exploit the molecular mass of a protein include: size exclusion chromatography (SEC) (see Chapter 7), dynamic light scattering (see Section 7.9), ultrafiltration (see Section 4.11) and denaturing (in the presence of the detergent) sodium dodecyl sulphate (SDS) polyacrylamide gel electrophoresis (SDS-PAGE) (see Chapter 8).

The list of the available techniques is not exhaustive and protein-specific variations abound in the literature.

2.9   SUMMARY

Amino acids are small zwitterionic molecules with many interesting characteristics. The genetic codes for twenty amino acids are used in the synthesis of eukaryotic proteins. These twenty amino acids have different functional groups; some have weak acid charges and others have hydrophobic properties. The biosynthetic enzymes involved in amino acid metabolism have evolved to use only the L-isomers of the twenty amino acids. The amino acids are joined sequentially adding only at the free carboxyl end of the polypeptide chain. To lower the thermodynamic energy associated with the polypeptide chain emerging from the ribosome, secondary structures (e.g., α-helix and β-sheet) are formed, broken and reformed until all the mRNA has been processed. The final tertiary structure of a protein is primarily driven by the thermodynamic need to accommodate the hydrophobic functional groups to keep them as far away from water as possible. The final shape of the protein has the majority of amino acids with hydrophobic functional groups in the core of the structure and the amino acids with charged and polar functional groups in contact with the watery cellular environment. There are limited physical properties associated with proteins to enable a successful purification protocol but an increasing number of chromatographic techniques to achieve success.

RECOMMENDED READING

Research papers

Cahn, R.S., Ingold, C.K. and Prelog, V. (1956) The specification of asymmetric configuration in organic chemistry. *Experientia* 12:81-124.

Rienders, J. and Sickman A. (2007) Modificomics: Posttranslational modifications beyond protein phosphorylation and glycosylation. *Biomol Eng* 24:169-177.

Solcum, D.W., Sugarman, D. and Tucker, S.P. (1971) The two faces of D- and L-nomenclature. *J Chem Educ* 48:597-600.

Books

Alberts, B., Johnson, A., Lewis, J., Raff, M., Roberts, K. and Walter, P. (2014) *Molecular Biology of the Cell.* 6th ed. Garland Science (Taylor & Francis Group), New York, USA.

Barrett, G.C. and Elmore, D.T. (2009) *Amino Acids and Peptides.* Cambridge University Press, Cambridge, UK.

Berg, J.M., Tymoczko, J.L. and Stryer, L. (2015) *Biochemistry.* 8th ed. W.H. Freeman, New York, USA.

Lesk, A. (2016) *Introduction to Protein Science: Architecture, Function, and Genomics.* Oxford University Press, Oxford, UK.

Nelson, D.L. and Cox, M.M. (2012) *Lehninger Principles of Biochemistry.* 6th ed. W.H. Freeman, New York, USA.

Petsko, G. and Ringe, D. (2008) *Protein Structure and Function.* Oxford University Press, Oxford, UK.

Williamson, M. (2011) *How Proteins Work.* Garland Science (Taylor & Francis Group), New York, USA.

Whitford, D. (2005) *Proteins: Structure and Function.* Wiley Blackwell, Chichester, UK.

Chromatography and the Strategy of Protein Purification

3

3.1 INTRODUCTION

At the turn of the 1900s, a Russian botanist named Mikhail Tswett separated plant pigments on a column of adsorbent material. He demonstrated that the pigments he extracted from plants are composed of more than one compound, some of which have colours other than green. "Chromatography" means "writing with colours" (from the Greek verb *graphein*, meaning "to write," and the noun *chroma*, meaning "colour"). The technique did not gain common usage in mainstream science until the 1930s, when paper and thin-layer chromatography (TLC) became popular techniques, when they were used to analyse the products of synthetic chemistry. Since then chromatography has blossomed into a wide variety of liquid- (e.g., high-performance liquid chromatography [HPLC]) and gas- (gas–liquid chromatography [GLC]) based separation techniques. The diversity of the chromatographic techniques available today means that there are methods to separate virtually any soluble (or volatile) molecule. Many of these techniques have been adapted or developed to provide the means to purify proteins from complex mixtures.

3.2 CHROMATOGRAPHY

Molecules within a complex mixture will have a variety of chemical structures with different properties. These properties can be grouped into four areas: (i) the presence of positive and/or negative charges on the molecule (surface charge); (ii) the molecule's polarity (either "water loving" [hydrophilic] or "water hating" [hydrophobic]); (iii) the ability of the molecule to enter the gas phase (volatility); and (iv) the size and shape of the molecule. If molecules have subtle differences in these properties, a chromatographic technique can be used in isolation (or in combination) to separate the molecules within a complex mixture.

Chromatography consists of two distinct immiscible phases (the mobile phase and the stationary phase) and molecules will interact differently with each of these immiscible phases depending on their properties. A familiar household example of two immiscible phases in close contact with each other is a beaker containing a volume of olive oil and water. The oil (hydrophobic) cannot dissolve in the water, so it remains floating on the surface of the water. However, the oil can be dispersed throughout the water by vigorous mixing, resulting in a cloudy emulsion. Immediately after the mixing has stopped, the oil droplets will fuse, and over a period of time the oil will once again float on the surface of water. The two immiscible phases will once again be evident (see Section 1.3).

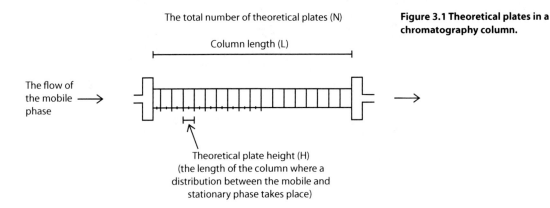

The total number of theoretical plates (N)

Column length (L)

The flow of
the mobile
phase

Theoretical plate height (H)
(the length of the column where a
distribution between the mobile and
stationary phase takes place)

Figure 3.1 Theoretical plates in a chromatography column.

If a molecule is introduced into the presence of two immiscible phases, it will preferentially reside in one or the other phases, depending on the properties of its structure. A completely hydrophobic molecule will prefer to reside in the oil phase and an extremely polar molecule will prefer to reside in the water phase. A molecule with both hydrophilic and hydrophobic features will distribute (or partition) between both phases. Using a separating funnel and two beakers, the extent of the distribution between the two phases can be measured and the equilibrium coefficient for the distribution between the two immiscible phases (K_D; see Section 3.3.1) determined.

In chromatography the two immiscible phases can be variety of liquid/liquid, liquid/gas or liquid/solid phases. When molecules are introduced into a chromatography column, they distribute between the two available immiscible phases; the mobile phase flows around (and sometimes through) the stationary phase, which may have a **ligand** covalently attached. The length of a chromatography column where a molecule forms a distribution between the two immiscible phases (analogous to the distribution using a separating funnel; see above) is called a theoretical plate (H = theoretical plate height). There will be a total number of theoretical plates in a column (N), which is related to the length of the column (L) (see Figure 3.1).

3.3   THE THEORIES OF CHROMATOGRAPHY

Two main theories have been proposed to explain aspects of chromatography. The plate theory describes the retention of molecules on the column and the rate theory covers the process of band broadening throughout the chromatographic run.

3.3.1   The plate theory of chromatography

Martin and Synge (1941) developed partition chromatography in liquid/liquid phases, for which they were awarded Nobel Prizes in 1952. The plate theory of chromatography describes the means by which molecules are retained on a chromatography column, proposing that the molecules introduced into the flow of the mobile phase when they encounter the stationary phase will distribute (partition) between the two phases according to their distribution coefficients (K_D). If there is a fixed flow rate through a column (of a set length) the retention time (t_r) and retention volume (V_r) can be determined and used to calculate K_D.

The distribution (or partition) coefficient (K_D) in chromatography

$$K_D = \frac{\text{the concentration of a compound in the stationary phase}}{\text{the concentration of a compound in the mobile phase}}$$

Separation of the different molecules in a complex mixture is only possible if the constituent molecules have different distribution coefficients (K_D). Molecules with a preference to distribute onto the stationary phase will migrate down the column at a slower rate than will the molecules with a preference to distribute into the mobile phase.

Imagine a sample that has been introduced into the mobile phase of a chromatographic column. Upon encountering the stationary phase, a distribution will occur according to the distribution coefficients of the molecules in the sample. The area within the column where an equilibrium takes place between the sample in the mobile phase and the sample in the stationary phase is called a theoretical plate. As the fresh mobile phase is introduced into the column, new equilibriums will take place. The more a molecule has the opportunity to form equilibria between the mobile and stationary phases, the greater the likelihood that it will be resolved from other molecules in a complex mixture. Chromatography columns with numerous theoretical plates will possess a superior ability to resolve complex mixtures.

3.3.2   The rate theory of chromatography

The plate theory of chromatography assumes that the molecules in the mobile phase interact immediately with the stationary phase and that progress of molecules down the column is by sequential transfer from one theoretical plate to the next theoretical plate. The rate theory of chromatography (van Deemter et al., 1956) encompasses aspects of chromatography that cannot be accounted for by the plate theory.

The van Deemter equation relates the theoretical plate height (H) with the linear flow rate (u) in a chromatography column (see Figure 3.2). Peak broadening as molecules progress down a chromatography column is influenced by:

(A) Eddy diffusion (see Figures 3.2 and 3.3)

   The molecules applied to a column will take a variety of random paths through the stationary phase. The molecules that take the shortest route will be at the front of the final peak and the molecules that progress through a longer path will be at the end of the peak. The contribution of Eddy diffusion to peak broadening is constant at all flow rates.

(B) Longitudinal diffusion (see Figures 3.2 and 3.3)

   The concentration of any molecule will be highest at centre of the peak. Molecules diffuse away from an area of high concentration to an area of low concentrate on (see Appendix 1), which contributes to peak broadening. The effect of longitudinal diffusion is increased at lower flow rates.

(C) Resistance to mass transfer (Cs transfer to the stationary phase and Cm transfer to the mobile phase) (see Figure 3.2)

   Molecules in the mobile phase do not necessarily interact with

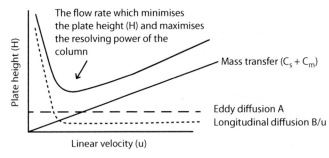

The flow rate which minimises the plate height (H) and maximises the resolving power of the column

Plate height (H)

Mass transfer ($C_s + C_m$)

Eddy diffusion A
Longitudinal diffusion B/u

Linear velocity (u)

Van Deemter equation $(H) = A + \dfrac{B}{u} + (C_s + C_m)u$

Figure 3.2 A van Deemter plot for a liquid chromatography column.

Factory A (Eddy diffusion) -peak broadening due to multiple paths through the resin. Molecule travels further.

Factory B/u (longitudinal diffusion) -peak broadening due to longitudinal diffusion molecule will always diffuse from an area of high concentration to an area of low concentration

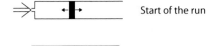

Start of the run

Towards the end of the run

Figure 3.3 The parameters that influence peak broadening in the progress of molecules down a chromatography column taken from the van Deemter equation.

the stationary phase instantly. They flow over and sometimes through the stationary phase before any interaction. If the flow rate of the mobile phase is too high, the molecules in the mobile phase that could have interacted with the stationary phase will be swept down the column with limited interaction with the stationary phase. This will contribute to broadening of the final peak. The effect of this resistance to mass transfer increases in a linear fashion as the flow rate increases.

There is an optimum flow rate for any chromatography column which minimizes the theoretical plate height (H) thereby maximising the theoretical plate number and the resolving power of the column (see Figure 3.2).

3.4   PARAMETERS IN CHROMATOGRAPHY

The emerging profile of all molecules (large or small) applied to a chromatographic column closely approximates a "normal" (Gaussian) distribution with a characteristic retention time (or volume). In the chromatography of small molecule (e.g., reversed-phase HPLC; see Section 3.7 and Section 8.8), the retention time can be used to tentatively identify the molecule in the sample by cross-reference to the retention time of a pure standard applied on the same column eluted with the same conditions. When the detection method utilises the **absorbance** of UV/visible light the area of the eluted peak can also be used to quantify (the **Beer-Lambert law**) how much of the sample contains the molecule of interest. This is achieved by applying increasing amounts of the pure sample standard and recording the changes in peak area to construct a calibration plot (peak area versus the amount of standard).

However, in the chromatography of proteins, these possible benefits are rarely used because the availability of pure standard protein can be limiting. The important parameters in protein chromatography include the *resolution* of the column (the ability of the column to provide baseline separation of molecules), the *capacity* (the amount of sample that can be applied before the column is overloaded and the resolution compromised) and the *yield* (the amount of biologically active protein that is eluted compared to the amount that has been applied). The resolution of a chromatography column is related to the theoretical plate number (N). The capacity of chromatography resin with adsorbent properties (see Chapter 5) used in protein purification is usually included in the information supplied by the manufacturers. It is usually expressed as the amount of a standard protein, such as bovine serum albumin (BSA) that binds per ml of resin. This should only be used as a guide, as the capacity of the resin will vary depending on the starting material. The yield of the target protein can be determined quantitatively and qualitatively (see Section 8.3).

3.5 THE STRATEGY OF PROTEIN PURIFICATION

3.5.1 Introduction

The theories of chromatography are applicable to the chromatography of small molecules and proteins, but special considerations have to be made when the purification of proteins is attempted. This is because proteins are polymers constructed from twenty different amino acids (see Chapter 2). The final biologically active structure of a protein is held together by a variety of relatively weak forces (hydrophobic, van der Waal, H-bonding and salt bridges) that can be disrupted if precautions are not put in place. For example, temperature and pH fluctuations, the presence of contaminating molecules (detergents, metal ions or solvents) and the activities of hydrolytic enzymes (**peptidases**) can result in the destabilisation of a protein's biologically active form (see Table 3.1).

Initially, protein purification (enrichment) can seem unnecessarily complex, with little or no strategy involved. However, with some background information and a little experience, protein purification can become an engrossing challenge. In addition, it is important to constantly bear in mind the purpose of starting the purification process in the first place. The process of purifying a protein can be time-consuming, so it is worth remembering that it can be difficult to produce a completely (100%) pure preparation of a protein. The process can expensive in terms of the equipment, the resins and the time required to run the columns and assay the fractions collected. A clear and specific target for the degree of purification required needs to be determined at the start of the purification process (see Table 3.2). For example, if the aim is to raise antibodies against the target protein or to measure the kinetics of an enzyme (free from conflicting activities), then it may not be necessary to purify the protein to homogeneity. One or two chromatographic procedures may produce the required level of purity to meet these targets. However, if the aim of

Table 3.1 Parameters that may impact upon the recovery of a target protein following extraction.	
Parameter	**Description**
Peptidase activity	Eukaryotic cells compartmentalise groups of proteins into distinct organelles. Upon extraction the proteins that are normally kept apart are mixed together. Some of these proteins will be peptidase enzymes present in the **lysosomes** of animal cells or the vacuoles of plant cells. It is important to establish the range of peptidase enzymes that are present in the extract (see Section 4.4.5) so that in subsequent extractions appropriate inhibitors can be added to reduce the endogenous peptidase activity. In the early stages of purification (when protein concentration is relatively high) the peptidase enzymes have a wide range of proteins to act upon and the damage done to the target protein may be minimal. But during the later stages of purification, when the protein of interest becomes a significant percentage of the total protein, any protease contamination will produce significant loss of yield. Bacterial contamination can be minimised by filtering chromatographic buffers through 0.2 μm membranes and by regularly centrifuging the extracts at 12,000 × g for 20 minutes (see Section 4.10). Co-purification of an endogenous peptidase can be checked by assaying the fractions from a chromatographic run using a peptidase assay (see Protocol 4.5). If this peptidase assay shows a positive signal, adjustments can be made to the chromatographic conditions to try to avoid co-elution, additional peptidase inhibitors can be added or other proteins (e.g., bovine serum albumin [BSA]) can be included as a preferential substrate to prevent proteolysis of the target protein.
Temperature and pH instability	Having determined the peptidase profile of the extract, the temperature stability of a protein can be established by incubation of the extract at different temperatures over a period of a week. This should be determined at the same time as buffer and pH compatibility (see Section 4.2). It may well be that the target protein can be stored at a different pH than the one required for maximal activity. The effect of different buffers on the activity can also be determined.
Irreversible denaturation on interfaces	Irreversible binding of the protein of interest may occur to the materials (glass, plastic and chromatographic resins) used in the purification process, particularly at the later stages of purification when the protein concentration is dilute. This unwelcome binding of protein to surfaces can be reduced by silanising the glassware and by the inclusion of a low level of a non-ionic detergent such as 0.01% (v/v) Triton X100. Microfuge tubes and pipette tips with low protein/peptide binding can be purchased and are recommended for use in the later stages of protein purification. In addition, protein will be lost at air/liquid interfaces; therefore great care must be taken to reduce the foaming of protein solutions.
Metal ions	Proteins that are exported from the cell can have a number of covalent disulphide bridges present to help stabilise their tertiary structure. Other proteins may have reduced sulphydryl groups present on the surface of the protein or at the active site of the protein. Divalent heavy metal ions can covalently bind with reduced sulphydryl groups altering the surface properties of a protein or causing an enzyme to be inactive. To avoid this problem the reagents and the water (ultrapure 18.2 MΩ·cm at 25°C) used to make up chromatographic buffers should be of the highest grade possible. In addition, the inclusion of a **chelating** agent (e.g., 1–5 mM EDTA) that can bind divalent metal ions will reduce the problem.

the purification procedure is to produce sufficient protein to grow a crystal or use as a therapeutic agent, then a **homogeneous** product must be produced.

The final level of purity to meet the desired target is an important parameter, determined in part by the yield of the protein at each stage of purification. The percentage recovery of the target protein is usually acceptable in the early stages of purification, when the total protein is high, but as the total protein decreases and the percentage of the target protein increases (relative to the total protein), large losses can occur. Protein will be lost at each stage of the purification process due to a variety of factors (see Table 3.1) and the mantra in any purification procedure must be "minimise the total number of steps to maximise the final yield." The phrase "steps" can

Table 3.2 Possible targets to warrant protein purification.

Target	Reasons	Stages required	See Sections and Protocols
Kinetic analysis	Removal of conflicting enzyme activities, inhibitors and activators	Extraction, clarification, concentration followed by initial capture (by IEX and or HIC).	Sections 4.2 and 4.4 Sections 5.2 and 5.5
Sequence data	Isolation of the gene. Searching for functionality by identifying motifs and domains	Extraction, clarification, concentration (possibly by acetone precipitation) followed by 2D-SDS-PAGE and MS/MS. Or further enrichment (by IEX and or HIC) prior to 2D-SDS-PAGE and MS/MS.	Sections 4.4–4.9; 4.11 Protocol 4.10 Sections 5.2 and 5.5; Section 8.3
Crystallography, Manufacturing: for the biotechnology or diagnostic industries	The production of substantial amounts of pure protein	An abundant protein can be purified; extraction, clarification, concentration; initial capture (by IEX and or HIC). A protein with low natural abundance can be purified as a recombinant protein overexpressed in, for example, *E. coli*. To produce relatively large amounts of protein which can be manufactured with an affinity tag (e.g., 6 His tag) to facilitate affinity purification. Polishing to remove aggregates or trace contaminants.	Sections 4.4–4.5 and 4.8; Sections 5.2 and 5.4 Sections 6.11 and 6.12 Section 7.5.2
Antibodies raised to the target protein for academic or industrial purposes	Partial purification to raise the antibodies. The antibodies could be used to determine cross-reactivity with other species and cellular location. Possibly as a diagnostic tool	Extraction, clarification, concentration followed by initial capture (by IEX and or HIC). **Polyclonal** and monoclonal antibodies purification by **protein A** or G. Alternatively, cation exchange, mixed modal and lectin affinity chromatography. Polishing to remove aggregates or trace contaminants.	Sections 4.4–4.5 and 4.8; Sections 5.2 and 5.4 Section 6.9 and Protocol 6.1 Sections 5.2 and 5.7; Protocol 6.2 Section 7.5.2

include both the handling stages (e.g., dialysis) and the chromatography procedures. The effect the number of steps in a purification schedule has on the final yield is illustrated in Figure 3.4. Assuming a 90% recovery at each stage of an 8-step purification schedule, the final yield will be 50% of the starting target protein. If the recovery is 75% at each stage, the final recovery will be as low as 25% after an 8-step schedule. It is not unrealistic to experience 80–90% recoveries in the early stages of a purification schedule, only for the recovery to plummet to below 25% recovery during the later stages. Consideration of this point will impact the overall purification strategy.

Having determined the level of purity sufficient to meet the proposed needs of the operator, one must determine a protein purification schedule. This does not necessarily have to be envisaged from scratch, as there will be a vast array of information already available in textbooks, academic

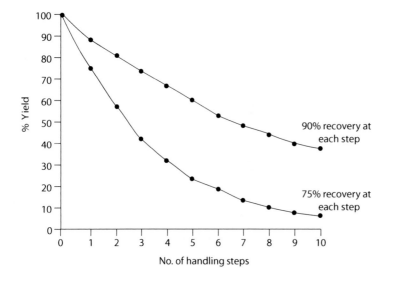

Figure 3.4 The decrease in overall yield in a protein purification schedule as a function of the number of handling steps (assuming either a 90% or 75% recovery at each step).

papers and the technical information provided by suppliers to support the use of the resins they manufacture. This published information does not necessarily have to be specifically about your target protein, as vital information can be gleaned from reading the efforts of other researchers who have been working on the same protein extracted from a different source. This information could include appropriate protein and enzyme assays, extraction and clarification procedures, and the pH and thermal stabilities of the target protein, as well as the starting and elution conditions for chromatographic resins (see Chapter 4). Previously printed information should also indicate the purity and yields that may be expected at each stage.

3.5.2   Strategy

The human genome contains approximately 30,000 different genes but there are more than 400,000 different proteins (the difference being due to alternative splicing of genes and the many post-translational modifications that can be present on proteins, e.g., glycosylation and phosphorylation). These different proteins have all been derived from the same pool of twenty amino acids (see Chapter 2). Included in those twenty amino acids are the four amino acids that have a charged functional group at physiological pH values (aspartate and glutamate, with a negatively charged functional group, and lysine and arginine, with a positively charged functional group). So, it is unlikely that there will be sufficient differences in the surface charge of proteins in a complex mixture to be able to isolate the target protein to homogeneity using this physical property alone.

Separating proteins based upon surface charge (e.g., ion exchange chromatography) will allow the operator to gather the target protein in a volume of buffer with proteins of similar charge. The target protein will be enriched relative to the new total protein pooled together based upon surface charge (see Chapter 5), and the other proteins eluted from the original complex mixture can be discarded. The next question will be "What should I do next?" The target protein is now in a less complex mixture of proteins with a similar surface charge, so another overlapping chromatography technique based upon a protein's surface charge (e.g., ion exchange chromatography with a diethylaminoethyl (-DEAE) functional group followed by ion exchange chromatography with a quaternary ammonium (-Q) functional group) is unlikely to be productive. However, there can be merit in switching to a smaller diameter of resin bead later in a purification schedule, as this can yield benefits in resolution. For example, an IEX resin with a 50 μm bead diameter may be used in the early stages of purification; then following the use of other chromatographic procedures, the use of an IEX resin with a 5 μm bead diameter will concentrate a dilute sample and should provide improved resolution of the eluted material due to its increased number of theoretical plates (see above). To further enrich the post-ion-exchange pooled fraction, another property of proteins that can be exploited to purify them (see Section 2.7) should be employed, because after being separated based upon surface charge, the proteins will still have subtle differences in hydrophobicity, biospecificity, size and possibly post-translational modifications.

A purification strategy based upon one physical property to the exclusion of the others is unlikely to be successful, whereas an **orthogonal** purification strategy that avoids overlapping methods but relies upon a combination of different techniques that exploit differences in the target protein's charge, biospecificity, hydrophobicity and/or size is more likely to be successful. In some instances, a one-step purification strategy based upon a protein's biospecificity (see Chapter 6) may provide the operator with a yield of the target protein with sufficient purity to fulfil the task aims.

3.5.3 The process of protein purification

Currently, protein purification can be roughly divided into two topics: the purification of recombinant proteins (see Chapter 6) and the purification of proteins from a natural source. Although initially these may seem distinct, they are not **mutually exclusive**. The purification of recombinant proteins relies on the operator engineering the target protein with an affinity label that facilitates a "straightforward" affinity-based purification procedure. This process has proven very successful but in a number of instances it has been found that the recombinant affinity procedure needs to be supplemented with other protein purification procedures to produce a homogeneous target protein. Additional steps may be needed to remove co-eluting proteins from the host organism used in the production of the target protein. These co-eluting proteins may also bind to the affinity resin or they may bind to the target protein. Awareness of other protein purification techniques, as well as when and how to use them, will provide the operator with a knowledge base to successfully complete the initial target requirement.

Whether the starting point is the purification of a recombinant protein or a protein purified from a natural source, the strategy for the purification of the target protein will follow a similar path. It is hoped that this book will provide some information to help in the purification process. Due care and attention to detail at each stage of the purification procedure (see Tables 3.3a and 3.3b; also Appendix 4) will enable the operator to maximise the amount of protein initially extracted and eventually recovered.

The cytoplasm of the cell is a reducing environment that is essentially oxygen-free and has a relatively high protein concentration. The extraction process is the first step in the purification of a target protein; this has to be efficient and sufficiently benign to obtain the maximum amount of the target protein in a biologically active form (if required). In the process of extraction there is a reversal of the cellular protein's natural environment, from a high protein concentration to a relatively low one (diluted usually five- to tenfold) and from a reducing to an oxidising environment (the aqueous buffer and extraction procedure; see Sections 4.5–4.9). Additional reagents may be required in the extraction buffer to help stabilise the extracted proteins in this initial extraction process. These reagents can include: (a) **reducing agents** to help overcome the deleterious effects of oxidation; (b) chelating reagents to reduce metal ions interacting with proteins, particularly those proteins with reduced sulphydryl groups. Particularly cysteine present on the surface of the protein or at its active site; and (c) peptidase inhibitors to inhibit the hydrolytic activity of peptidases that may be released during the extraction process, thus minimising the damage to the target protein in the extraction process (see Table 3.1 and Section 4.4). The initial extraction will contain the target protein, but it will also contain unbroken cells and metabolites. Therefore, the next step in the purification process should be a clarification step.

In the laboratory, differential centrifugation is the most common procedure used to clarify an extract. Incremental increases in the relative centrifugal force (g) and the time the force is applied to the extract can be used to sequentially fractionate the contents of disrupted eukaryotic cells and to remove the debris from **prokaryotic** cells (see Section 4.10). In industry, the initial extraction process may generate large volumes of the extract, which will require the use of specialised centrifuges, ultrafiltration or fluidised bed setups (see Sections 4.11 and 4.12) to clarify the extract. When the extract has been clarified free from debris the dilute extract will require concentration to remove water and unwanted cellular metabolites which can be considered the major contaminants at this stage of the purification process.

A variety of techniques can be used to concentrate the clarified extract prior to its application to a chromatographic resin (see Section 4.11). In the early stages of protein purification, a precipitation step (e.g., using ammonium sulphate, polyethylene glycol [PEG] or a solvent) is favoured in the laboratory due to the low cost of the materials and the relatively easy recovery of the precipitated protein by centrifugation. Ultrafiltration (see Section 4.11.10) may be preferred in an industrial setting because large amount of salts, PEG and solvents would present unacceptable problems in terms of safe disposal of waste and in the case of solvents, fire risk. Protein precipitation by salts and ultrafiltration are relatively easy-to-use techniques and they produce a good yield, but they usually have low resolving power. However, the clarified and concentrated extract will have been prepared for application to a chromatographic resin.

It is difficult to generalise on the route any purification process would take after the clarification stage. However, some chromatographic techniques are best employed at different stages of the schedule. (Table 3.3a provides a list of techniques that favour employment at different stages of the purification process and Figure 3.5 provides a general overview of purification schedules with reminders to examine the level of purity at each stage.) The information in Table 3.3 and Figure 3.5 remains suggestive because the overriding maxim of any purification process is to be pragmatic and complete the task at hand. So, if a technique works, then stick with it, even if it is being used in a different area of the purification process. The choice and order of chromatographic steps depend upon the target protein. For example, a protein produced by recombinant technology can be purified using two or three chromatographic steps (see Chapter 6), whereas more than two chromatographic steps are typically required for the purification of non-recombinant proteins extracted from cellular material.

Table 3.3a The different stages of protein purification and some suggested techniques that may be appropriate in a laboratory protein purification protocol with some industrial scale alternatives.

Stage	Target	Lab scale	Industrial scale
Extraction	Maximise the amount of target protein extracted into an appropriate buffer	(a) There are many different extraction procedures depending on the source material (see Section 4.5 and Table 4.6) (b) Peptidase inhibitors or other additives (see Section 4.4.5) may be included to minimise the loss of target protein	(a) Ball mill (b) Liquid shear (e.g., French press) (see Section 4.8.2) (c) Additives may be used but this can drive up costs. The speed of extraction at a reduced temperature is used to control the initial loss of the target protein.
Clarification	Removal of eukaryotic organelles and cellular debris	Typically centrifugation (e.g., differential centrifugation of eukaryotic cell extracts) (see Section 4.10.1)	(a) Industrial centrifuges (e.g., solid bowl scroll or stacked disc) (b) Tangential or cross-flow ultrafiltration (c) The clarification and capture can be combined using expanded bed chromatography (see Section 4.12)
Concentration	Removal of water	Typically ammonium sulphate precipitation followed by centrifugation to capture the precipitate (see Section 4.11)	(a) Tangential or cross-flow ultrafiltration (b) Precipitation using polyethylene glycol (PEG), followed by centrifugation to capture the precipitate (c) Ion exchange chromatography
Initial contaminant removal	High capacity for binding the target protein. Excellent recovery of the target protein and good resolution from contaminants	Column chromatography on short fat columns (IEX, HIC) using gradient elution (see Sections 5.2–5.5)	(a) Batch purification (see Sections 4.12–4.13) (b) Large-scale column chromatography using **isocratic** elution (see Section 3.6.7) (c) Membrane filters are available with ion exchange properties (see Section 4.13)
Affinity	Excellent resolution	(a) Manufacturer-supplied affinity resin (e.g., Cibacron blue agarose) (b) Bespoke affinity resin (c) Immobilised metal ion affinity chromatography (IMAC) (d) A series of different chromatography resins determined experimentally (see Chapter 6)	(a) Manufacturer supplied affinity resin (e.g., protein G-agarose) (b) Bespoke affinity resin (c) Immobilised metal ion affinity chromatography (IMAC) (d) A series of different chromatography resins determined experimentally (see Chapter 6) (e) Ultrafiltration (see Section 4.11.10)

(Continued)

Table 3.3a (Continued) The different stages of protein purification and some suggested techniques that may be appropriate in a laboratory protein purification protocol with some industrial scale alternatives

Stage	Target	Lab scale	Industrial scale
polishing	Removal of minor contaminants	(a) Long thin columns are used for size exclusion chromatography (see Section 7.2) (b) Native PAGE (see Section 8.3.6.1) (c) IEF (see Section 8.6) (d) Ultrafiltration (see Section 4.11.10)	(a) Ultrafiltration (see Section 4.11.10)

Pre-purification planning for both laboratory (see Section 3.5 and Section 4.4) and industrial scale protein purification:
(a) Set purification goals.
(b) Plan the putative purification procedure.
(c) Check that the appropriate instruments are available and the funding is in place to cover possible contingencies.
(d) Establish a convenient assay for the target protein.
(e) Establish thermal and pH stability of the target protein (see Section 4.2)
(f) Undertake small scale chromatographic resin experiments to screen for appropriate resins and the conditions to bind and elute the target protein (see Section 4.2 and Protocol 5.1).
(g) Undertake a screen to identify the best source of the target protein (tissue, cell or recombinant organism; see Section 4.4).
(h) Undertake a screen to identify the best method of extracting the target protein (tissue, cell or recombinant organism; see Sections 4.5–4.9).

Table 3.3b Laboratory and industrial scale techniques which may be used throughout a protein purification protocol.

Procedures used throughout the Purification process	Lab scale	Industrial scale
Buffer exchange	(a) Dialysis (see Protocol 4.9) (b) SEC using Sephadex G-25 or G-50 or **Biogel** P6-10; see Section 7.5.3 and Protocol 7.1) (c) Centrifugal concentrators (see Section 4.11.10.2)	(a) Size exclusion chromatography (SEC) (see Section 7.2)
Purification check	(a) Enzyme and protein assays (see Section 4.2) (b) Electrophoresis (e.g., SDS-PAGE; see Section 8.2) (c) HPLC (e.g., Reversed-phase chromatography; see Chapter 3 and Section 8.8) (d) Amino acid composition (e.g., MALDI MS/MS or RP-HPLC ESI MS/MS)	(a) Enzyme and protein assay in the QC lab (see Section 4.2) (b) Electrophoresis (e.g., SDS-PAGE, see Section 8.2) in the QC lab (c) HPLC (e.g., reversed-phase chromatography, see Section 8.8) (d) Immunoassays to (i) check for the presence of host proteins in a target protein produced in a recombinant system and (ii) check for the presence of proteins leaking from an immunoaffinity resin, see Sections 6.9 and 8.8) (e) Amino acid composition (e.g., MALDI MS/MS or RP-HPLC ESI MS/MS)
Resin or membrane cleaning and regeneration	Washing and storage according to the manufacturer's instructions	Typically a wash with 1.0 M NaOH (hot) to cleanse and sanitise the membrane or resin prior to reuse
Process validation	May not be required	Stringent attention to the validity of the methods used may be required

Selection of the starting material (tissue or cells)[1] (see Section 4.4)
Selection of the disruption technique (see Sections 4.5–4.9)
Clarification of the **homogenate** (see Section 4.10)

(A) Concentrate the extract
(Note: after ammonium sulphate precipitation, dialysis
[B] may be required prior to IEX but not prior to HIC)

(B) Dialysis (see Protocol 4.9) prior to chromatography

(C) Chromatography[2]
Try IEX (see Section 5.2)
  or HIC (see Section 5.5)
  or IMAC (see Section 6.11)

Chromatography for recombinant
  proteins (see Section 6.12)
if 6 His tag uses IMAC (see Section 6.11)
if a fusion protein uses affinity
  chromatography (see Section 6.12.3)

Chromatography for antibodies
Try affinity chromatography on
  protein A or G (Protocol 6.1)
Try HCIC (see Section 3.5)
Try MMC (see Section 5.7)
Try lectin affinity chromatography
  (see Section 6.10)

Assay for increases in activity and yield (see Section 8.2)
Observe the purity using SDS-PAGE (see Section 8.3 and Protocol 8.1)

(D) Chromatography[3]
  e.g., Affinity chromatography (see Section 6.1) or dye ligand chromatography (see Section 6.8) or
  chromatofocusing (see Section 5.3) or preparative IEF (see Section 8.6.1)
If an antibody is available to the target protein try immunoaffinity chromatography (see Section 6.9)
If the target protein has an accessible **thiol** group try covalent chromatography (see Section 6.7)
If the target is glycosylated try lectin affinity chromatography (see Section 6.10)

Assay for increases in activity and yield (see Section 8.1)
Observe the purity using SDS-PAGE (see Section 8.3 and Protocol 8.1)

(E) Chromatography[4]
  e.g., SEC (see Section 7.1) or hydroxyapatite (see Section 5.4) or MMC (see Section 5.7) or preparative
  PAGE/electroelution (see Section 8.4)
If activity is required try switching to an IEX or HIC resin with a smaller bead size (see Section 3.4) and
  collect only the peak fraction
If activity is not required try RP-HPLC (see Section 8.8)

Assay for increases in activity and yield (see Section 8.1)
Observe the purity using SDS-PAGE (see Section 8.3 and Protocol 8.1)

There are no proscribed routes through a protein purification procedure and at every stage **empirical**
  determination of the procedure's efficacy should be undertaken.
Understand the aims of the experiment and stop once those aims have been achieved (see Section 3.5).
If a technique does not produce the desired increase in yield or specific activity, stop using the technique and
  move to a different one.

[1]Likely to be a convenient and abundant source of the target protein yielding the largest total activity.
[2]In the initial stages, a chromatographic procedure will typically have excellent capacity with good resolution
  and will produce excellent yield of the target protein. Combinations of techniques can be used,
  e.g., HIC followed by IEX or IEX followed by IMAC.
[3]At this stage, a highly resolving technique can be used; the downside is that this may have variable capacity
  and yield. It may be possible to use a combination of techniques.
[4]At this stage, removal of contaminants, aggregates or resolution of hard-to-remove components may be required.

**Figure 3.5 A flowchart of a generic
protein purification strategy.**

Having clarified and concentrated the protein from the initial extract, it is prudent to employ a chromatography technique that has a high-binding capacity (i.e., a lot of starting material can be applied before the resolution of the column is compromised), good resolution and excellent yield. There are several techniques that demonstrate these properties, including: ion exchange chromatography (IEX), hydrophobic interaction chromatography (HIC) and immobilised metal ion affinity chromatography (IMAC) (see Chapters 5 and 6). Combinations of these techniques, in columns of decreasing volume (as the total protein decreases) and possibly of decreasing resin bead size (see Section 3.5.2), may produce a preparation that satisfies the initial aims of the purification process.

However, if the above techniques in combination have not provided the resolving power necessary to produce a homogeneous target protein, it will be necessary to introduce a technique that exploits the unique biospecific character of the target protein. The following techniques with high resolution can be considered, including: affinity chromatography (see Chapter 6), immunoaffinity chromatography (see Section 6.9), chromatofocusing (see Section 5.3), preparative polyacrylamide gel electrophoresis (see Section 8.4) or preparative isoelectric focusing (IEF) (see Section 8.6). The resolving power of these techniques is high, but in some instances the methods used to elute the bound target proteins from affinity resins (see Sections 6.4 and 6.9.2) can be harsh. This may result in the irreversible denaturation of the majority of the target protein and hence a significant reduction in the yield of biologically active material. This may be a problem if the purification goal is kinetic analysis of the target protein, as kinetic experiments can require a lot of active enzyme. If, on the other hand, the purification goal is to raise antibodies to the target protein, the presence of relatively pure protein with little activity may not be a problem.

Ideally, towards the end of the purification schedule, the sole goal will be to remove only small amounts of contaminating protein, which may appear as additional faint bands on a polyacrylamide gel (see Chapter 8) or small additional peaks on a size exclusion chromatography readout (see Section 7.5.2) from a greatly enriched preparation of the target protein. It is at this stage that as the total protein concentration starts to drop, the loss of the target protein as a percentage of the units originally extracted can easily reach double figures. If this is the case, the initial aims of the purification process (i.e., what level of purity is required) may have to be reviewed. If a compromise position is not acceptable, techniques that can be employed to remove the trace contaminants include: analytical size exclusion chromatography (SEC) (see Section 7.5.1), hydroxyapatite (see Section 5.4), reversed-phase chromatography (RPC) (note that RPC may denature the target protein; see Section 8.8) and polyacrylamide gel electrophoresis (PAGE; see Section 8.4). It is to be hoped that after all the effort expended during the purification process the initial goals will have been met.

3.6   THE EQUIPMENT REQUIRED FOR PROTEIN PURIFICATION

The equipment required to undertake column chromatography does not need to be complicated or expensive. If protein purification is not a high priority in a laboratory, it is pointless to spend a lot of money on specialised equipment. However, money spent on good columns, pumps,

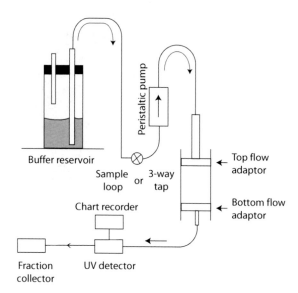

Figure 3.6 A typical protein purification chromatographic setup.

monitors and fraction collectors will improve reproducibility and assist the operator throughout the experimental procedures (see Appendix 8; list of chromatographic equipment suppliers). A typical chromatography setup is shown in Figure 3.6.

3.6.1   Columns

The choice of column depends on the technique to be used and the amount of sample to be applied. In general, techniques such as IEX or HIC require short fat columns (with a length to diameter ratio of up to 20:1), whereas size exclusion chromatography works best with long thin columns (with a length to diameter ratio of about 100:1). Affinity techniques are usually conducted in small volume columns (short and fat if the affinity between the target protein and the ligand attached to the column is high, and long and thin if the affinity is low). The columns can be purchased from a number of different manufacturers (Appendix 7; the list of chromatography equipment suppliers). Flow adaptors will increase the versatility of the column purchased by completely enclosing the resin bed volume. This means that the sample will be applied directly onto the top of the resin, preventing dilution of the sample, which is important in size exclusion chromatography experiments.

Small-volume, low-cost alternative columns can be constructed relatively easily using plastic syringes (up to 50 ml) and/or glass Pasteur pipettes. The solvent exit can be blocked with glass wool (to prevent the chromatography resin from leaving the column) and the mobile phase can be introduced manually or with a rubber bung that has a syringe needle pushed through (see Figure 3.7). For larger volumes (>50 ml) a commercial column is recommended, but glass tubing cut to the required length and then drawn to a taper can be used.

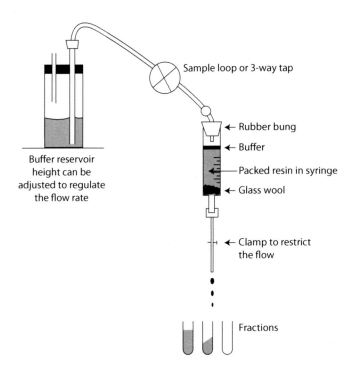

Sample loop or 3-way tap

Buffer reservoir
height can be
adjusted to regulate
the flow rate

← Rubber bung

← Buffer

— Packed resin in syringe

← Glass wool

← Clamp to restrict
the flow

Fractions

Figure 3.7 A simple to construct protein purification chromatographic setup using a syringe body, a rubber bung and a syringe needle.

3.6.2   Tubing

Flexible plastic tubing is required to connect the column to the chromatography setup. In low pressure systems, polyethylene tubing (internal diameter [i.d.] 1.0 mm) can be used to transport the majority of the liquid around the system, and a range of tubing of different i.d.'s can be used to connect the polyethylene tubing to the equipment or to other lengths of tubing. In medium- to high-pressure systems (see Section 3.7), PEEK (polyether ether ketone) tubing (i.d. 0.15–2.0 mm, outer diameter 1.59 mm and 3.18 mm), plastic ferules and/or finger tight connectors are required.

3.6.3   Pumps

When the stationary phase particles are relatively large (e.g., 50 µm), it is possible to move the mobile phase through the stationary phase using **hydrostatic pressure** (see Figures 3.6 and 3.7). The flow rate of the mobile phase can be regulated by adjusting the height of the buffer reservoir relative to the column outlet. However, for ease of use and consistently delivered variable flow rates, a peristaltic or a piston pump is recommended. At smaller bead diameters (≤20\µm), medium- to high-pressure pumps are required to move the stationary phase through the column (see Section 3.7).

3.6.4   Fraction collectors

When a complex protein mixture is applied to the resin in a column, it will be fractionated during the chromatographic run. The volume of the chromatographic run emerging from the column outlet can be divided into fractions of a suitable volume. Manually collecting 50 ml fractions from a 500 ml total volume is not too onerous a task, but the same cannot be said if the same volume is to be divided into 5.0 ml fractions or less. Fraction collectors are available that will collect more than 100 fractions on a volume or time basis. In addition, there is usually the facility to collect the chromatographic run into tubes of different sizes and formats (0.25 ml [96 well] microtitre plates, 1.5 ml **microfuge tubes**, 15–50 ml test tubes and bottles). In automated protein purification systems, the fraction collector can be set to collect only when protein peaks appear ($Abs_{280\ nm} > 0.1$) or in a well-characterised purification schedule, the fraction collector can be set to collect one peak (target protein), discarding the volume that contains the proteins of no interest to waste.

3.6.5   Detectors

Most proteins absorb light at 280 nm due to the presence of the amino acids tyrosine and tryptophan in their structure. An inline spectrophotometer placed after the exit from the column and set to detect the absorbance of ultra violet light at 280 nm provides a convenient method to monitor the progress of a chromatography experiment. Alternatively, the fractions collected throughout a chromatographic run can be analysed for the protein by manually measuring the absorbance of each fraction at 280 nm ($A_{280\ nm}$) against an appropriate buffer blank using a desktop UV/visible spectrophotometer. Diode array detectors can be purchased to continuously monitor UV and visible light at a variety of wavelengths.

3.6.6   Gradient makers

A number of chromatographic procedures (including IEX and HIC; see Chapter 5) require changes in salt concentration to elute bound protein. This can be accomplished by passing a buffer with one concentration of salt through the column and collecting the eluted protein. The salt concentration can then be altered and the process repeated. Fractions are then collected throughout this isocratic elution of the column (see Figure 3.9). The isocratic elution (see Section 3.6.7) of columns is often used during the industrial purification of proteins (see Table 3.3).

A gradient maker can be used to generate a continuously changing salt concentration presented to the proteins bound to a chromatography column. These can be purchased (or constructed; see Figure 3.8) and consist of two reservoirs of equal diameter connected by a clamped tube in the middle. The tube with the starting conditions is stirred, and when the flow rate starts, the clamp connecting the two reservoirs is removed. As liquid is pumped from the reservoir with the starting conditions, it is replaced by liquid from the end conditions reservoir. Thus the salt concentration in the starting conditions reservoir gradually changes in a linear fashion. Alternatively, medium- to high-pressure protein chromatography systems (see Table 3.4 and Figure 3.8) with a binary pump will generate a gradient by proportionally mixing the starting and end condition buffers prior to pumping the buffer onto the resin. This is controlled by the data management systems used to control the use of the equipment.

3.6.7   Different elution procedures

There are three basic elution procedures that can be used in isolation or in combination to elute compounds applied to a chromatography column.

Table 3.4 The differences between a high-pressure liquid chromatography (HPLC) system and an automated protein purification system.

Component	HPLC	Protein purification system	Comments
Operating pressure	6000 psi	Typically <100 psi	The resins used in protein purification are generally not as robust as the silica based resins used in HPLC.
Tubing	Stainless steel	Peek or plastic tubing	
Injection system	Typically small volumes (5–100 µl) using a fixed volume loop. This can be a single injection loop or typically using an automatic sample injection system.	Small volumes (0.05–1.0 ml) using a fixed volume loop. Large volumes using a variable volume (1–20 ml) loop.	Large volumes of dilute protein sample can be applied to a high capacity resin (e.g., IEX or HIC) by loading the sample into a buffer reservoir and pumping the sample liquid through the column. For larger volumes/amounts of peptides or metabolites preparative "Flash" chromatography columns are required
Pumps	Usually two pumps to allow a gradient elution	If one pump is used a gradient maker can be incorporated into the system (see Section 3.6.6). If two pumps are available for the starting and end condition buffers, they are instructed to deliver the correct proportion of each and then there is post-column mixing.	In protein purification when salt buffers are left in the tubing in contact with the pump heads, there is a chance that the salts will crystallise and damage the pump heads. A regular washing procedure (provided by the manufacturer) to wash behind the pump heads with water (or water /solvent) to remove any buffer salt that may accumulate.
Detection	Variable wavelength 200–800 nm	Fixed wavelength 260 nm and 280 nm	Additional detectors can be bought to detect peptides in the low UV (e.g., 215 nm). (see Section 3.6.5)
Fraction collection	Typically an analytical system	Sample collection systems from small to large (µl-litre) volumes	HPLCs can be used as a preparative system with fraction collectors but other method of scale up (e.g., flash chromatography) are available (see Section 3.9)

In general: (a) Protein purification systems can be run in a cold room/cabinet if a temperature-labile protein is to be separated. (b) If protein purification systems are not in constant use, the pumps, tubing and columns should be left in 20% (v/v) ethanol to restrict the growth of bacteria and fungi (c) to prevent salt precipitating in the ethanol-water mix, a wash with water prior to parking the system in 20% (v/v) ethanol will be required.

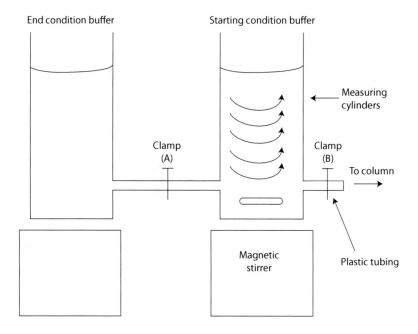

End condition buffer

Starting condition buffer

Measuring cylinders

Clamp (A)

Clamp (B)

To column

Magnetic stirrer

Plastic tubing

(i) Add the liquid and start the stirrer
(ii) Release clamp (A) and then clamp (B)

Figure 3.8 An easy-to-construct gradient former for use in the gradient elution of protein from a chromatographic resin. This would typically be used in conjunction with a peristaltic pump.

3.6.7.1   Isocratic elution

When the mobile phase is constant throughout a chromatography run, this is described as isocratic elution of the components in the applied sample (see Figure 3.9A). Size exclusion chromatography (SEC; see Chapter 7) provides a good example of isocratic elution, where proteins do not bind to the SEC resin within the column but partition into the spaces of the porous beads. In SEC, the buffer of the mobile phase remains constant throughout and does not influence the elution of the components in the applied sample. In isocratic elution, a long thin column and a slow flow rate will help maximise the possible interactions between the components in the mobile and the stationary phase.

3.6.7.2   Stepped isocratic elution

When components of the applied sample interact and bind to the chromatography resin, they will remain bound to the resin while the starting buffer conditions remain constant. To elute the bound components, the salt concentration in the buffer needs to be increased (e.g., with ion exchange chromatography [IEX] [see Section 5.2]) or decreased (e.g., with hydrophobic interaction chromatography [HIC] [see Section 5.5]). In IEX, this can be achieved using a gradient of increasing salt concentration (see Section 3.6.7.3) or by adding additional salt to the starting buffer and running this elevated buffered salt solution through the column for two column volumes. Protein will elute as a peak and will represent all the proteins that would elute between the starting and end conditions of this

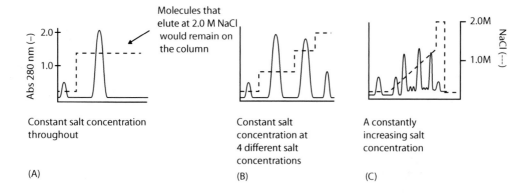

Molecules that elute at 2.0 M NaCl would remain on the column

Constant salt concentration throughout

(A)

Constant salt concentration at 4 different salt concentrations

(B)

A constantly increasing salt concentration

(C)

Figure 3.9 The different mobile phase profiles that can be utilised to elute components applied to a chromatography column. (A) Isocratic elution. (B) Stepped isocratic elution. (C) Gradient elution.

elution (e.g., 0–0.5 M NaCl). This process can be repeated by increasing the salt in the buffer (e.g., 0.5–1.0 M NaCl followed by 1.0–1.5 M NaCl) until the final salt conditions (e.g., 1.5–2.0 M NaCl) have flowed through the column. The protein applied to the IEX column will fractionate into four separate peaks, representing the increasing charge on the proteins eluted (see Figure 3.9B).

3.6.7.3   Gradient elution

The components of the sample bound to a chromatography resin can be eluted from the column by gradually changing the elution conditions using a gradient (normally a linear gradient) from the starting conditions to the end conditions over 5–20 column volumes. By gradually altering the mobile phase, components with different partition coefficients will move from the stationary phase into the mobile phase when the appropriate mobile phase flows over the resin in the column. Components will be separated on the basis of their partition coefficients and will elute from the column in different volumes. The ever-changing elution conditions cause a multitude of partitions to be established within the column (see Figure 3.9C).

When two components do not show baseline separation, an isocratic step can be introduced into the profile of a gradient column elution. This isocratic stage will maximise the subtly different partition coefficients the components have in their interaction with the stationary phase and the constant mobile phase.

3.6.8   Regeneration and storage of chromatographic resins (media)

At the end of a chromatography run, if the resin is to be used again, it can be regenerated according to the manufacturer's instructions and then re-equilibrated in the starting conditions.. If the column is not to be immediately reused, the resin can be regenerated within the column (according to the manufacturer's instructions), and then washed with two column volumes of water followed by two column volumes of a preservative (e.g., 20% (v/v) ethanol; 0.01% (w/v) thimerosal or sodium azide). (Please follow the manufacturer's recommendations on the most appropriate preservative for the particular resin. Also consult the local Health and Safety adviser about the use and disposal of these preservatives.) Please remember to always pay attention to the pressure readout when washing. If the pressure starts to increase, drop the flow rate down and continue with the washing procedure. Alternatively, the column may be eluted in the opposite direction to the flow down the column, this will elute the bound contamination away from the resin in the column and the detector. The column can also be dismantled and, the resin washed before storage in a preservative in the fridge.

3.7   AUTOMATED PROTEIN PURIFICATION CHROMATOGRAPHY SYSTEMS

There are a number of different commercial systems developed for the purification of proteins (see Figure 3.8), including those manufactured by the GE Healthcare Ltd (AKTA range) and Bio-Rad Laboratories, Inc (NGC) systems. The equipment is modular, allowing easy removal and addition of components, which facilitates system flexibility. These systems are derived from and have many similar components to high-performance liquid chromatography (HPLC) systems, which are primarily used to separate small molecules rather than proteins. Both protein chromatography and HPLC systems consist of precision pumps (one or two), an injection device (usually an autosampler), a chromatographic column (variable depending on the technique), a detection device (e.g., UV/visible spectrophotometer) and a fraction collector. The whole system is usually controlled by software running on a computer, which additionally allows for data collection and analysis of the run. It is possible to convert a stainless steel HPLC system into a protein purification system by replacing the metal tubing for plastic PEEK tubing, which should allow for the successful separation of labile protein molecules. The use of aqueous buffers in protein chromatography means that there is always a danger that salts will come out of solution and build up on a component within the chromatography system. The operator should wash the solvent flow path with water throughout the entire instrument on a regular basis, paying particular attention to the pumps to prevent salt build up.

Figure 3.10 (1) Buffer reservoirs: (a) start conditions buffer; (b) end conditions buffer; (c) additional buffers or wash solutions can be included. (2) Buffer selection valve (controlled by data management system). (3) Twin precision pumps (including a process to clean behind the pump heads). (4) Precolumn buffer mixing chamber (there may also be an inline filter to prevent particles from coming into contact with the column). **(5a)** The injection valve usually has three settings (controlled by the data management system): (i) LOAD: When the liquid flows from the pump onto the column allowing the operator to load the sample into the loop. (ii) INJECT: The liquid flows from the pump through the loop onto the column. (iii) PURGE: The liquid flows straight to waste. **(5b)** The variable flow path of the injection system. (A) The liquid flows from the valve onto the column (B) the liquid flows into the valve. (C and D) between C and D is situated an injection loop (various sizes) (E) waste from over filling the loop (F) the liquid flow can be diverted from the column and sent straight to the waste. This would occur when the pumps are being washed or when the buffer conditions are changed (purge). **(6)** The column of choice. **(7)** The waste reservoir. **(8)** The detector (typically UV detection set at 280 nm for proteins or 214/220 nm for peptides). **(9)** The fraction collector (variable volumes can be collected). **(10)** The data management system

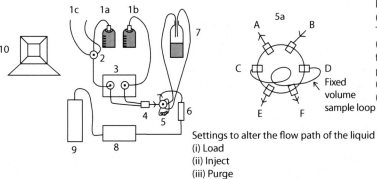

Settings to alter the flow path of the liquid
(i) Load
(ii) Inject
(iii) Purge

3.8 SIMULATED MOVING BED CHROMATOGRAPHY (SMBC)

In simulated moving bed chromatography (SMBC), the process of sample application and recovery are continuous. This is achieved by a system of valves and interlinked columns that creates a chromatographic system with an apparently endless stationary phase. SMBC has been in use for many years in industrial chromatography for the preparation of many different molecules, and a commercially available laboratory system has recently been adapted for use in the biotechnology industry. The Semba Bioscience (Octave) continuous flow chromatography system (Semba Bioscience Inc, USA) provides a means to continuously purify proteins, with applications in the production of monoclonal antibodies or recombinant proteins. The stationary phase comprises eight columns connected in series with the valves between the columns used to introduce and remove the flow of liquid from column to column. In SMBC, an isocratic elution relies on the different migration rates of the components in the applied **feedstock** throughout the entire stationary phase. By experimentally establishing the appropriate flow rate, the elution conditions and the valve timing (open or closed), a method can be determined that allows the continuous application of sample and the purification of the target protein. Separations that require multiple buffers (binding, washing elution and regeneration), such as affinity chromatography, can also be established using SMBC.

3.9 PROTEIN PURIFICATION CHROMATOGRAPHIC RUNS

Regardless of the equipment involved or the chromatographic technique that will be employed in the purification strategy, all chromatographic runs follow a set of separate but interrelated stages (see Appendix 4).

Prior to embarking on a chromatographic run, it is a good idea to spend some time getting to know the protein you are working with (see Section 4.4). Properties such as the pH optimum for catalytic activity, pH optimum for storage, thermal stability, the peptidase enzyme profile of the extract used and the effect of activators and inhibitors on these properties can be evaluated in small scale experiments to provide a guide to the starting conditions for a chromatographic run (see Protocol 5.1).

3.9.1 Pre-packed chromatographic columns

These will be purchased from the manufacturer containing a preservative and accompanied by appropriate handling instructions (e.g., pressure limits, solvent compatibility and the regeneration procedures). Protocol 3.1 outlines some general procedures to employ when using an automated protein purification system. When the buffers have been prepared and the pumps have been primed with the buffers, attach the column to the automated protein purification setup, check that the upper pressure limit setting has been adjusted, and then wash the column with distilled water (or follow the procedures outlined in the manufacturer's instructions) at a low flow rate to remove the preservative on the column (2–5 column volumes should suffice). Then (also at a low flow rate) pump the starting conditions buffer through the column. Gradually increase the flow rate until the required flow rate for the proposed run is achieved.

3.9.2   Empty chromatography columns

These columns can be purchased and packed with chromatographic media, which are usually stored at 4°C in a **bactericide/fungicide** (e.g., 0.1% (w/v) thiomersal; 0.05% (w/v) sodium azide or 20% (v/v) ethanol). The preservative needs to be removed and the resin equilibrated in a buffer that encourages the protein of interest to bind to the resin (e.g., a low salt buffer for IEX or a high salt buffer for HIC [see Chapter 5]). This can be conveniently achieved by using a Buchner flask connected to a vacuum to which a funnel with a sintered glass mesh is attached.

The chromatographic resin can be poured onto the glass mesh and the vacuum started. The preservative is quickly removed, and the resin can then be washed in distilled water, followed by the start buffer, for the chromatography experiment. Allow the vacuum to remove most of the buffer and then switch off the vacuum.

Resuspend the resin in start buffer (2× the resin volume) and allow the resin to settle. Particles that do not settle ("**fines**") should be removed by **aspiration**. If the fines are not removed before the column is packed, they can lodge themselves into spaces in and between the resin. This will increase the back pressure and may block the flow of the mobile phase. Once the fines have been removed the resin can be degassed under vacuum (to remove dissolved gas from the buffer/resin **slurry**) before being packed into the column.

Prior to the assembly of the column, it is recommended that the mesh at the ends of the column (or flow adaptors), which prevents the resin from leaving the column, are checked for tears and then cleaned by placing the adaptors in a beaker of water, followed by **sonication** in an ultrasound cleaning bath (or if the mesh is visibly dirty, you can ultrasound clean first in 0.1 M NaOH containing 5% (w/v) SDS followed by a water wash) for 5 min.

The assembled chromatographic column should be checked for leaks at the seals and the connections to the tubing using water. Once the integrity of the column has been verified, a small volume of start buffer should be placed in the bottom of the column and run from the outlet to liberate trapped air beneath the mesh. Additional start buffer can then be added to cover the end mesh.

The column should be tilted at an angle (approximately 30–45° from the vertical) and the degassed resin in a buffer slurry introduced to the column by running the slurry down the sides of the column until the column is full. The column should be placed in a vertical position (check with a spirit level) and the resin packed into the column at a flow rate marginally faster than the anticipated flow rate for the experimental run. (This will prevent a reduction in the column's volume when the sample is applied.) Remember that the resin has been introduced to the column as a slurry (i.e., there is more liquid than resin) and this will require the introduction of more resin from the slurry to achieve the required bed volume.

When the required bed volume has been packed, the flow of liquid can be stopped and the upper column connector can be attached. Take care at this stage to ensure that there is no air trapped within the system.

The resin within the column can then be equilibrated with the starting buffer (5–10 column volumes) at a flow just above the required experimental flow rate. At the end of this equilibration, check that the upper end adaptor is only in contact with the chromatographic resin. Small changes in volume of the column can then be adjusted before the run.

The column should ideally be packed at the temperature at which the chromatographic run is to be conducted. Remember the concentration of gas in liquid increases as the temperature decreases. If a column is packed with buffer from the fridge and then run at room temperature gas bubbles will emerge in the resin. The choice of the experimental temperature will be guided by the thermal stability of the target protein, the estimated run time and the possible presence of peptidase enzymes, particularly in crude extracts. Most modern resins have been manufactured to withstand increased pressures, which allows for relatively high flow rates (>5.0 ml min^{-1}). This significantly reduces chromatographic run times and a lot of protein purification experiments can be conducted at room temperature. If the target protein is particularly unstable, the chromatographic run should be conducted in a cold environment, or, alternatively, the fractions from the run can be immediately placed on ice.

After the resin has been equilibrated with the starting buffer, and if there are no leaks, the sample can be applied either through an inline three-way valve or using a sample loop (see Figure 3.8). If a large volume of sample is to be applied, stop the pump delivering the start buffer, transfer the tube leading from the starting conditions buffer to the sample and use the pump to apply the sample to the column (taking care to avoid air bubbles when transferring the tube between buffer and sample). When the sample has been applied, stop the pump and reconnect the system to the starting conditions buffer. As soon as the sample has been applied to the top of the column, fractions from the column outlet should be collected throughout the chromatographic run.

In general, smaller diameter (3–15 μm) resin beads will improve the resolution. This is because as the diameter of the bead decreases, more beads can be packed into the column, which increases the number of available **theoretical plates**. The columns with smaller diameter beads need higher pressures to move the liquid through the column and require medium- to high-pressure pumping systems (see Table 3.4).

3.9.3 Flow rates and elution of the sample

Flow rates in protein chromatography are usually measured in ml min^{-1}, which is fine for individual experiments but to compare chromatographic runs made with the same sample on different columns, a linear flow rate is used (cm h^{-1}).

$$\text{Linear flow rate (cm h}^{-1}) = \frac{\text{Flow rate (ml min}^{-1})}{\text{Cross-sectional area of the column (cm}^2).}$$

As a result of the starting conditions selected, some proteins will bind to the resin while other proteins will fail to interact and will percolate through the resin to the end of the column as unbound material. The unbound material should be eluted from the column using the start buffer until the absorbance at 280 nm of the unbound eluate reaches a background level. The elution conditions can then be applied and the eluted protein should be collected in fractions.

In adsorptive protein chromatographic procedures (e.g., IEX, HIC, and affinity chromatography; see Chapters 5 and 6), the shape and width of the eluting protein peaks can often be improved by inverting the column before applying the elution conditions (i.e., running the elution conditions in the opposite direction to the application conditions).

> **Note:** Never assume that the chromatographic run has worked, even if it has worked for the previous ten runs. Please remember to keep all the fractions (including the unbound fractions) until you are absolutely sure which fraction(s) contain the target protein.

3.10 SCALING UP THE PURIFICATION AND SOME CONSIDERATIONS ABOUT INDUSTRIAL PROTEIN PURIFICATION

In general, there are no differences in the principles behind the use of a chromatographic resin in an academic laboratory compared to its use in an industrial setting. However, there are obvious differences in scale, both in the volume of extract to be processed and the volume of resin used throughout the purification procedures.

Setting a target for the degree of purification required at the outset is applicable to both laboratory- and industrial-scale protein purification schemes. Many pre-purification considerations are also common (see Table 3.3b). In the early stages, the laboratory-scale operator will need to ensure that the required reagents are in place and the necessary time is pre-booked to use appropriate centrifuges and possibly an automated protein purification system. Depending on the target protein, "scaling up" could mean using the automated purification system to repeat the same run many times or using several automated systems to repeat the run several times. However, if the target requirements outstrip the limitations of these suggestions, the industrial-scale operator will require the help of additional people in the planning stage. Process engineers will be needed to provide information on the availability and use of industrial-scale chromatography columns and equipment; manufacturers will need to be consulted on the availability of resins; and throughout the planning process, considerations will have to be made as to the budget and the paperwork required for validation. This is particularly important if the target protein is to be utilised as a therapeutic agent. Documented data on the purification process will be required throughout the purification process, including evidence of the purity of the final target protein (a variety of methods may be needed to demonstrate the final purity; see Chapters 7 and 8). Additional information will be required on the sanitisation procedures used and the number of times the resins are used before they are replaced.

3.11 SUMMARY

There are a large number of techniques that can be used to purify proteins, and these can be used in a variety of ways to reach the original target set at the commencement of purification. Of course, improvements can always be introduced into a protocol as new ideas or chromatography appear. Many factors (yield, capacity and percent recovery) have to be taken into account, including the cost of implementing any change.

PROTOCOL FOR CHAPTER 3

Protocol 3.1 The preparation of a sample and buffers for a protein purification chromatographic run using an automated protein purification system

(a) Always use water with the highest level of purity (e.g., 18.2 MΩ·cm at 25°C) available to prepare the buffers.

(b) The buffers should be equilibrated to the temperature at which the chromatographic run will be conducted (buffers stored at 4°C will release dissolved gas as they warm up).

(c) After they has reached the required temperature, check the pH.

(d) Filter the buffers through a 0.2 μm filter to remove particulate material and bacteria (to prevent blocking the pores in the chromatographic resin contained in the columns and reducing the back pressure in the system).

(e) Centrifuge the sample at 12,000 × g for 20 min to clarify the sample of any protein precipitate, particulate matter or bacteria prior to its application to the chromatographic resin (this will help prevent the resin in the column becoming blocked; see above).

(f) Check that the pump heads are free from salt deposits (different machines have different system washing procedures).

(g) If the chromatographic system has been parked in 20% (v/v) ethanol, prime both pumps with water without the flow going through the column according to the manufacturer's instructions. (In the pump washing process the system will vent the liquid to waste at an elevated flow rate circumventing the column.)

(h) Set a low flow rate and flush the entire system with water until the ethanol has been removed.

(i) Prime the pumps with the starting buffer (e.g., low salt for IEX) and eluting buffer (e.g., high salt for IEX) according to the manufacturer's instructions. (This usually pumps the buffers to waste at an elevated flow rate, circumventing the column.)

(j) To protect the column from adverse pressure surges, set a maximum pressure limit (below the maximum allowed for the resin within the column) on the chromatographic system's software.

(k) Set the starting conditions buffer to flow through the column at a low flow rate and check for leaks in the system (tighten the connections where applicable).

(l) Check that the flow moves through the column to the detector and onto the fraction collector.

(m) Check that the fraction collector moves from tube to tube at the correct interval (time or volume) and is not impaired in its movements by stray tubing.

(n) Gradually increase the flow rate to an acceptable level (a level that generates less than the maximum backpressure).

(o) Allow at least two column volumes of the staring conditions buffer to flow through the column and then zero the absorbance on the detector.

(p) Load the sample into the injection loop (fixed volume loops from 0.05–10.0 ml; variable volume loops 0–20 ml). Large volumes of sample can be loaded onto the column using the pump used to deliver the starting conditions buffer.

(q) Start the appropriate programme for the separation procedure undertaken.

(r) As protein elutes form the column, it may be appropriate to take the tubes from the fraction collector, number them and place them on ice (or in the fridge).

(s) After the run, a quick assay of every other tube (or one in three) will give the location of the target protein. The fractions containing the target protein can be pooled. Use the pooled fractions to determine the volume, activity and protein concentration (see Section 4.10) and include this information in the experimental protein purification table (see Section 8.1).

RECOMMENDED READING

Research papers

Martin, A.J.P. and Synge, R.L.M. (1941) A new form of chromatogram employing two liquid phases. *Biochem J* 35:1358-1368.

Martin A.J.P. and Synge, R.L.M. (1941) Separation of the higher monoamino-acids by counter-current liquid-liquid extraction: the amino-acid composition of wool. *Biochem J* 35:91-121.

van Deemter, J.J., Zuiderweg, F.J. and Klinkenberg, A. (1956) Longitudinal diffusion and resistance to mass transfer as causes of nonideality in chromatography. *Chem Eng Sci* 5:271-289.

Books

Carta, G. and Jungbauer, A. (2010) *Protein Chromatography: Process Development and Scale-Up.* Wiley Blackwell, Chichester, UK.

Lundanes, E., Reubsaet, L. and Greibrokk, T. (2014) *Chromatography: Basic Principles, Sample Preparations and Related Methods.* Wiley-VCH, Wienheim, Germany.

Meyer, V.R. (2010) *Practical High-Performance Liquid Chromatography.* 5th ed. Wiley Blackwell, Chichester, UK.

The Groundwork

4

4.1 INTRODUCTION

The earlier chapters in this book have dealt with the properties of water, buffers, amino acids and proteins. This theoretical background will be useful throughout any purification procedure, providing a framework of knowledge to help answer some of the problems that may arise. The knowledge that is specific to your protein of interest can be acquired by reading the relevant scientific papers. However, the best way to become acquainted with your target protein is to undertake a number of small scale procedures before embarking on the purification process. This holds true for the operator enriching a target from a cellular extract as well as the operator using a recombinant protein expression and purification kit. The information obtained from this ground work will pay dividends when decisions have to be made on the choice of resin and starting/elution conditions for chromatography.

A convenient protein assay and a suitable assay for the target protein are two fundamentals that have to be addressed early. Bearing in mind that a chromatographic run may generate many tens of fractions, an assay that is easy to perform will allow speedy processing of results and limit the sample storage time between chromatographic runs. The choice of assay will depend on the target protein/enzyme, but it is possible to use an indicative assay to focus in on the fractions containing the target protein and then use a more complex assay to assay the pooled fractions in preparation of the purification table (see Chapter 8). The assay does not need to be based upon biological activity, for example an antibody can be used to identify a protein of interest in the fractions eluted from a chromatographic resin.

4.2 ASSAY TO IDENTIFY A TARGET PROTEIN

There is a wealth of information in the published literature detailing assays for a wide range of enzymes. This can be supplemented with information from reputable web pages such as the enzyme database BRENDA (http://www.brenda-enzymes.info/). Older references may suggest using assays volumes suitable for either test tubes (15.0 ml) or microfuge tubes (1.5 ml). These volumes will consume relatively large amounts of enzyme and reagents. Fortunately, these days most enzyme assays can be miniaturised into a microplate format, significantly reducing the amount of reagent and target protein that have to be sacrificed for the assay. The most common microplate formats are plates with 96 wells made from polycarbonate or polypropylene, with a well volume of 0.3 ml. At the end of the assay the change in absorbance in the visible spectrum of light, (plastic 96 well microplates compatible with UV light are available), relative fluorescence or relative luminescence can be read in a microplate reader providing data within minutes. There are other formats of microplates containing 6, 24, 384 and 1586 wells to increase the throughput of data.

If the target protein is an enzyme then a few factors have to be taken into account when designing or using an assay. If the enzyme requires cofactors (e.g., metal ions) these should always be included in the assay in excess.

4.2.1   Temperature

The rate of any chemical reaction will double by a 10°C rise in temperature. In the context of chemistry elevating the temperature of a reaction beyond body temperature makes good sense. Biochemical reactions within living systems are also governed by this reaction rate doubling as the temperature increases. Thus, the biochemical reactions that occur in plant cells in the winter will be slower than the same reactions in the same cells in the summer months. Insects (arthropods) and lizards (reptiles) are considered to be "cold blooded." They are often viewed laying in the sun to elevate their body temperatures eventually enabling them to move quickly. However, the insects and lizards do not lay in the sun all day as there is a limit to the amount of heat their bodies can tolerate and when this temperature limit has been reached they move into the shade. Mammals, on the other hand, are "warm blooded" and have evolved their body temperature to 37°C, facilitating rapid metabolism that is independent of the environmental temperature.

Why 37°C and not 50°C or 60°C? This is because the forces that hold a protein together (hydrogen bonding, ionic bridging, van der Waal interactions and hydrophobic interactions see Chapter 2) are individually relatively weak forces and these forces can be compromised when the temperature rises above a critical level. This critical temperature can be determined experimentally but most proteins (bacteria, arthropod, reptile, plant or mammal) start to unravel and lose their biological integrity between 40–60°C. Most enzymes are thermally semi stable between 30–40°C, that is, protein structure can tolerate temperatures up to 40°C enabling increased reaction rates, but above 40°C the protein structure starts to unravel. The choice of temperature for an enzyme assay is a balance between a temperature that enables an efficient rate of reaction but does not immediately denature the target enzyme. The chosen temperature must also allow the enzyme to be active throughout the duration of the assay.

To enable the fractions from a chromatographic run to be processed quickly, an enzyme assay should be performed at the highest temperature the target enzyme can tolerate. In general, bacterial, plant and animal enzymes all perform well at 37°C. However, the temperature tolerance for the target protein can be determined experimentally by incubating a clarified (centrifugation at $12,000 \times g$ for 30 min) protein extract at different temperatures (e.g., 10°C, 20°C, 30°C, 40°C, 50°C, 60°C and 70°C) for 5–10 min before cooling the extract to be assayed at the normal assay temperature (37°C). A plot of specific activity (see Chapter 8) against temperature (°C) will indicate the temperature above at which the target enzyme becomes terminally inactivated (see Figure 4.1A).

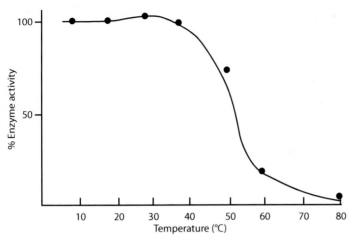

(A)

Figure 4.1 (A) A typical temperature inactivation profile for an enzyme. (B) A typical pH activity profile for an enzyme.

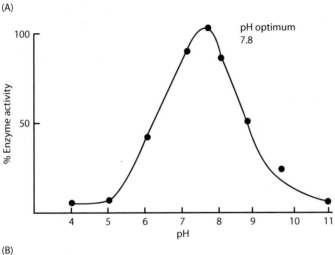

(B)

4.2.2   Substrate concentration

For a single substrate reaction plotting the rate of an enzyme cata-lysed reaction against substrate concentration results in a characteristic Michaelis–Menten plot. This plot informs the researcher that no matter how much substrate is added to the assay it is impossible to reach maxi-mum velocity in an enzyme catalysed reaction (see below and Table 4.1).

Michaelis – Menten equation $$v_0 = \frac{V_{max}[S_0]}{[S_0] + K_m}$$

When the substrate concentration $[S_0]$ is equal to is equal to the $\mathbf{K_m}$ value

$$v_0 = \frac{V_{max}[K_m]}{[K_m] + [K_m]}$$

$$v_0 = \frac{V_{max}[K_m]}{2K_m}$$

Table 4.1 The percentage of V_{max} in an enzyme catalysed reaction as a function of the substrate concentration (S_0).

Substrate concentration (S_0)	% V_{max}
$S_0 = K_m$	50.0
$S_0 = 5\ K_m$	83.3
$S_0 = 10\ K_m$	90.1
$S_0 = 25\ K_m$	96.1
$S_0 = 100\ K_m$	99.0
$S_0 = 500\ K_m$	99.8

$$v_0 = \frac{V_{max}}{2}$$

that is, the velocity (v_0) is 50% of V_{max} when the substrate concentration [S_0] is equal to the K_m value.

When the substrate concentration [S_0] is equal to a concentration 10 times the K_m value.

$$v_0 = \frac{V_{max}[10\ K_m]}{[K_m]+[10\ K_m]}$$

$$v_0 = \frac{V_{max}[10\ K_m]}{11\ K_m}$$

$$v_0 = \frac{10\ V_{max}}{11}$$

That is, the velocity (v_0) is 90.1% of V_{max} when the substrate concentration [S_0] is equal to the 10 times the K_m value.

The Michaelis–Menten equation demonstrates that the maximum velocity of any enzyme reaction cannot be reached (see Table 4.1). In practise it is impossible to feed high substrate concentrations into a reaction mixture due to solubility problems and expense. Substrate concentrations set at 5–20 fold higher than the K_m value (83–95% of the maximum velocity) will ensure efficient catalysis without great expense.

When the substrate concentration in an assay is fixed at values near to saturating levels the initial rate of an enzyme catalysed reaction is directly proportional to the enzyme concentration. Ideally, there should be a linear relationship between the enzyme concentration and the rate of reaction.

Enzyme activity is measured in **international units (I.U.)** this is equal to 1 μmol of product formed (or substrate consumed) min^{-1} at a given temperature (usually 25°C). Another measure of enzyme activity is the S.I. unit (**katal**), which is defined as 1 mol of the product formed (or substrate consumed) sec^{-1} at a given temperature (usually 25°C). For a UV/colourimetric assay the amount of product formed (or consumed) per minute can be calculated using the Beer-Lambert law (see Exercise 8.1), providing a **molar absorptivity** coefficient (ε) at a given wavelength is available. In general, the international units of enzyme activity (I.U.) are more popular because they produce more workable numbers.

For some enzymes international units (or katals) are not always appropriate and in this case it is usual for the operator to define the unit of activity. For example, some proteolytic enzyme activities are quoted as a change in absorbance at a given wavelength at a given temperature (e.g., 1 unit of enzyme activity is defined as ΔA_{440nm} of 0.001 min^{-1} at 25°C). The value of the absorbance change over unit time is immaterial as long as the unit is clearly defined.

4.2.3   pH

The pH that an enzyme is maximally active *in vitro* may not match the pH that the enzyme normally experiences *in vivo*. The *in vitro* pH maximum can be determined across a wide pH range, most enzymes will show a specific pH optimum and then a range of activities (<100%) across a range of pH values (see Figure 4.1B). To help monitor the activity from a chromatographic column the conditions that encourage maximum activity should be employed. This is important particularly in the latter stages of a purification schedule when the protein concentration will drop dramatically. Different buffers (see Section 1.7) may suit different enzymes and a range of buffers at different molarities (see Table 4.2) should be tested at the target enzyme's pH optimum. In addition, the pH that an enzyme is maximally active may not be the ideal pH to retain activity during storage (e.g., pepsin is maximally active at pH 2–3 but is should be stored at pH 7.0). In a separate series of experiments the ideal pH for storage can be determined (see Section 4.14).

4.3   PROTEIN ASSAYS

During a protein purification schedule along with the means to specifically detect the protein of interest it is important to routinely measure the protein concentration (mg ml^{-1}) present in the sample. This provides a means to determine the efficiency of each chromatographic method employed (see Chapter 8) and the means to determine the correct loadings for electrophoretic analysis. At all stages in a purification schedule it is desirable to have as much of the target protein as possible (high total activity) while at the same time limiting the amount of other proteins present in the sample relative to the target protein (high specific activity) (see Sections 8.1 and 8.3). To limit the amount of sample sacrificed during a protein assay a microplate version of the protein assays in Table 4.2 can be used (see Protocol 4.2).

There are a number of different protein assays (Table 4.2; Protocols 4.1–4.4) available for the routine measurement of protein in a sample, using bovine serum albumin (BSA) as a standard protein to construct a standard calibration graph. The unknown samples are treated in the same manner as the standards and the colour generated is converted into a protein concentration by reference to the standard calibration graph. The results obtained will not be completely accurate, because the readings for the samples are in reference to a standard protein (BSA). This implies that all the proteins in the sample have the same number of reactive amino acids as BSA, which is not true for all proteins. However, this small loss in accuracy is traded off for the convenience of the methods used.

Table 4.2 Popular protein assays.

Protein assay	Based on	Detection range	Disadvantages	Advantages	Comments	References
Absorbance of UV light at 280 nm	The amino acids tyrosine and tryptophan present in a protein's structure absorb UV light at 280 nm	0.2–2.0 mg ml^{-1} To increase the sensitivity tyrosine and tryptophan exhibit fluorescence. (excitation 280 nm; emission 340 nm)	In crude extracts other compounds absorb light at 280 nm, e.g., amino acids, nucleic acids and nucleotides	Quick and non-destructive	UV transparent cuvettes required The content of trp and try varies between different proteins. Protocol 4.1	Warburg and Christian (1941)
Coomassie blue dye binding	Dye binding to basic amino acids within a protein's structure (arginine, lysine and histidine)	Std assay 0.1–1.0 mg ml^{-1} Micro assay 0.05–0.1 mg ml^{-1}	(a) Detergents can interfere with the colour development	Quick and relatively inexpensive	The content of lys varies between different proteins; Protocol 4.4	Bradford (1976) **Modification** Shu-Sheng and Lundahl (2000)
Biuret	Reduction of Cu^{2+} to Cu^{+} by the peptide bond in alkaline conditions	1.0–5.0 mg ml^{-1}	(a) Insensitive. (b) Ammonia and Tris buffers can interfere	Inexpensive	Ammonia and Tris ions can interfere	Gornall et al. (1949)
Lowry	Reduction of Folin–Ciocalteau reagent by oxidised aromatic amino acids generated in the Biuret reaction	0.1–1.0 mg ml^{-1}	Many compounds interfere with the colour development	Popular		Lowry et al. (1951) **Modifications** Raghupathi and Diwan (1994); Harrington (1989); Rodriguez-Vico et al. (1989)
Bicinchoninic acid (BCA)	BCA chelates Cu^{+} to enhance the colour development of the Biuret reaction. The colour development in BCA is influenced by the presence of cysteine, cysteine, tyrosine and tryptophan	Std assay (microfuge tube and microplate format) 0.1–1.0 mg ml^{-1} Micro assay 0.05–0.1 mg ml^{-1}	(a) Ammonia and Tris can interfere (b) Compounds that can reduce Cu^{2+} ions will interfere, e.g., reducing sugars, e.g., glucose	Can be used in the presence of a detergent	Protocols 4.2a, 4.2b and 4.3 Useful for peptides and proteins	Smith et al. (1985) **Modification** Brown et al. (1989) **Peptides** Kapoor et al. (2006)

All protein assays have drawbacks and the one you use will largely depend on the one that is routinely used in the laboratory at the time you are working. Standardisation is important when results are compared between workers in the same and different laboratories. The bicinchoninic acid (BCA) protein assay (see Protocol 4.2) is sensitive (see Protocol 4.3) and can be used in the presence of detergents, whereas the Coomassie blue dye binding assay (see Protocol 4.4) is quick and easy to use. However, every protein assay has limitations that need to be appreciated (see Table 4.2). In most cases these limitations can be overcome by the use of appropriate buffer controls treated in the same manner as the standards and samples. There are many proprietary protein assays most are based on the reactions and reagents outlined in Table 4.2.

When using the BCA assay (see Protocol 4.2) interference can be avoided by precipitating the protein from the contaminating buffer using 7% (w/v) trichloroacetic acid (final concentration) and collecting the precipitate by centrifugation at $12,000 \times g$ for 15 min. The resulting protein precipitate may or may not be visible so mark the top of the tube on the side where the precipitate will reside after centrifugation (see Section 4.10). The precipitate can then be dissolved in 5% (w/v) SDS in 0.1M NaOH before the addition of the BCA standard working reagent (Brown et al., 1989). Interference in the Coomassie blue dye binding assay can be overcome by adsorbing proteins onto a calcium phosphate resin (hydroxyapatite: see Section 5.4) in ethanol (Shu-Sheng and Lundahl 2000).

4.4 THE EXTRACTION OF PROTEIN FROM CELLS OR TISSUE

4.4.1 Introduction

The initial groundwork will lay the foundations for subsequent experiments; during this process the operator will gain knowledge about a suitable assay and the storage conditions to use with the target protein. The stage is set for the first challenge, how to maximise the total amount of active biological material extracted from the target tissue or cellular pellet. This will represent the total protein and activity with which to subsequently endeavour to purify the target protein (see Section 8.1). This initial extraction stage is crucial and warrants investigation to help maximise the amount of the target protein to subsequently work up. The purification starts with the extraction and allows the removal of the target protein from the host cells or tissue. This requires a means of disrupting the tissue/cells into a suitable buffer in a protein-friendly manner.

The concentration of protein within a cell is high (approximately 180 mg ml^{-1}) and these inter cellular proteins are bathed in a reducing liquid environment. The increase in protein concentration also increases the viscosity of the cytoplasm relative to water. This is to be expected as the cytoplasm of a eukaryotic cell must support the organelles within the cell. Viscosity is a measurement of a liquids resistance to flow. A protein in solution influences the viscosity of the solution by its concentration and its inherent shape and size. The cytoplasm is approximately 8 times the viscosity of water (blood serum at 70.0 mg ml^{-1} is approximately twice the viscosity of water) and marginally more viscose than the nucleoplasm. The increased viscosity of the cytoplasm will influence how molecules flow in the cellular fluid. Small metabolites will diffuse slower in the cytoplasm compared to a buffer solution. These localised small spheres (diffusion in 3D) of metabolites at a relatively high concentration of will help promote the progress of an intermediate metabolite through a metabolic pathway.

When the extraction process is initiated an environment is generated that is exactly the opposite of the environment contained within the cell. The cellular disruption process empties the contents of the cell into a suitable buffer, thus diluting the protein concentration approximately tenfold. Prolonged mechanical processing to ensure complete disruption of the cells (or tissue) subjects the extracted protein to an oxidising environment (air bubbles). Consequently, at the start of an extraction process the target protein is experiencing a novel environment. The detrimental effects of this novel environment and the subsequent loss of the target protein can be minimised by addressing a few factors.

The extraction buffer (50–250 mM) should be set at a pH which is ideal for the target protein usually between pH 7.0 and 8.5, into which can be added a range of reagents which will promote protein well-being. Some of these reagents will help stabilise the target protein and others will help to inhibit unwanted hydrolytic activities. The inclusion of these additional reagents and their effective concentrations should be determined experimentally for an extraction from different cells or tissue.

4.4.2 Reducing agents

Any disulphide bridges present in a protein help to stabilise the tertiary structure of the protein (see Chapters 2 and 8). These disulphide bonds are usually present only in proteins that are exported from the cell. Cytoplasmic proteins do not contain disulphide bridges but proteins resident within the eukaryotic endomembrane system (see Chapter 2) or destined for cellular export may contain disulphide bridges. During the extraction of eukaryotic cells these endomembrane proteins may be released into the extraction buffer. Cytoplasmic proteins may be missing disulphide bridges but they may contain reduced sulphydryl groups from the functional group of cysteine (see Table 2.1) on the surface of their structure. The oxidation state of these surface sulphydryl groups may be important in properties of a target protein. The extraction process launches proteins into an oxidising environment which will have a direct effect on the oxidation state of these sulphydryl groups. Protection of these surface sulphydryl groups during the extraction and purification process will be essential to maintain their structure and functionality. In addition, some enzymes possess a reduced sulphydryl group at their active site and the oxidation of this active site sulphydryl will result in an inactive enzyme.

To overcome the problems of the reducing environment during the extraction process reducing agents such as dithiothreitol (DTT), 2-mercaptoethanol (2-ME), Tris(2-carboxylethyl)phosphine/HCl (TCEP/HCl), cysteine or reduced glutathione can be added to the extraction buffer to prevent oxidation of sulphydryl residues (2-ME is the cheapest option but also the most pungent). Tris(2-carboxylethyl)phosphine/HCl is a useful reducing agent that is odourless and stable in solution. If a target protein does contain vulnerable sulphydryl groups the inclusion of a reducing agent in the buffers used throughout the purification process is recommended.

The choice of reducing agent can be determined experimentally but it is worth remembering that they have a variable half-lives in solution.

Dithiothreitol has a half-life of 40 h in 0.1 M potassium phosphate buffer pH 6.5 at 20°C but at pH 8.5 in the same conditions the half-life decreases to 1.5 h. Whereas, 2-mercaptoethanol is stable for 100 hours at pH 6.5 and 4 hours at pH 8.5. Fresh buffers prepared prior to extraction or chromatography will help overcome this problem. Alternatively, a fresh reducing agent can be supplemented to the buffer prior to use at any time during the purification process.

4.4.3 Chelating agents

Sulphydryl groups within a protein's structure are not only prone to oxidation (see above) but they are reactive towards divalent heavy metal ions (e.g., Pb^{2+}) present in the buffers. These heavy metal ions may be present only at low concentrations within the water or the powders used to prepare the buffers but their interaction with sulphydryl groups in the structure of a protein is essentially irreversible. The use of ultrapure reagents and water ($18.2 \ M\Omega \ cm^{-1}$) will limited the concentration of contaminating ions and the addition of a chelating agent, e.g., 1–5 mM ethylenediaminetetraacetic acid (EDTA) will limit the remaining metal ions from interacting with the target protein. Chelating agents (see Table 4.3) are compounds containing electron rich molecules (nitrogen, oxygen or sulphur) that interact with the heavy metal ions via co-ordinate covalent bonds, donating 2 electrons to vacant orbitals in the metal ions electronic configuration (see Sections 6.11 and 6.12). These co-ordinate covalent bonds in the reducing agents effectively trap the metal ion in an electron rich cage. Thus preventing the metal ion from interacting with any free reduced sulphydryl groups

Table 4.3 Common chelating agents.

Chelating agent	Chelating ion	Uses
Citric acid	Variety of metal ions	Used in the softening of water by entrapping metal ions. Used to control the pH and as a flavouring in soft drinks
Diethyldithiocarbamic acid (DIECA)	Copper ions	Used in the extraction of plant material to limit the activity of copper dependent poly phenol oxidase enzymes (see Protocol 4.6)
Diethylenetriaminepentaacetic acid (DPTA)	Most divalent metal ions	Used in paper making
Dimercaprol	Variety of heavy metals	Used as an antidote for arsenic, cadmium and mercury poisoning
Ethylenediaminetetraacetic acid (EDTA)	Most divalent metal ions	Widely used in biological buffers to chelate any metal ions present at low levels in buffers. Used in the treatment of metal ion toxicity
Ethylene glycol tetraacetic acid (EGTA)	Primarily Ca^{2+}	Used in biological buffers to control the free calcium concentration. This is important in calcium activated enzymes
Nitrilotriacetic acid (NTA)	Most divalent metal ions	Used in detergents, also attached to agarose resins in immobilised metal ion affinity chromatography (see Sections 6.11 and 6.12)
Vitamin B_{12} (Vit B_{12})	Cobalt ions	Important cofactor in cellular metabolism

present in a protein's structure. It is worth remembering that many of the chelating agents are acidic and they should be dissolved in the buffer prior to adjusting the final pH of the buffer.

In addition, there are many naturally occurring metal ion chelation complexes including; the haem porphyrin rings in haemoglobin/myoglobin (chelating Fe^{2+}), the cytochrome proteins (chelating Fe^{2+}) and in green plants the light harvesting molecule chlorophyll (chelating Mg^{2+}). Other metalloproteins that chelate metal ions include: carbonic anhydrase (Zn^{2+}), calmodulin (Ca^{2+}) and the zinc finger transcription factors (Zn^{2+}). If the target protein requires metal ions for biological activity chelating agents should be used with caution. Although after extraction the essential ions can be added in excess to the assay buffer to reveal the biological activity.

4.4.4   Enzyme substrates/Inhibitors/Activators/ Cofactors

The addition of low concentrations of enzyme substrates, inhibitors, activators and cofactors into the extraction buffer may shift a protein into a compact or stable conformation that may improve the recovery during the extraction or purification process. These low molecular weight components can be removed at a later date by precipitation of the protein (see Sections 4.11.2–4.11.4), ultrafiltration (see Section 4.11.10), dialysis (see Protocol 4.9) or size exclusion chromatography (see Protocol 7.1).

4.4.5   Inhibitors of peptidase enzymes

In eukaryotic cells hydrolase enzymes (including peptidase enzymes) are compartmentalised into discrete organelles (the lysosomes in animal cells and vacuoles in plant cells). After initiating the extraction process these organelles will be disrupted releasing the peptidase enzymes to freely mix with and hydrolyse the cellular proteins. The pH optimum of these naturally occurring hydrolytic enzymes is around pH 5.5 so by carefully maintaining the extraction buffer at a pH value above pH 5.5 will help to minimise the deleterious effects of these naturally occurring protein hydrolase enzymes.

Peptidase (endoproteases) cleave internal peptide bonds unravelling the tertiary structure of the cleaved protein. If a protein is exposed to peptidase for an extended time period, the correctly folded protein will be fragmented into a mixture of peptides with a wide range of relative molecular masses (M_r). Peptidase can be divided into different subgroups; serine peptidase have a serine residue at their active site (e.g., chymotrypsin and trypsin), sulphydryl peptidase have a sulphydryl group at their active site (e.g., calpain, bromelain and papain), acid peptidase have aspartate residues at their active site (e.g., pepsin, cathepsin and renin) and metallo-peptidase II require metal ions for activity (e.g., thermolysin). Peptidases (exopeptidase) cleave single amino acids from either the N- or -C terminus of a protein/peptide, e.g., bovine carboxy-peptidase A (metallo-peptidase) or porcine leucine amino-peptidase.

The activity and type of peptidase in an extract can be determined experimentally by using azocasein (see Protocol 4.5) in the presence and absence of specific inhibitors (see Table 4.4). The appropriate levels of inhibitors can then be included in the extraction medium to minimise any unnecessary damage to the target protein. If the level of peptidase activity is low in the crude extract the damage to the target protein will be negligible as

Table 4.4 Common proteolytic inhibitors and some of their properties.

Proteinase/peptidase	Inhibitor	Working range	Comments
Serine	**Phenylmethylsulphonyl fluoride (PMSF)**	0.1–1 mM	Esterase inhibitor which is soluble in isopropanol and ethanol. Quickly broken down in water (approximate half-life in water: pH 7.0 = 120 min at pH 8.0 = 30 min).
Serine	Soybean trypsin inhibitor	Equimolar with proteinase	Stable at –20°C. The inhibitor dissociates from the target proteinase at low pH values.
Serine	di-isopropylfluorophosphate (DFP)	100 μM	Soluble in isopropanol. Stable for 1 month at –70°C.
Serine and some sulphydryl	Antipain	1–100 μM	Soluble in water. Stable for 1 month at –20°C.
Serine and some sulphydryl	**Leupeptin**	10–100 μM	Soluble in water but prepare fresh
Sulphydryl	**E64**	1–10 μM	Soluble in water. Stable at –20°.
Sulphydryl	Iodoacetimide	10–100 μM	Soluble in water. An alkylating reagent which will also target free surface sulphydryl groups on many proteins.
Acidic	**Pepstatin**	1 μM	Soluble in methanol or DMSO. Stable at –20°C.
Metallo	EDTA	1–10 mM	Soluble in water. Store at 4°C.
Amino-peptidases	Bestatin	1–10 μM	Soluble in methanol. Stable for 1 month at –20°C.
All groups	α_2-macroglobulin	Equimolar with proteinase	Stable at –20°C pH 6.0–7.0.

the target protein concentration is initially low relative to the other proteins. Problems can occur later in a purification schedule (when the target protein concentration increases relative to the other proteins) especially if a peptidase enzyme co-purifies with the target protein. Alternatively, cocktails of peptidase inhibitors can be purchased (e.g., Sigma, UK or ThermoFisher Scientific, UK) and added to the initial extract to prevent proteolysis. Some peptidase inhibitors are not specific and care must be taken to check that any inhibitors added do not inhibit the activity of the target protein (this can be determined experimentally).

4.4.6 Phosphatase inhibitors

Phosphorylation of proteins by kinases represents a common post-translational event within cells. The addition of a phosphate group to protein bound serine, threonine or tyrosine functional group temporarily imparts a large negatively charged structure to a protein. The additional negative charge results in a conformational change in the phosphorylated proteins structure as any charged groups in the vicinity of the phosphate moiety will be repelled or attracted depending on their own charge. The change in the proteins conformation may initiate the activity of the phosphorylated protein and possibly its interaction with other proteins. The addition of a phosphate group may be transient as cellular phosphatases rapidly remove the additional phosphate group returning proteins to their original conformation. If the phosphorylation state of a target protein is of interest then a cocktail of phosphatases inhibitors with broad specificity can be included in the extraction buffer (e.g., sodium fluoride 1–20 mM, sodium vanadate, sodium pyrophosphate and β-glycerophosphate at 1–100 mM). Cocktails of phosphates inhibitors are available (e.g., Sigma, UK or ThermoFisher Scientific, UK) to be added to extraction buffers.

4.4.7   Removal of nucleic acids and nucleoproteins

The process of extracting proteins from cells (eukaryotic or prokaryotic cultured cells) can sometimes result in a rapid increase in viscosity due to the liberation of nucleic acids into the extraction buffer. These nucleic acids can be fragmented by the addition of nucleic acid degrading enzymes, e.g., **DNase** (25–50 μg ml^{-1}) and RNase (50 μg ml^{-1}) into the extraction buffer. Incubation with these enzymes for a short period of time will help to restore the viscosity of the extract to normal levels.

Nucleic acids have a negative charge and the addition of positively charged material, for example, 1% (w/v) protamine sulphate or 0.1% (w/v) polyethyeneimine will combine with the nucleic acids forming a precipitate that can be removed from the soluble protein by centrifugation (see Section 4.10.1). If sonication is part of the extraction procedure (see Section 4.6.5) nuclease treatment is not usually required as the high energy sound waves generated by the sonicators are known to fragment polymeric DNA.

4.4.8   Removal of lipoproteins

If an extract is suspected to be rich in lipoproteins (e.g., ascites fluid) the addition of dextran sulphate and $CaCl_2$ to a final concentration of 0.2% (w/v) and 500 mM, respectively, will aggregate the lipoproteins which can then be removed by centrifugation (see Section 4.10.1).

4.4.9   Additions for the extraction of plant tissue

The extraction of proteins from plant material presents additional problems to that experienced in the extraction of proteins from animal sources (see Protocol 4.6). The choice of starting material will also influence the extraction method as young green tissue (see Section 4.5.2; mortar and pestle) will be easier to extract than older mature green tissue (see Section 4.5.2; Waring-style blender). If the target protein from plant tissue is not part of the plants photosystem it may be prudent to start the extraction with plant material which has been grown in the dark (etiolated). The plant tissue will be a pale yellow in colour and the polyphenol oxidase activity will be reduced. Appropriate experiments will determine if etiolated tissue is a good source for the target protein.

Once a plant extraction process has started the extract will almost immediately begin to discolour. Visibly changing from a green to a brown colour within minutes of starting the extraction. This is because plants contain secondary metabolites some of which (phenols and tannins) can bind to proteins causing them to aggregate and precipitate. They also have polyphenol oxidase enzymes which convert the phenols into reactive quinones which also interact with proteins increasing the problems of protein aggregation and precipitation. The activity of phenol oxidases enzymes can be moderated by restoring the reducing environment that would be present within the intact plant cell (see Section 4.4.2). This can be achieved by increasing the concentration of reducing agents (DTT, 2-ME or TCEP) in the extraction buffer to 10–15 mM and by the inclusion of oxygen scavengers such as vitamin C (5 mM).

Polyphenol oxidase enzymes have a requirement for copper ions so the inclusion of a copper chelating agent (see Section 4.4.3) such as diethyldithiocarbamate (DIECA) that will help to inhibit their activity (see Protocol 4.6, which describes the isolation of an enzyme from plant material). Polyphenol oxidases have a relatively acidic pH optimum so increasing the pH of the extraction buffer to pH 8.5 and then immediately re-adjusting the pH after extraction will also limit the activity of these enzymes. In addition, providing an excess of an alternative substrate for polyphenol oxidase enzymes will also limit the damage to extracted plant proteins. A convenient alternative polyphenol oxidase substrate is insoluble polyvinylpolypyrrolidone (PVPP), which can be added as a solid powder after the initial extraction process to a final concentration of 5% (w/v). The insoluble PVPP can then be removed at the clarification stage by centrifugation or filtration (see Section 4.10.1). Working efficiently and keeping the extract on ice (or at 4°C) will also help to minimise the activity of polyphenol oxidases, peptidase and phosphatase enzymes.

4.4.10 Additions for the extraction of membrane proteins

Significant enrichment of membrane proteins can be achieved by isolating the organelle/membrane of interest by differential centrifugation (see Protocol 4.6, which outlines the preparation of membranes from plant tissue; the process is comparable to membrane isolation from animal tissue). Throughout the extraction and clarification process buffers should contain either 0.2 M sucrose (0.15 M NaCl can be used as an alternative but it may elicit the removal of peripheral membrane proteins; see below) to help maintain the integrity of eukaryotic organelles. Membrane proteins can be approximately divided into two types either peripheral proteins (attached to a phospholipid bilayer by non-covalent interactions) or integral proteins (embedded in or attached to the phospholipid bilayer by a hydrophobic appendage). Following centrifugation the proteins described as peripheral can be removed from a membrane preparation by washing the membrane pellet in a low (or high) pH buffer, a buffer with a high salt concentration or by the addition of a chelating agent such as EDTA (5 mM). The peripheral membrane proteins washed from the membranes can be separated by centrifugation (see Section 4.10.1) and purified as soluble proteins. The integral membrane proteins can be subdivided into a number of different types including the intrinsic integral proteins that span both leaflets of the phospholipid bilayer and extrinsic integral proteins whose structure is associated with only one leaflet of the phospholipid bilayer (see Figure 4.2). These integral membrane proteins have regions of hydrophobic amino acid sequences within their structure which allows them to associate with the hydrophobic core of a phospholipid bilayer. As such, they cannot be removed by a simple ionic or pH washing procedure. To solubilise a biological membrane requires reagents (detergents or solvents) that can solubilise both the phospholipid and proteins that make up the membrane structure.

In general, solvent mixtures (e.g., chloroform:methanol:HCl mixed in a ratio of 2000:1000:2) are used only if the membrane lipids are of interest. The solvents have a detrimental effect on the structure of proteins

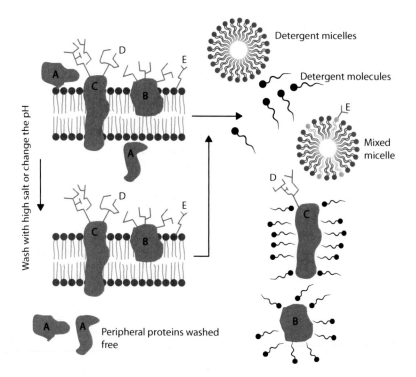

Figure 4.2 The use of salt to remove peripheral membrane proteins and detergents to solubilise membrane proteins and lipids. A = peripheral membrane protein; A′ = peripheral membrane protein washed from the membrane by a change in pH or by a wash with a buffer containing a high concentration of salt; B = extrinsic membrane protein (shaded hydrophobic region present in one leaflet of the membrane); B′ = extrinsic membrane protein with the shaded hydrophobic region covered by the hydrophobic tails of the detergent; C = intrinsic membrane protein spanning both leaflets of the membrane bilayer. The alpha helix spanning the membrane contains hydrophobic amino acids; C′ = the intrinsic membrane protein with the hydrophobic alpha helix region covered by the hydrophobic tails of the detergents preventing water molecules from interacting with the hydrophobic area; D = sugar residues attached to proteins (glycoproteins) present in the outer leaflet (away from the cytoplasm) of the membrane; E = sugar residues attached to lipids (glycolipids) present in the outer leaflet of the membrane.

(see Chapter 2) making the recovery of activity virtually impossible. However, solvents (e.g., acetone) can be a very useful method for concentrating small amounts of protein (see Section 4.11.3)—for example, prior to electrophoresis (either 1D- or 2D-PAGE; see Chapter 8 and Protocol 8.1).

Detergents are used to solubilise membrane lipids and proteins by effectively masking the hydrophobic areas within their structure with the detergents molecules thus preventing water molecules from interacting with their hydrophobic areas (see Figure 4.2). The physical properties of all detergents will work to solubilise all membrane proteins but some proteins will only remain biologically active in the presence of a limited number of detergents. This would have to be determined empirically by determining the biological activity of the target protein in the presence of a wide range of available detergents (see Table 4.5). An important property of detergents is the concentration above which they start to form micelles, called the **critical micelle concentration** (CMC), which is dependent upon on the temperature and ionic detergents are also influenced by the concentration of salt. The aggregation number (number of detergent monomers in a micelle which determines the micelle relative molecular mass) also has implications, as detergents which form large micelles are hard to remove from the solubilised proteins.

Table 4.5 The properties of common detergents.

Detergent	Classification	M$_r$ of monomer	CMC* (mM)	Aggregation number	Micelle M$_r$	Removal by dialysis or desalting
Tween 80	Non-ionic	1310	0.012	58	76,000	No
Triton X100	Non-ionic	650	0.3	140	90,000	No
Triton X114	Non-ionic	537	0.21	Not determined	Not determined	No
Bridj 35	Non-ionic	1225	0.09	40	49,000	No
Bridj 38	Non-ionic	1120	0.077	70	82,000	No
Nonidet P40	Non-ionic	603.0	0.05–0.3	100–155	60,000–93,500	No
Lubrol PX	Non-ionic	582	0.006	110	64,000	No
Octyl-β-glycoside	Non-ionic	292	23–25	27	8000	Yes
Octyl-β-thioglycopyranoside	Non-ionic	308	9	Not determined	Not determined	Yes
SDS	Anionic	288.5	2.3	84	24,200	Yes
Sodium deoxycholate	Anionic	414.6	1.5	5	2000	Yes
CTAB	Cationic	364	1.0	170	62,000	Yes
CHAPSO	Zwitterionic	630.9	8.0	11	9960	Yes
CHAPS	Zwitterionic	614.9	6–10	10	6150	Yes

*Critical micelle concentrations (CMCs) in the presence of 50 mM Na$^+$ ions.

Throughout the purification of a membrane protein by chromatography, low concentrations (below the detergents CMC) of the correct detergent may help to maintain the solubility of the target membrane protein. This can be a problem as some detergents absorb ultraviolet light at the same wavelength as proteins (see Chapter 2; the amino acids tyrosine and tryptophan in a protein's structure absorb light at 280 nm), which makes monitoring of the purification procedure using a UV detector difficult. The concentration of membrane proteins in the fractions collected during a chromatographic run can be quantified using a protein assay that is compatible with the presence of detergents (see Table 4.5).

The presence of detergents can also be a problem when selecting chromatographic techniques to purify a membrane protein. In ion exchange chromatography (IEX) (see Section 5.1) a detergent with the same charge as the resin or a neutrally charged detergent would be required to avoid the detergent molecules binding to the IEX resin. However, the presence of detergents is not a problem for size exclusion chromatography (SEC) (see Sections 7.1–7.5), making this chromatographic technique a popular first purification step for membrane proteins. Many membrane proteins are glycoproteins and lectin affinity chromatography (see Section 6.10) using a lectin protein which tolerates the presence of detergents can also be used. At any point in the purification of membrane proteins the detergent may need to be removed, dialysis (see Protocol 4.9) and group desalting using size exclusion chromatography (SEC) (see Protocol 7.1) can be used for some detergents (see Table 4.5). During the planning of the membrane protein purification procedure choose a detergent with a high CMC and a low relative molecular mass (M_r), e.g., octyl-β-glycoside to ensure efficient detergent removal via SEC.

Triton-X114 is a detergent with useful properties for enriching an extract containing hydrophobic proteins. At low temperatures during the extraction phase the detergent is **homogenous** but then separates into immiscible phases at temperatures above 22°C. The relatively dense detergent phase enriched in membrane proteins can be separated from the upper detergent depleted phase by centrifugation (see Section 4.10.1). This procedure can also be used to deplete endotoxins (**lipopolysaccharides** (LPS) derived from the outer membrane of Gram negative bacteria) from a bacterial extract before purification commences. *Escherichia coli* (Gram negative) is a popular bacterial host for the production of recombinant proteins (see Section 6.12) and Triton-X114 can be used to deplete LPS prior to purification of the recombinant protein of interest.

4.5   TECHNIQUES USED TO DISRUPT TISSUE OR CELLS

Having established the ideal buffer and pH for an extraction, which also contains the appropriate additions of peptidase and phosphatase inhibitors (see above, Sections 4.4.5–4.4.6), it is worth examining the method of tissue/cell disruption to maximise the amount of active target protein isolated. Remember this stage is the starting point for the purification process and the protein extracted represents 100% of the material that can be subsequently purified (see Chapter 8).

The cells from animal, plant, bacterial and fungal sources have different physical properties, e.g., cell diameters and surface properties. Consequently, different extraction techniques or combinations of extraction techniques may be required to maximise the yield of any target protein.

4.5.1   Animal cells or tissue

Animal cells (approximate diameter 10–20 μm) are surrounded by a thin (6.0 nm) plasma membrane which can be easily broken by the shear forces generated by tissue grinders, **homogenisers** (see Section 4.6.4) or sonicators (see Section 4.6.5). In addition, the integrity of animal cell membranes can be broken by the inclusion of membrane destabilising compounds (e.g., detergents and solvents) or by osmotic shock.

If a target protein is to be extracted from animal tissue (e.g., liver or lung), the tissue should be washed and trimmed free of surrounding cartilaginous and fatty tissue. The tissue should be cut into small pieces with scissors (or a knife) before being disrupted by the shear forces generated during homogenisation (see Section 4.6.4). Small amounts of animal cells or tissue can be fragmented in a tissue grinder or a small hand held homogeniser (e.g., **Dounce** (glass-glass) or **Potter–Elvehjem** (glass-Teflon) (see Figures 4.3A and 4.3B). Larger amounts of animal tissue with or without attached fibrous tissue can be homogenised using a Waring blender or a Polytron/Ultra-Turrax disruptor (see Figure 4.4).

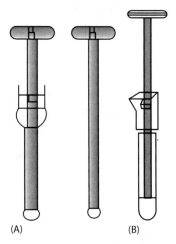

(A)   (B)

Figure 4.3 (A) Dounce tissue grinder. (B) Potter–Elvehjem homogeniser. (Courtesy of GPE Scientific Limited. Adapted from homogeniser manufacturers's website: http://www.gpelimited.co.uk.)

4.5.2   Plant cells (typically 100 μm in diameter)

Plant cells have a carbohydrate based cell wall surrounding the plasma membrane. The problems associated with this additional fibrous material will depend upon the plant tissue used (e.g., young or older tissue). Grinding with acid washed sand in a mortar and pestle can be used for small amounts of tissue and homogenisation in a Waring-style blender can be used for larger amounts of tissue. Dry seeds and grains from plants will probably require more vigorous disruption methods (e.g., "coffee" grinder, bead blender or ball mill) prior to extraction in an appropriate buffer.

4.5.3   Bacterial cells (0.7–4.0 μm in diameter)

Bacteria can be divided into two groups Gram positive and Gram negative (bacteria that stain positive or not with crystal violet and iodine). Gram positive bacteria have a plasma membrane surrounded by a **peptidoglycan** coating (20–50 nm) whereas Gram negative bacteria have a periplasmic space (7.0 nm) separating a peptidoglycan coat (3.0 nm) covered in lipopolysaccharide polymers (7.0 nm) held together by divalent metal ions. These cell coatings and the relatively small diameter of bacterial cells make them difficult to break open by conventional homogenisation techniques. Other disruption techniques such as liquid extrusion under pressure, sonication and enzymic lysis also can be used (or combinations of these techniques) (see Table 4.6).

Table 4.6 A summary of extraction methods which are best used with different tissue.

Method	Animal tissue	Animal cell culture	Plant tissue	Plant cell cultures	Bacteria	Yeast	Fungi (filamentous)
Osmotic shock		п					
Grind in liquid N_2	п	п	п	п	п	п	п
Grind with acid washed sand	п	п	п	п	п		
Homogeniser, e.g., Dounce	п	п	п	п			
Ultra sonicator		п		п	п	п	
Blenders	п	п	п	п			
Blenders with beads	п	п	п	п	п	п	п
Polytron	п	п	п	п			
Ballotini beads		п		п	п	п	п
Compression/Expansion		п		п	п		
Freezing/Thawing		п		п	п	п	
Enzyme treatment, e.g., **lysozyme** or lysozyme + detergents					п		
Enzyme treatment, e.g., Lyticase						п	

4.5.4   Fungal cells

Fungal cells have a plasma membrane surrounded by a cell wall composed mainly of **polysaccharide** (80–90%). This is typically chitin (a polymer of *N*-acetyl glucosamine) and cellulose. Filamentous fungi (2–7 µm in diameter) are susceptible to agitation with abrasive materials and yeast (*Saccharomyces cerevisiae*; 5–10 µm in diameter) can be disrupted by liquid extrusion, sonication and agitation with abrasive materials (see Table 4.6).

The cells from different sources have different properties and will require different extraction procedures. Table 4.6 summarises suitable extraction procedures for different tissues but the most appropriate extraction procedure would have to be determined experimentally and analysed for their efficacy (e.g., see Exercise 8.1).

4.6   THE EXTRACTION METHODS USED WITH SMALL AMOUNTS OF TISSUE OR CELLS

Heat can denature a protein's structure and mechanical extraction procedures that generate heat should be performed on ice or in a cold environment. A reduced temperature will also help to minimise the activity of any peptidase enzymes present in the extract (see Section 4.4.5).

4.6.1   Liquid nitrogen

Tissue (animal or plant) should be cut into small pieces and placed into a suitable container. Taking appropriate safety precautions the liquid nitrogen should be added slowly to the tissue in an appropriate container to rapidly freeze the tissue. The frozen tissue should be transferred into a precooled mortar and ground into a fine powder with a pestle (for plant tissue acid washed sand can be added to aid the extraction process). Chilled extraction buffer can then be added to solubilise the proteins.

4.6.2   Acid washed sand

Tissue should be cut into small pieces and placed into a precooled mortar. The tissue can be ground with a mortar in the presence of acid washed sand, chilled extraction buffer and appropriate additions for the tissue being worked on (e.g., insoluble PVPP for green plant tissue; see Section 4.4.9).

4.6.3   Osmotic shock

Animal cells from tissue culture can be disrupted by placing the cells in a suitable hypotonic buffer (≤50 mM). The cells will take up water and burst, disgorging the cellular content into the buffer. This technique can be used in conjunction with sonication (see below, Section 4.6.5) or in the presence of a detergent to improve the yield of the target protein.

4.6.4   Homogenisers/Tissue grinders

Homogenisers come in a variety of different sizes and configurations to accommodate volumes in the range of 0.1–100.0 ml. Dounce tissue grinders (see Figure 4.3A) have a borosilicate glass mortar that can be used with a glass pestle with a large clearance (0.5–0.11 mm) for the initial reduction of soft tissue or cellular based sample. This can be followed by a glass pestle with a smaller clearance (0.025–0.055 mm) to fragment the cells but leaving the nuclei and **mitochondria** intact. Potter–Elvehjem homogenisers (see Figure 4.3B and Protocol 4.7, which outlines the use of a Potter–Elvehjem homogeniser in the extraction of animal tissue) have a borosilicate glass mortar to be used with a Teflon pestle, which can be rotated mechanically at 600 rpm or used as hand held unit. The Teflon pestle provides an increased level of safety compared to the Dounce glass/glass homogenisers.

When using either a Dounce or Potter–Elvehjem homogeniser the tissue should be cut into small pieces (or tissue culture cell pellet collected after centrifugation) and placed into the glass mortar. Chilled extraction buffer can be added, and the pestle is used to provide the shear forces necessary to fragment the tissue. During the homogenisation process, the mortar should be periodically chilled using ice to moderate the damage to proteins caused by the heat generated during the homogenisation process.

4.6.5 Sonicators

The tissue culture cell pastes collected after centrifugation (12,000 × *g* for 15 min) should be suspended (<20% w/v) in a chilled extraction buffer. The suspended cell culture should be surrounded with ice and secured, before the titanium probe is lowered into the liquid (typically just touching the surface of the liquid). The probe should not touch the bottom or the sides of the sample vessel. Ear defenders should be worn before the instrument is started. The supplied electrical signal is used to cause oscillations in a piezo-electric crystal that is transferred to a titanium probe. The probe rapidly moves the liquid forward but retreats faster than the liquid. During the backwards step the pressure drops below the vapour pressure of the liquid which causes bubbles to form. As the liquid returns the gas bubbles collapse causing shock waves which can perforate the membranes of animal/plant cells from culture and some bacterial cells. Typically, 170 watts acoustic power at 20 kHz for short bursts of 30 seconds provides cell disruption, but the exact conditions for each cell type needs to be determined experimentally. Cooling cycles (15–30 secs disruption followed by 1 min on ice with no disruption) can be used to prevent proteins from being **denatured**.

4.7 EXTRACTION METHODS FOR LARGE AMOUNTS OF ANIMAL/PLANT TISSUE OR CELLS

4.7.1 Blenders

Domestic or Waring blenders can be used to quickly fragment animal and plant tissue (see Protocol 4.6 which outlines the use of a blender to isolate plant proteins). The chilled tissue should be placed in the bowl of the blender (chilled stainless steel bowls will quickly conduct away any heat produced) along with chilled extraction buffer. The lid should be attached and the blender set to operate in short (15–30 secs) bursts interspersed with cooling time until the tissue is fragmented. When the blender starts the liquid should be circulated in a vortex to ensure efficient homogenisation. Additional chilled liquid may be added to ensure the homogenate moves in a vortex.

4.7.2   Blenders with beads

A variety of instruments from different manufacturers offer the use of either glass (Ballotini; see below, Section 4.7) or ceramic (zirconium oxide) beads (0.1–0.15 mm dia.) in conjunction with a rapidly vibrating platform (different devices can be obtained to suit the target tissue or cell of choice see Appendix 7) to disrupt a variety of tissue or cells from bacteria, plant, fungus or animals. The efficiency of disruption can be adjusted by altering the time the tissue/cells are in contact with the vibrating beads.

4.7.3   Ultra-Turrax/Polytron homogenisers

Animal or plant tissue can be dispersed efficiently using a Polytron homogeniser (Kinematica, CZ) (see Figure 4.4A) which acts in a similar manner to domestic hand held blenders. The tissue to be fragmented is first cut into small pieces and then placed into a beaker with sufficient chilled buffer on ice. Start the homogeniser when it is immersed in the buffer, the tissue is torn between the probe's rotor moving at up to 27,000 rpm and the stationary stator surrounding the rotor (see Figure 4.4B). Different units can be purchased for different volume throughputs and different probes can be purchased to deal with a variety of different tissues.

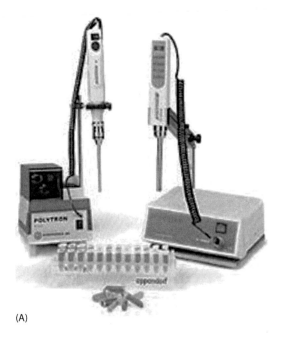

(A)

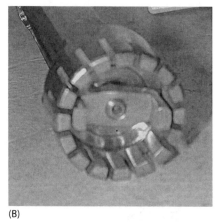

(B)

Figure 4.4 (A) Handheld Polytron units. (B) The tip of a Ultra-Turrax/Polytron probe. (Courtesy of Metrohm AG. Taken from https://www.fishersci.co.uk/shop/products/kinematica-polytron-pt1200e-handheld-homogenizer-3/13160633.)

4.8   THE EXTRACTION METHODS USED WITH BACTERIAL OR YEAST CELLS

4.8.1   Abrasive materials

Small amounts of bacterial or yeast cells can be disrupted by first freezing the cell pellet in liquid nitrogen and then grinding the frozen material to a powder with acid washed sand in a mortar and pestle (see Section 4.6.1). Alternatively, cells can be suspended in extraction buffer with glass ("Ballotini") or ceramic (zirconium oxide) beads (0.1–0.15 mm dia.) and shaken vigorously. The cells are disrupted by collision with the beads and the method is most effective against cells with large diameters, e.g., filamentous fungi or plant cell cultures. In addition, a large number of small diameter beads are more effective than a small number of large beads because of the increase in the number of collisions. The shaking can take place using specialist equipment (proprietary device, e.g., ball mill; see Appendix 4.7) or using a vortex mixer, but the exact conditions need to be determined experimentally.

4.8.2   Compression/Expansion

Cell pellets of bacterial or animal cells collected by centrifugation (12,000 × g 15 min) can be placed in a thick metal cylinder with an accompanying piston ("French press"). Pressure (10,000–40,000 psi) is then applied using a mechanical press and released by a valve at the bottom of the cylinder. The sudden release of pressure and shear forces generated at the valve opening tears the majority of the cells apart. Between 2 to 4 passes through the press is usually required for maximum cell lysis. Another type of mechanical device is an "X-press" which extracts bacterial protein from cells under pressure using a frozen paste of cells and extrusion through a disc. The "Parr" disruption bomb uses nitrogen gas to pressurise a stainless steel vessel, when the pressure is released the nitrogen gas dissolved in the cells explodes the cells providing efficient cell disruption. The equipment for compression and expansion/extraction can be expensive but it is versatile and can be also applied to pellets of animal/plant cell cultures. Pre-treatment of bacterial cells with lysozyme (degrades the bacterial the cell wall) and detergents (see Table 4.5 and Section 4.8.4) prior to compression/expansion extraction techniques will increase the effectiveness of the extraction process. Pretreatment of yeast cells with Lyticase will weaken the yeast cell wall prior to extraction but compression/expansion is not suitable for filamentous fungi or spores. If the production of recombinant proteins is routinely used it will be worth investing in the purchase of a "Press," otherwise the use of detergent and enzyme mixtures should suffice.

4.8.3   Freezing and thawing

Freezing bacteria and mammalian cells in a freezer causes the cells to swell and break as ice crystals form in the cytoplasm. The cellular contents can be collected during the thawing cycle at 37°C. Several freeze/thaw cycles are required for efficient lysis which can be very detrimental to the recovery of many proteins. The process is dependent on the age and type of cell as well as the rates of freezing and thawing. These factors would need to be determined experimentally.

4.8.4   Enzyme treatment

The plasma membranes of bacterial cells are covered in a peptidoglycan matrix (see Section 4.5.3) making them susceptible to enzymic hydrolysis. Lysozyme can be used to breakdown the peptidoglycan complex surrounding Gram-positive bacteria. Gram-negative bacteria require the disruption of the lipopolysaccharide coating by EDTA prior to lysozyme treatment. The cell walls surrounding yeast cells can be broken down with β-1,3-glucanases (e.g., Lyticase or Zymolyase) to produce spheroplasts (yeast cells without a cell wall). The use of these glucosidase enzymes degrades the cell walls surrounding the bacterial or yeast cells and their cellular contents can be accessed by combining the enzyme treatment with another procedure such as osmotic shock, detergents, chelating agents, freezing and thawing or compression and expansion. Premixed solutions of enzyme and detergent can be purchased from suppliers (e.g., ThermoFisher Scientific, UK). The cost of the reagents may make this enzymic method inappropriate for large scale extractions and a "Press" (see above Section 4.8.2) may be the method of choice.

4.9   POINTS TO REMEMBER ABOUT EXTRACTION PROCEDURES

- Remember to cool the items of equipment and buffers before extraction to minimise the heat damage to proteins.
- Where possible include cooling cycles to minimise the damage to proteins caused by the heat generated in the extraction process, e.g., 15–60–15 seconds (cooling-extraction-cooling).
- Add the appropriate additives (e.g., peptidase or phosphatase inhibitors).
- Always check the pH of the extract after extraction and adjust as necessary.
- After the initial extraction the mixture will contain debris and unbroken cells stored on ice. This debris can be removed by centrifugation (see Section 4.10.1) forming the first precipitate. Normally this is discarded but it can be re-extracted to maximise the yield of the target protein. However, repeated re-extraction of the initial debris precipitate rarely justifies the time and cost in terms of the yield of the target protein.
- Not all techniques will be an appropriate extraction method for every tissue or cell. The efficacy of an extraction method would have to be determined empirically for the target tissue (cell).
- In eukaryotic cells if the target protein is located in an organelle, the extraction process should be engineered to leave the sub-cellular organelles intact. This will be assisted by the inclusion of 0.2 M sucrose and/or 0.15 M NaCl in the extraction buffer and differential centrifugation (see below, Section 4.10.1).
- If the target protein is a peripheral membrane protein (see Figure 4.2) use a low molarity buffer throughout the extraction process. Isolate the appropriate enriched membrane fraction and then increase the molarity of the buffer (and/or the NaCl

concentration) to wash the peripheral membrane protein from the membranes fraction. Centrifuge (80,000 × g 60 min) to precipitate the membrane fraction and use the supernatant as the starting fraction for the purification process.

* Combining different extraction methods may produce an improved extraction procedure, e.g., the use of a Polytron blender followed by sonication, or the use of lytic enzymes followed by freezing and thawing.

4.10 THE TECHNIQUES USED TO CLARIFY HOMOGENISED EXTRACTS

4.10.1 Centrifugation

After the conversion of the target tissue or cell suspension into a homogenate the insoluble debris will have to be removed prior to chromatography. A eukaryotic cell homogenate will contain clumps of cells, cellular organelles, fragments of membranes and soluble cellular components in the extraction buffer. Large clumps of fibrous plant or animal material can be filtered out using four layers of muslin prior to centrifugation.

The viscosity of the buffer that particles are suspended in is important is determining the rate of centrifugation. In general, particles sediment under the influence of **gravity** as a function of their size and density, with the larger and denser particles forming the first sediment. In a rotating centrifuge rotor, particles are subjected to a centrifugal field with an elevated g force which increases the rate of sedimentation. The applied g force is a combination of rate of rotation (RPM) and the distance from the centre of the rotor to the furthest point in the centrifuge tube (r_{max}) present in the rotor. Particles suspended in a liquid will be subjected to different g forces depending on the rotor shape (see Figure 4.4).

Different rotors have variable distances from the centre of the rotor to the furthest point in the centrifuge tube (r_{max}). To standardise centrifugation conditions and to enable researchers to accurately reproduce centrifuge conditions, values for centrifugation are quoted in g (average) rather than rev min^{-1} (RPM). Most modern centrifuges allow the experiment to be run in relative centrifugal force (RCF) and rpm but RCF should be the conditions of choice for any laboratory scientist. If the facility to run the experiment in RCF is not available then the calculation below can be used to convert RPM into RCF (see Exercise 4.1). Alternatively, if the rpm and the average radial distances are known a **nomogram** (see Figure 4.5) can be used to calculate the RCF in that experiment.

$$\text{The applied centrifugal field (G)} = \omega^2 r \qquad (4.1)$$

r = radial distance from the centre of the axis rotor to the particle being centrifuged (cm)

ω = angular velocity (**radians** sec^{-1})

1 radian is the angle subtended at the centre of a circle by an arc with an equal length to the radius of the circle. One revolution of the rotor is equivalent to 360° = 2π radians.

$$\omega = \frac{2\pi \text{ rev min}^{-1}}{60}$$

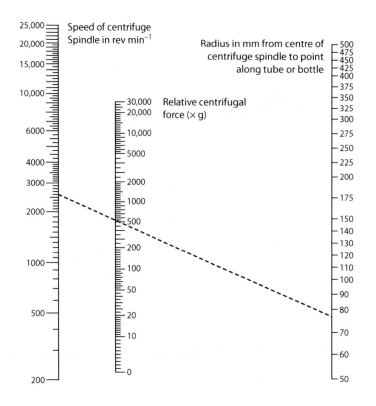

Figure 4.5 Nomogram for calculating relative centrifugal force. (Adapted from Corning website: http://www.corning.com /lifesciences/technical_information /techdocs/nomogram.asp.)

Substitute into (Equation 4.1)

$$(G) = \frac{4\pi^2 (\text{rev min}^{-1})^2 r}{3600}$$

A more user-friendly version of the RPM to RCF is shown below and also in Exercise 4.1.

Where (r) is the distance from the centre of the rotor to the furthest point in the centrifuge tube sitting in the rotor in mm (r_{max}). Revolutions min^{-1} (RPM)

Thus, RCF = $1.118\, r \left[\dfrac{\text{RPM}}{1000} \right]^2$

To use the nomogram measure the radius (mm) from the centre of the centrifuge rotor to a point on the centrifuge tube (see Figure 4.4; the average distance is usually quoted). Draw a line from the right-hand column (radius value) to the left-hand column (rotor speed in rpm). The relative centrifugal force (RCF) is where the line crosses on the centre column.

Fixed angle rotors come in a variety of different sizes but large rotors capable of accommodating larger volumes have a lower maximum speed limit and hence a lower maximum RCF. The K-factor of a rotor (supplied in the rotor data sheet) determines the pelleting efficiency of a rotor (a low K-factor indicates a higher pelleting efficiency) and this can be a useful parameter when comparing the efficacy of different rotors. It is an expression of the time taken for a particle to band in a particular rotor. Efficient rotors have a high RCF and a low sedimentation path length therefore a low K-factor. This can be useful particularly in density gradient centrifugation (see Section 4.10.1.3).

The time (t_1 and t_2) taken for a particle to band in 2 different rotors (K_1 and K_2) is given by

$$t_1 = K_1 t_2 / K_2$$

4.10.1.1   Differential centrifugation

In general, the densities of the organelles in eukaryotic cells are very similar but they do vary in size (see Table 4.7 and Figure 4.6) and as such can be separated by differential centrifugation with the largest particles being the first to sediment. The eukaryotic cell or tissue homogenate is placed into a centrifuge tube and accurately balanced against another tube with more sample or against water. The tube are placed into an angle rotor (see Figure 4.4A) and

Table 4.7 The size and density of common eukaryotic cell components and suggested marker enzymes and proteins[a].

Organelle	Diameter (μm)	Density (g cm^{-3})	Centrifugation speed required to sediment	Example of marker enzyme (detected using an activity assay)	Example of marker protein (detected using an antibody)
Nuclei	5–10	1.4	Low speed (1000 × g 10 min)	DNA dependent RNA polymerase	Lamin or cyclins
Mitochondria	1–2	1.19	Medium speed (20,000 × g for 20 min)	**Outer membrane** Monoamine oxidase B **Inner membrane** Cytochrome C oxidase	**Outer membrane:** Monoamine oxidase B **Inner membrane:** Cytochrome C oxidase
Lysosomes	0.2–2	1.12	Medium speed (20,000 × g for 20 min)	Acid phosphatase β-N-acetylglucosaminidase	Protein LAMP1
Peroxisomes	0.7 (variable)	1.07	Medium speed (20,000 × g for 20 min)	catalase	Protein PEX14
Golgi	(variable)	1.03–1.06	High speed spin (80,000 × g for 60 min)	NADP$^+$ phosphatase	**Animal:** 58K Golgi specific protein Protein GM130 **Plant:** Arf ADP ribosylation factor 1
Tonoplast	(variable)	1.10	High-speed spin (80,000 × g for 60 min)	**Plant:** Nitrate sensitive ATPase	**Plant:** Tonoplast intrinsic protein (TIP)
Plasma membrane	(variable)	1.02–1.04 Plant: 1.165–1.175	High-speed spin (80,000 × g for 60 min)	Na$^+$/K$^+$ ATPase **Plant:** Vanadate sensitive ATPase	Na$^+$/K$^+$ ATPase Cadherin **Plant:** Plasma membrane H+ ATPase
Ribosomes	0.02	1.6	Very high speed (150,000 × g for 180 min)		**Plant:** 60S ribosomal protein L13-1

[a]Specific organelle marker protein antibodies can be purchased in a kit for animal and plant tissue (see Appendix 7).

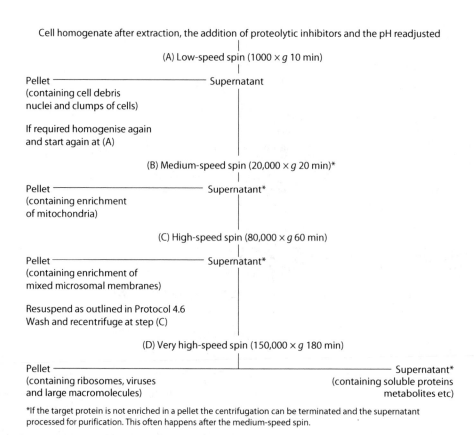

Figure 4.6 Cell fractionation by differential centrifugation flowchart.

then subjected to increasing *g* force for extended time periods (see Figure 4.5) The pellets at each stage of the differential centrifugation can be collected and suspended in a small volume of sucrose buffer using a Dounce or Potter–Elvehjem homogeniser (see Section 4.6.4). The samples can be stored as aliquots at −25°C. When the samples are to be used, after thawing it is recommended that they are again suspended using a Dounce or Potter–Elvehjem homogeniser to disperse any aggregates form during freezing and thawing.

4.10.1.2   Density gradient centrifugation

If the target protein is located in a particular organelle or membrane at the appropriate stage (see Table 4.7 and Figure 4.6) the pellet can be suspended in buffer containing 2–5% (w/v) sucrose. This can either be used as the starting point of a purification (e.g., chromatography) protocol or the sample can be enriched further using density gradient centrifugation. In density gradient centrifugation the sample (in 2–5% w/v sucrose) after differential centrifugation is layered onto a gradient of sucrose, e.g., 5–40% (w/v) sucrose (Ficol, Percoll or metrizamide can be also be used at different concentrations). The gradient of sucrose can be generated using a gradient maker (see Section 3.6.6) and a peristaltic pump. Alternatively, the gradient can be generated as a series of different sucrose concentrations, e.g., 40, 35, 30, 25, 20, 15, 5% (w/v) sucrose sequentially layered on top of each other using a pipette. This method needs to be performed with care to avoid to any mixing at the interfaces between the different sucrose concentrations. When the gradients have been poured and the sample (a small volume of concentrated membrane sample) has been layered onto of the sucrose gradient with care, make sure that the tubes remain upright. Carefully balance the tubes and store them in an ice bucket until they are placed into the buckets of a high speed swing out rotor (see Figure 4.4A). This rotor is preferred for density gradient centrifugation because the RCF impacts on the sample with consistent force through the centrifuge tube during the experimental run time. During centrifugation the particles will migrate through the sucrose according to density, size and shape. When the particles reach a density boundary that they cannot cross they will gather at the interface. The bands of different components are sharpened by the fact that the leading edge of each component encounters a sucrose boundary with increasing denser material during its progress down the sucrose gradient. The trailing membrane components in a fraction (with equal density) will move towards the boundary but cannot pass. This allows the components to focus as sharp bands provided the experiment is allowed to run to completion. At the end of a differential centrifugation experiment a slow deceleration of the rotor is recommended (without any braking >10 min) to prevent any disturbance and mixing of the focused membrane samples at the sucrose boundary interfaces. The enriched membrane samples can be recovered by carefully puncturing the bottom of the centrifuge tube with a syringe and using a peristaltic pump to flow the liquid into the tubes in a fraction collector (see Figure 4.7). The denser membrane samples will elute first.

Alternatively, the tip of a glass Pasteur pipette can be heated in a Bunsen burner flame until soft, using tweezers the tip can be extended and bent to an angle of approximately 110°. When the modified Pasteur pipette is cool it can be carefully inserted down the side of the centrifuge tube held in a vertical clamp and the membrane components removed. The samples with less density will be removed first. Marker enzyme activity (see Table 4.7) and/or SDS-PAGE combined with Western blotting can be used to determine the components identify and enrichment (see Section 4.10.1.4).

4.10.1.3   Equilibrium density centrifugation

Alternatively, after differential centrifugation the sample can be layered onto or into a 20–70% (w/v) continuous gradient of sucrose (Ficol, Percoll or metrizamide can be used as an alternative) generated using a

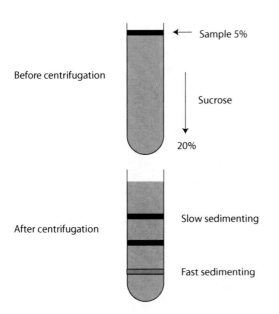

Sample 5%

Before centrifugation

Sucrose

20%

After centrifugation

Slow sedimenting

Fast sedimenting

Figure 4.7 Density gradient centrifugation.

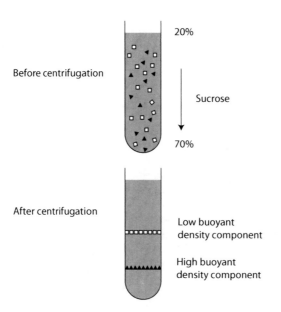

Before centrifugation

20%

Sucrose

70%

After centrifugation

Low buoyant
density component

High buoyant
density component

Figure 4.8 Equilibrium density gradient centrifugation.

gradient maker and a peristaltic pump. During ultracentrifugation using a swing out rotor (see Figure 4.4A) the particles will migrate up or down the density gradient until they reach a point in the gradient where their density matches that of the density of sucrose. This technique is referred to as equilibrium density gradient centrifugation (see Figure 4.8). The bands can be collected by puncturing the centrifuge tubes with a syringe, attached to a peristaltic pump. The fractions can be collected and identified using the suggested procedures outlined above and below (see Sections 4.10.1.2 and 4.10.1.4).

4.10.1.4   Membrane fraction identification

The identity of the membranes isolated during a centrifugation experiment and the enrichment factor can be determined using either marker enzymes (see Table 4.7). Alternatively, after measuring the protein concentration (see Protocols 4.1–4.4) the samples can be analysed by SDS-PAGE and transferred onto nitrocellulose membrane (see Protocols 8.1 and 8.3) to be probed for the presence of a marker protein with an appropriate antibody (see Table 4.5). If a sample of the crude extract (pre-centrifugation extract) is loaded onto the gel at the same time the enrichment factor in the purified membrane fraction can be estimated. It is important to remember that differential and density gradient centrifugation produce enriched membrane fractions (containing some contamination by the presence of other membranes) not homogenous membrane fractions.

4.10.2   Aqueous two-phase partitioning

Immiscible phases are the basis of chromatography (see Chapter 3) and can be formed when solutions of two polymers (e.g., polyethylene glycol (PEG) and dextran), or a polymer and a high salt solution (e.g., PEG and phosphate buffer) are mixed (see Table 4.8). When the proportions are correct separate immiscible phases will form. These phase compositions can be used to separate proteins from cell debris (clarification) or to fractionate and concentrate proteins. The majority of the particulate matter will partition into the polar lower layer (dextran) and the protein will partition into the less polar upper layer (PEG). The proteins interact with the molecules in the phases by weak interactions (H-bonding, hydrophobic, van der Waal and ionic interactions) and will partition into a phase where the overall free energy (ΔG; see Section 1.3, Section 4.11.2 and Appendix 1) is lowest. The partitioning event is not destructive to protein's structure and will generally result in the good recovery of biologically active proteins.

The exact conditions required to enrich a protein by two-phase partitioning needs to be determined experimentally. The manipulation of different parameters such as the concentration and type of polymer used, the ionic strength and pH of the buffer or the presence of hydrophobic groups on the polymers can be altered to achieve enrichment of a target protein into the upper phase. In addition, ligands can be attached to the polymers to facilitate an affinity separation by selective isolation of a target protein (see Chapter 6).

In the laboratory, stock solutions of the polymer (PEG and Dextran) are used to construct the phases in a centrifuge tube. The sample can be added to the phases in the centrifuge tube and mixed. The phases can be easily separated by centrifugation ($2000 \times g$ for 5 min) using a swing out rotor (see Figure 4.9) or the phases can be allowed to settle under gravity (10–20 min). The two phases can then be separated and assayed for protein, activity and volume. If required the upper PEG layer can be added to more Dextran (or a different polymer) and the process repeated to improve the enrichment. The protein can be recovered from the PEG by ultrafiltration (see Section 4.11.10) using a filter with an appropriate molecular weight cutoff or salt can be added to the PEG (see Section 4.11.3) rich phase to establish a new phase into which the protein will preferentially partition into.

4.11   THE TECHNIQUES THAT CAN BE USED TO CONCENTRATE PROTEINS FROM DILUTE SOLUTIONS (LABORATORY SCALE)

Proteins are present within the cell in a reducing environment at a relatively high concentration (>50 mml^{-1}). After extraction the cellular proteins are disgorged into an oxidising buffer, which also dilutes the protein

Table 4.8 Polymers used in aqueous phase partitioning.		
Polymer	**Composition**	**M$_r$**
Polyethylene glycol (PEG)	Polymer of ethylene glycol	600–20,000; usually 4,000–8,000
Dextran	(1–6) polymer of glucose	500,000
Ficoll	Copolymer of sucrose and epichlorohydrin	400,000
Reppal PES	Hydroxypropyl derivative of starch	100,000–200,000
Aquaphase PPT	Hydroxypropyl derivative of starch	
Source: Roe, S. (Ed.) (2001) *Protein Purification Techniques.* 2nd ed. Oxford University Press, Oxford, UK. p. 146, Table 3.		

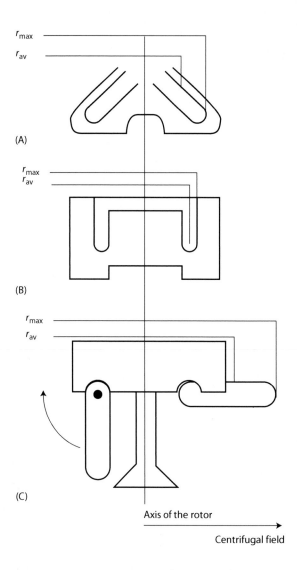

r_{max}

r_{av}

(A)

r_{max}
r_{av}

(B)

r_{max}

r_{av}

(C)

Axis of the rotor

Centrifugal field

Figure 4.9 The design of three main types of centrifuge rotors and the radial measurements for the minimum: (A) Fixed angle rotor, (B) vertical tube rotor and (C) swing out rotor. (r_{min}) average ($r_{average}$) and maximum (r_{max}) distances from the centre of the rotor.

several fold. The buffer is present to facilitate successful extraction of the target protein but at the initial stages of purification, the excess water can be viewed as a major contaminant. This is particularly true for industries where pumping large volumes of dilute feedstock can be expensive. A concentration step is often needed that may also have the benefit of removing low molecular weight inhibitors/contaminants (e.g., metal ions) from the extract containing the target protein.

After extraction and clarification (see above, Sections 4.4–4.10) the next step in a purification schedule is usually the concentration of the extracted protein. In addition, concentration steps may also be required throughout the purification schedule, e.g., prior to a chromatographic step or prior to electrophoresis, and there are a variety of techniques that can be used.

4.11.1 Salt precipitation

The solubility of proteins in an aqueous environment depends on the temperature, pH and the concentration and composition of the solution the protein is dissolved in. Proteins have a surface that is covered in a patchwork of different functional groups (ionisable, polar and hydrophobic) the arrangement of which is dictated by the protein's sequence of amino acids. This variable surface distribution of functional groups makes it difficult to predict how a protein will interact with the constituents of a solution and empirical determinations of the solubility of a target protein is usually undertaken, initially on a small scale before being scaled up.

Water interacts with the surface of a protein forming dipole interactions with the polar and ionisable groups. Whereas water forms clathrate ("caged") structures when in contact with any hydrophobic groups (see Chapter 1.3 and Appendix 1). When a protein in solution experiences an increasing salt concentration (i.e., salt added to the protein solution) the water molecules surrounding the proteins surface (solvation shell) are gradually stripped away. At the same time the hydrophobic patches become more exposed increasing the number of clathrate water molecules in the system. This increase in ordered water molecules is thermodynamically unfavourable because the entropy (S; see Appendix 1) decreases. The second law of thermodynamics states that entropy (S) of a system(measure of the randomness of a system) tends to increase over time. The presence of the clathrate water molecules decreases the entropy of the system conating the protein solution.

Gibbs free energy equation $\Delta G = \Delta H - T\Delta S$

In the Gibbs free energy equation, a decrease in entropy results in a positive free energy change ($+\Delta G$), which is thermodynamically unfavourable. To release the clathrate water molecules and increase the entropy (S) the hydrophobic patches on the surface of the protein interact with each other to form inter-protein complexes. When these complexes become large they can no longer be held in solution by the remaining water molecules surrounding the surface of the protein complex. They start to come out of solution and visible as a cloudy dispersion that can be collected by centrifugation ($12,000 \times g$ for 30 min). Proteins with a large complement of surface hydrophobic groups will precipitate first and those with the least surface hydrophobic groups will precipitate at higher salt concentrations. The differences in the hydrophobic amino acid content and surface distribution of these hydrophobic surface patches can be utilised as a means to fractionate complex protein mixtures (see Section 5.5, Protocol 4.8 and Appendix 1).

In the laboratory the most common method for concentrating proteins from solutions is by increasing the salt concentration, which results in protein precipitation. Proteins usually demonstrate increased solubility at low salt concentrations ("salting in") and decreased solubility at high salt concentrations ("salting out"). The Hofmeister series of ions (see Figure 4.10) was determined by the ability of ions to precipitate a mixture of chicken egg proteins. The anions with multiple charges appear to be more effective at "salting out" proteins than cations.

The ideal salts for precipitating proteins are on the left of the Hofmeister series, but in practise ammonium sulphate is used for the routine precipitation of proteins because:

Anions: $PO_4^{3-} > SO_4^{2-} > CH_3COO^- > Cl^- > NO_3^- > ClO_4^- > SCN^-$

Cations: $NH_4^+ > K^+, Na^+ > Mg^{2+} > Ca^{2+} > Ba^{2+}$

Lyotropic	*Chaotropic*
salts	*salts*

Figure 4.10 The Hofmeister series.

- Ammonium sulphate dissolves at high concentrations (0.76 g ml^{-1}; approximately about 4 M at 0°C) generating little heat. The amount of solid ammonium sulphate to add to achieve to appropriate percentage saturation is given in Table 4.9.
- The density of saturated ammonium sulphate solution (1.235 g ml^{-1}) is less than the density of aggregated protein (1.29 g ml^{-1}), which allows collection of the precipitated protein by centrifugation (typically 12,000 × g for 15–30 min).
- Ammonium sulphate precipitation is a mild method of concentrating proteins giving very good recovery of biological activity.
- Proteins can be stored as an ammonium sulphate precipitate pellet (covered in a volume of saturated ammonium sulphate) at −25°C for long periods with little loss of activity. When the protein is required the liquid saturated ammonium sulphate can be poured away, the precipitate pellet can be dissolved in buffer and dialysed (see Protocol 4.9) or subjected to size exclusion chromatography (see Protocol 7.1) if required to remove the majority of the remaining ammonium ions.

Some points to note about using ammonium sulphate:

- Fractionation of complex protein mixtures can be achieved by incrementally increasing the percentage ammonium sulphate concentration and collecting the precipitates that form by centrifugation (see Protocol 4.8, which describes the total and fractional precipitation of proteins using ammonium sulphate).
- Ammonium sulphate precipitation is not a highly resolving technique, for this reason there is little to be gained in using small incremental additions of the salt to try and produce a highly purified fraction containing the target protein. Broad incremental additions are usually used to capture all of the target protein in one fraction. After the precipitate has been collected and dissolved in a buffer the extract is then moved onto chromatographic fractionation techniques (see the example extractions in Protocols 4.6–4.8, which use ammonium sulphate to concentrate extracted protein).
- Ammonium sulphate precipitation is not usually used in industry as it has a corrosive effect on stainless steel.
- Ammonium sulphate will acidify the extract; check the pH after the addition of the salt and adjust if required.
- Traces contamination of the extract by heavy metal ions in the ammonium sulphate can be a problem. Use the highest quality reagents available and include 5 mM EDTA as a protective chelating agent (see Section 4.4.3) if the target protein is particularly sensitive to metal ions.
- The formation of protein aggregates can be problematic at protein concentrations below 1.0 mg ml^{-1}. At the latter stages of purification other techniques to concentrate proteins are recommended (see below).

Table 4.9 The amount of solid ammonium sulphate (gram L^{-1}) to achieve the required % saturation at 0°C.

Initial % sat at 0°C	Target % saturation at 0°C																
	20	25	30	35	40	45	50	55	60	65	70	75	80	85	90	95	100
0	106	134	164	194	226	258	291	326	361	398	436	476	516	559	603	650	697
5	79	108	137	166	197	229	262	296	331	368	405	444	484	526	570	615	662
10	53	81	109	139	169	200	233	266	301	337	374	412	452	493	536	581	627
15	26	54	82	111	141	172	204	237	271	306	343	381	420	460	503	547	592
20		27	55	83	113	143	175	207	241	276	312	349	387	427	469	512	557
25			27	56	84	115	146	179	211	245	280	317	355	395	436	478	522
30				28	56	86	117	148	181	214	249	285	323	362	402	445	488
35					28	57	87	118	151	184	218	254	291	329	369	410	453
40						29	58	89	120	153	187	222	258	296	335	376	418
45							29	59	90	123	156	190	226	263	302	342	383
50								30	60	92	125	159	194	230	268	308	348
55									30	61	93	127	161	197	235	273	313
60										31	62	95	129	164	201	239	279
65											31	63	97	132	168	205	244
70												32	65	99	134	171	209
75													32	66	101	137	174
80														33	67	103	139
85															34	68	105
90																34	70
95																	35

4.11.2 Organic solvent precipitation

The dielectric constant of a solvent is the ability of the solvent to repel the attractive forces between 2 charged particles. Water has a dipole (see Section 1.3), which makes water a good solvent to dissolve ionic material resulting in water having a large dielectric constant (80.4). The addition of solvents such as ethanol or acetone can lower the dielectric constant of water reducing its ability to prevent oppositely charged groups on the surface of proteins from interacting. In addition, water starts to hydrate the solvent molecules, which strips the solvation shell from around the protein exposing more polar and charged groups. Aggregation occurs via these ionic interactions with the most highly charged precipitating first.

Cold acetone (−25°C) added to a protein solution in a ratio of (9:1) initiates precipitation which concludes if the protein:acetone mixture is stored overnight at −25°C. The precipitate can be collected by centrifugation ($12,000 \times g$ for 30 min at 4°C). In general this method of protein concentration does not allow for the correct refolding of proteins and as such any biological activity is not usually recovered. However, the technique works well even at low protein concentrations and it is a convenient method of preparing samples prior to 2D-PAGE or immunisation to create antibodies (see Protocol 4.10). At very low protein concentrations a precipitate may not be visible at the bottom or side of the centrifuge tube. It is important to treat the area where the precipitate is expected to be as if a precipitate is there. Carefully wash the area of the centrifuge tube corresponding to r_{max} (see Figure 4.4) with a small volume of buffer (e.g., SDS-PAGE or IEF sample buffer prior to 1D or 2D PAGE respectively) to prepare the sample for further analysis. Solvent precipitation of proteins would not be used on an industrial scale because of the obvious fire risks.

4.11.3 Polymer precipitation

Polyethylene glycol (PEG: M_r 6,000–20,000) is a **hygroscopic** compound, if the solid is added to a protein solution at concentrations up to 25% (w/v) it strips the solvation shell surrounding the surface of the protein resulting in protein precipitation that can be subsequently collected by centrifugation. The precipitation of proteins by PEG occurs in a similar fashion to solvent precipitation (see above, Section 4.11.2) but the lower concentrations of PEG used result in improved recovery of biological activity.

4.11.4 Aqueous two-phase partitioning

Proteins can be selectively partitioned into a phase by using mixtures of Polyethylene glycol and dextran polymers (see Section 4.10.2). Protein being less polar than other biological molecules tends to partition into the upper layer (PEG). By altering the phase composition where there is proportionally less PEG than dextran, protein can then be concentrated into the smaller volume of the PEG layer. The exact conditions to effect a successful partition needs to be determined experimentally.

4.11.5 Isoelectric precipitation

The isoelectric point (pI) of a protein is the pH value where the protein has no net charge and minimum solubility (see Chapter 2 and Sections 5.2 and 8.6). When the pH of a protein solution is adjusted towards the pI of the target protein a precipitate can form. This can be collected by centrifugation ($12,000 \times g$ for 30 min; see Section 4.9). However, the recovery of any biological activity can be very low. This may not be a problem if the precipitate is to be used for electrophoresis (e.g., 1D- or 2D-PAGE) or to be used to immunise a rabbit/mouse to raise antibodies against the target. However, in general isoelectric precipitation should be used with caution.

4.11.6 Chromatography

Ion exchange chromatography (see Section 5.2) and hydrophobic interaction chromatography (see Section 5.5) possess high protein–binding characteristics (typically 10–100 mg of protein ml^{-1} of resin). Relatively small resin volumes can be used to concentrate proteins from large volumes of dilute feedstocks. The binding of proteins to these resins does not depend on the protein concentration of the initial stock, it is reproducible and the binding can be easily reversed with good recoveries of active material. This concentration technique can be used in both the early and later stages of a purification protocol and fits well into industrial applications.

4.11.7 Hygroscopic material

In the later stages of a purification protocol when the total protein concentration is low and the volume is manageable: The sample can be placed in a prepared dialysis bag (see Protocol 4.9) and held in a measuring cylinder. Powdered hygroscopic material such as sucrose, Sephadex (G25 or G50) or polyethylene glycol (8000–20,000) can be packed around the dialysis bag to withdraw the water through the dialysis membrane. This method can be very efficient and the sample must be continually observed to prevent the sample in the dialysis bag from drying out. When the desired level of concentration has been achieved the sample can be removed and the inside of the dialysis bag rinsed with a small volume of buffer to maximise the recover the target material.

4.11.8 Dried acrylamide

A high percentage ($\geq$12%) acrylamide can be polymerised at (see Protocol 8.1) and dried in an oven for several days before being stored at room temperature. If a fragment of dried acrylamide is added to a protein extract the acrylamide will swell back to normal size taking up the liquid from the sample. This technique is best used in the later stages of purification to concentrate small volumes (<1.0 ml) of dilute sample.

4.11.9 Lyophilisation (freeze drying)

The solution of the target protein should be rapidly frozen in liquid nitrogen to avoid any deleterious effects of slow freezing (e.g., pH changes and ice crystal formation) and placed into a suitable freeze dryer to remove the water in the sample under a vacuum. Water in the frozen protein solution is removed by **sublimation** under reduced pressure. If the target protein is to be rehydrated for an assay after storage, the protein can be lyophilised in the buffer components and stored at −25°C. For long-term storage at −25°C the air in the glass vessel can be displaced by nitrogen gas before the glass vessel is sealed with a gastight lid. When required for an assay ultrapure water can be added to rehydrate the protein in the buffer components.

If the target protein is to be stored as a lyophilised powder free from buffer components then the last chromatographic step (e.g., size exclusion chromatography; see Sections 7.1–7.5) should be conducted in a volatile buffer (see Table 4.10) before freeze drying. Nonreducing sugars (e.g., sorbitol, sucrose, and trehalose), cyclodextrin derivatives, enzyme substrates and lyotropic salts (see Section 4.11.2; e.g., ammonium sulphate) can be added to help stabilise the target protein during lyophilisation. The effects of these additives on the stability of the target protein would have to be determined empirically. Lyophilisation can be a convenient method of concentrating large volumes of dilute sample and as a method for the long term storage of proteins. There are a large variety of freeze dryers available for academic and industrial applications. The efficacy of lyophilisation with the target protein would need to be determined experimentally.

Table 4.10 Volatile buffers (both the acids and bases that are used to adjust the pH should be volatile).

pH range	Buffer system
2.0	Formic acid
2.3–3.5	Pyridine/formic acid
3.3–4.3	Formic acid/trimethylamine
3.3–4.3	Formic acid/ammonia
3.3–4.3	Acetic acid/ammonia
3.0–6.0	Pyridine/acetic acid
4.3–5.3	Acetic acid/trimethylamine
4.3–5.3	Acetic acid/ammonia
6.8–8.8	Trimethylamine/HCl[a]
7.0–8.5	Ammonia/formic acid
8.5–10.0	Ammonia/acetic acid
7.0–12.0	Trimethylamine/carbonate
7.9	Ammonium bicarbonate
8.0–9.5	Ammonium carbonate/ammonia
8.5	Ammonium carbonate
8.8–9.8	Ammonia/formic acid
8.8–9.8	Ammonia/acetic acid
9.3–10.3	Trimethylamine/formic acid Trimethylamine/acetic acid Trimethylamine/ammonium carbonate
10.7	Dimethylamine/ammonia
10.6	Methylamine

*Take care trimethylamine has a strong smell of rotting fish.
Source: Applichem "Biological Buffers" (https://www.applichem.com/fileadmin /Broschueren/BioBuffer.pdf).

4.11.10   Ultrafiltration

Ultrafiltration is a versatile technique with many formats. Protein solutions are concentrated by filtration under pressure through semi permeable membrane filters. Ultrafiltration is capable of concentrating bacteria and proteins by using membranes with different molecular weight cutoff values. The technique is only marginally dependent upon the charge of the particle and is more dependent on the size and shape of the particle. Elevated temperatures improve filtration rates by lowering the **viscosity** of the liquid but elevated temperatures may also cause protein denaturation.

4.11.10.1   Stirred cells

A membrane (see Figure 4.11) with the appropriate MWCO (e.g., 10,000 will retain all molecules with a mass above 10,000) is placed at the bottom of the stirred cell (sizes range from 3–2000 ml). After the sample has been placed into the ultrafiltration cell, the lid is replaced and the apparatus is placed on a magnetic stirrer (or shaken) to reduce membrane fouling as the sample concentrates (see Figure 4.12). The concentration begins when the stirred

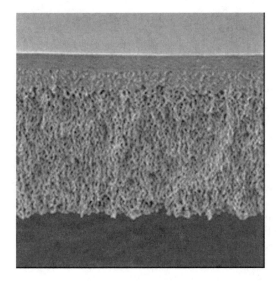

Figure 4.11 A cross-section through a Millipore ultracell regenerated cellulose membrane showing the porous structure of the membrane.

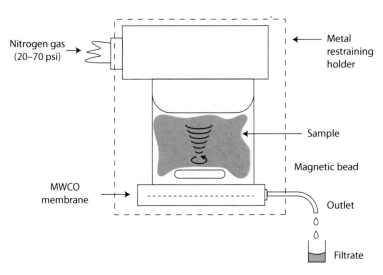

Nitrogen gas
(20–70 psi)

Metal
restraining
holder

Sample

Magnetic bead

MWCO
membrane

Outlet

Filtrate

Figure 4.12 Stirred cell ultrafiltration concentrator.
MWCO, molecular weight cutoff.

cell is connected to a source of pressurised nitrogen gas (70 psi). The pressure of the gas forces the liquid through the membrane, concentrating the sample. The technique can also be used to exchange buffers by repeatedly topping up the stirred cell with the new buffer and repeating the concentration step.

4.11.10.2   Centrifugal concentrators

In the laboratory centrifugal concentrators have all but replaced stirred cells for a number of reasons (a) Most laboratories will have a both a bench top centrifuge (5–50 ml) and a microfuge tube (1.5–2.0 ml) centrifuge. (b) A stirred cell can process only one sample at a time whereas a centrifuge can process many samples together (c) The centrifugal concentrators come in a range of sizes (0.5–50 ml) and with a variety of MWCO (or IEX) options (see Figure 4.13).

The upper chamber of the concentrator has MWCO filter on one face that is placed *towards* the axis of the centrifuge rotor. The sample is placed into the upper chamber and centrifugal force is used to force the liquid through the MWCO filter. This concentration technique works best with dilute (<5.0 mg ml^{-1}) protein samples because membrane fouling with crude extracts (>5.0 mgm ml^{-1}) greatly increases the time taken to concentrate a sample. Crude extracts can be concentrated by other methods such as salt precipitation (see above, Section 4.11.1).

4.11.10.3   Static concentrators

The sample is loaded into the static concentrator using a pipette and an absorbent pad mounted behind the ultrafiltration (MWCO) membrane draws the liquid through the membrane. The molecules above the molecular weight cutoff are retained and will concentrate into the bottom of the sample container. The advantages of these concentrators are that they are available in different sizes (0.5–20.0 ml) and no additional equipment is required (see Figure 4.14).

4.11.10.4   Tangential flow (cross-flow) concentrators

The large surface areas offered by tangential flow concentrators make them a viable alternative to stirred cell ultrafiltration concentrators for the concentration of large volumes of protein solutions. In a flat plate system (see Figure 4.15), the solution to be concentrated (retentate) flows continuously across a membrane (or stacks of membranes). As the filtrate passes through the membrane under pressure the retentate becomes concentrated because water and molecules smaller than the MWCO pass through the membrane. In hollow fibre concentrators the ultrafiltration membrane is manufactured as a tube (internal diameter 0.5–3.0 mm) with the MWCO filter on the inside of the tube. The feedstock is pumped through the fibres (connected in series) with the filtrate passing through the hollow fibres and the retentate becomes more concentrated. Elevated flow rates improve the rates of filtration but increased flow rates can also increase protein denaturation. This concentration technique can be used in both the early and later stages of a purification protocol and fits well into industrial applications.

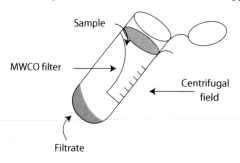

Sample

MWCO filter

Centrifugal field

Filtrate

Figure 4.13 Micron® centrifugal concentration unit.

Sample application and retrieval

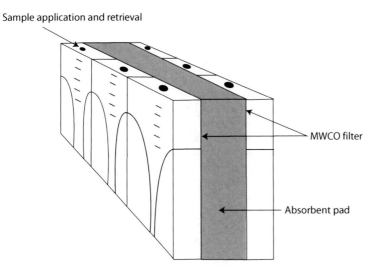

Figure 4.14 A static ultrafiltration concentrator.

MWCO filter

Absorbent pad

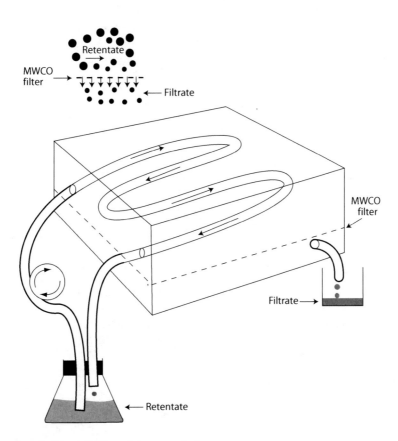

Retentate

MWCO filter

Filtrate

MWCO filter

Filtrate

Retentate

Figure 4.15 Diagram of a tangential flow plate concentrator.

4.12   CLARIFICATION OF PROCESS SCALE EXTRACTS

4.12.1 Process scale centrifugation

In the production of proteins for commercial use there will be a need to collect the cells producing targets proteins and then the removal of cellular debris after extraction. This will be on a different scale to processing extracts within a laboratory requiring modified centrifuges to collect and clarify cellular extracts in a continuous process. Disc stack (also known as conical plate or disc bowl) centrifuges/separators are routinely employed to clarify the extracts generated in the biotechnology industry. The liquid flows into the disc stack centrifuge near to the axis of rotation and is allowed to flow up through a series of angled plates resting on top of each other (see Figure 4.16). The plates split the flowing liquid into a large number of thin streams. Under the influence of the centrifugal field, the larger and denser particles contact the angled plates and move down the plate to be gathered in a collecting area. The collecting area is periodically vented to prevent a build up of these particles halting the clarification process. The liquid and smaller particles flow up though the centrifuge and exit at the top near to the axis of rotation. The maximum g-force generated in disc centrifuges varies between 5000–15,000 × g depending on the size of the disc bowl and the rotational speed of the rotor.

Tubular centrifuges have a relatively simple robust design (see Figure 4.17) and can be used to separate immiscible liquids with a density difference. The liquid flows in from the bottom of the centrifuge and baffles direct the flow into the main rapidly rotating bowl. The larger and denser fraction travels to the outer edge of the bowl and is removed from the lighter fraction at the top of the device. Tubular centrifuges can generate up to 100,000 × g at the periphery of the rotating bowl. They are designed for continuous flow but can be used as a batch device where the larger and denser particles (e.g., cells) gather as a pellet on the outer walls of the

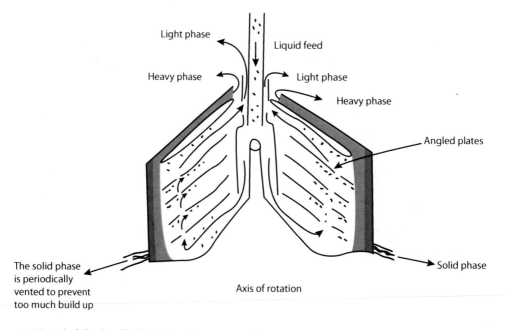

Figure 4.16 A typical disc bowl industrial continuous centrifuge.

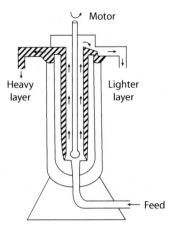

Figure 4.17 The flow path through a typical tubular centrifuge.

rotating bowl. The device is periodically stopped and the pelleted material removed.

Several passes through the system may be required to effect an acceptable separation of the solid from the liquid. Any imperfection in the fabrication of the continuous centrifuge will become a focal point for the collection of debris so these centrifuges are constructed of polished steel and regular maintenance/washing is required to ensure trouble free operation.

Centrifugation clarifies a cell homogenate by exploiting the differences between particle size and density, but the high viscosity of some cell extracts, the small differences in particle size and the large volumes of liquid can make centrifugation an inappropriate technique for the clarification of process scale extracts. Ultrafiltration (see Section 4.11.10) can be used to produce particle free extracts as the problems associated with viscosity can be overcome by dilution. The downside of this strategy is that the increase in process time can result in a decreases in the yield of the target protein. The ultrafiltration setups used in the process industry include flat plate tangential flow devices, hollow fibre tubes and spirally wound membranes. A typical large scale purification will combine centrifugation and ultrafiltration in the collection and clarification of process scale extracts endeavouring to utilise the advantages of both techniques to maximise the amount of the target protein prior to the purification of the target protein.

4.12.2 Stirred bed

The tissue or cell extract can be stirred with a resin (e.g., ion exchange) after which the resin is separated from the particulate liquid by filtration or sedimentation. The resin can then be washed and the target protein eluted using a batch process with an isocratic elution (see Section 3.6.7) or the resin can be packed into a column and then eluted with a salt wash. However, the adsorption efficiency of this technique is poor because there is only one adsorption equilibrium this results in a larger volume of resin required to bind the same amount of sample when this is compared to a resin packed into a column. The larger volume of resin also presents greater handling problems.

4.12.3 Fluidised bed

The particulate extract can be pumped through a suspension of resin and liquid known as a fluidised bed. However, turbulence and channelling in the fluidised bed can be extensive, resulting in the poor adsorption of any protein. Time-consuming recycling of the feedstock would be required to achieve the maximum amount of target protein binding to the resin. To improve the operation of fluidised beds the resin particles need to be fixed in the liquid stream, baffles and magnetic particles have been used to achieve this with some success.

4.12.4 Expanded bed

A resin with particles of different sizes and densities become suspended in a liquid flow. The largest dense particles remain at the bottom of the column and the lighter smaller particles are held in suspension by the upward flow of the liquid resulting in a stable (expanded) bed of resin. The particles have been constructed with agarose containing a quartz core (GE Healthcare) and a gel within ceramic zirconium bead (Pall) to which a variety of functional groups can be attached (IEX, HIC, affinity or IMAC). The crude feedstock is applied with an upward flow that expands the resin particle bed (see Figure 4.18). The cell debris passes through the expanded bed unimpaired and the cellular protein binds to the resin.

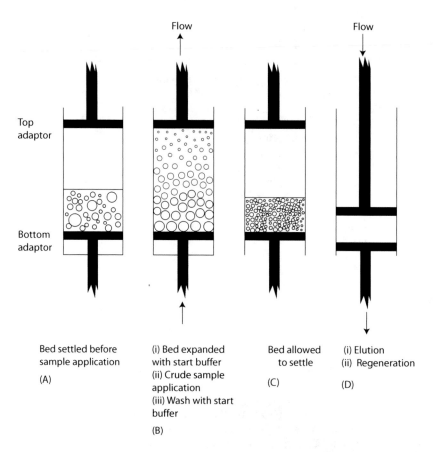

Figure 4.18 At the start of the expanded bed process: (A) large and small beads rest together. (B) The mobile phase is introduced from below the beads which separate according to their size and density (i). The crude sample is applied and flows over the beads in the moving liquid (ii). The required interaction takes place, e.g., IEX and the crude debris are washed free from the bed (iii). (C) The bed is allowed to settle after the initial wash. (D) The target protein is eluted free from debris by eluting in the reverse direction to the flow, e.g., high salt (i). After a sanitation wash (e.g., hot NaOH) the resin is re-equilibrated in the start buffer (ii).

After a wash step the upward flow of liquid is stopped to allow the bed to settle. The upper adaptor is lowered to the bed surface and the elution conditions applied. These robust resins also allow the stringent washing procedures required by the biotechnology industry.

4.13   MEMBRANE CHROMATOGRAPHY

Column chromatography using resins is not always an ideal medium for processing the large volumes of viscous feedstocks experienced in the biotechnology industry. Micro and macroporous adsorptive membranes (2–3 mm thickness) can be used instead of conventional bead based resins. These membranes are easy to scale up and may have better flow properties than the equivalent conventional columns, which also speeds up the process of washing, binding, elution and sanitation. This decrease in process time should reduce the costs and the possible denaturation of the target protein.

The membranes (thin discs, hollow fibres and spiral wound membranes) can be constructed of a variety of materials including; cellulose and cellulose derivatives, inert polymers (polymethacrylate, polystyrene, polyethylene nylon and polyamide) as well as chitin and chitosan. In addition, a variety of functional groups (IEX, HIC, reversed-phase and affinity) can be attached to the membranes as a means to fractionate and purify complex protein mixtures.

The use of membranes to process samples in the laboratory is also becoming popular. Ion exchange membranes and affinity membranes (e.g., **protein A** for the purification of IgG; see Protocol 6.1) are now available to rapidly process small volume samples.

4.14   THE STORAGE OF PROTEIN SAMPLES

Some of the amino acid functional groups present in a protein structure are prone to alteration on storage (see Chapter 2). Amide nitrogen will be lost from glutamine and asparagine residues at most pH values. The functional groups of the amino acids cysteine, methionine and tryptophan are prone to oxidation. The non-enzymic addition of reducing sugars to the free amino groups at the N-terminus or lysine residues in a protein's structure can occur in crude non-dialysed extracts. In addition, protein aggregation or proteolysis can also occur at most temperatures. The stability of proteins during storage is not easy to predict and has to be determined empirically, preferably before embarking on chromatographic analysis.

This can be undertaken by incubating aliquots of the target protein after clarification or following dialysis after ammonium sulphate concentration under different storage conditions in the presence of different compounds (see Section 4.11.1 and Protocols 4.8–4.9). The sample can be periodically assayed for activity and protein concentration (every day for the first week, then weekly for the first month, followed by monthly for the next 2 months) to assess the suitability of the storage conditions. The rate at which the sample is frozen can affect the stability of stored protein. So it is advisable to freeze the protein sample in liquid nitrogen before storing the sample aliquots at the different storage temperatures.

The storage containers should ideally have low protein–binding characteristics, and be pre-sterilised or autoclaved. The reagents (highest grade possible) should be filtered through 0.2 μm membranes to remove bacterial and particulate contamination. Alternatively, the samples can be centrifuged at 12,000 × *g* for 30 min to remove any aggregates or bacteria. After centrifugation the clarified supernatant should transferred to a suitable storage vessel.

Suggested storage temperatures: Liquid nitrogen (–196°C), freezer (–80°C), freezer (–25°C), fridge (4–8°C) and room temperature (RT).

Suggested conditions:

- Different buffers at one pH to determine an ideal storage buffer.
- Different pH values in the ideal storage buffer.
- The ideal storage buffer at the ideal pH in the presence of the following at different concentrations; substrate(s), reversible inhibitors/activators, cofactors, reducing agents, proteolytic inhibitors, lyotropic salts (e.g., ammonium sulphate at a concentration below the concentration that causes the target protein to precipitate), anti-microbial agents (e.g., 0.05% (w/v) sodium azide or 0.01% (w/v) thiomersal), non-reducing sugars (e.g., sucrose, trehalose or sorbitol), cyclodextrin, glycerol (this will increase the viscosity of the medium) or ethanediol (this will increase the viscosity of the medium but not as much as glycerol).
- Combinations of these different conditions (e.g., reducing agents in the presence of ethanediol) may eventually provide the ideal storage conditions for the target protein.

Antibodies with a recommended storage temperature of –25°C can be mixed with an equal volume of glycerol and stored as a cold liquid at –25°C to improve their storage properties (don't forget the dilution when the antibody is to be used). Protein extracts precipitated and collected as an ammonium sulphate pellet (see Section 4.11.1) or after lyophilisation (see Section 4.11.9) will provide the ideal storage environment for many proteins.

4.15 SUMMARY

The time spent in preparation for protein purification is an investment. This is true in the purification of proteins from a natural or recombinant source. It will cultivate familiarity with the protein and this will reap rewards when the chromatography steps are set in motion. Most of the suggested procedures outlined in this chapter can be conducted in small volumes, and although this will not exactly match how a larger volume will behave, it will alert the operator to be cautious at critical stages. The techniques identified in this chapter are by no means an exhaustive list and the operator should look in the literature for any technique pertinent to the target protein.

EXERCISE 4.1 CENTRIFUGATION: THE CONVERSION OF REVOLUTIONS PER MINUTE (RPM) TO RELATIVE CENTRIFUGAL FORCE (RCF)

In the centrifugation of biological material, it is important to quote relative centrifugal force (RCF), not revolutions per minute (rpm). This is because increases in rpm and RCF are not related in a linear fashion (see the equation below).

The acceleration of a centrifuge is normally expressed as a multiple of the acceleration due to gravity (g), which is 9.80 m s^{-2}.

Relative centrifugal force (RCF) depends upon the speed of the rotor (n) in RPM (*revolutions per minute*) and the radius of the rotor (r; *in mm*).

Thus, RCF = 1.118 r $(n/1000)^2$

For example: A bench centrifuge at 3000 RPM with a rotor that had a radius of 95 mm. What is the RCF?

$$RCF = 1.118 \times 95 \times (3000/1000)^2$$
$$RCF = 1.118 \times 95 \times (3)^2$$
$$= 956 \ g$$

This value can now be duplicated on another centrifuge.

Q. Calculate the RCF in the same centrifuge when the rpm was increased to 5000. (Answer in Appendix 6.)

PROTOCOLS FOR CHAPTER 4

Protocol 4.1 The measurement of protein concentration using the absorbance of light at 280 nm

Proteins absorb light maximally at 280 nm, mainly due to the presence of the aromatic residues in the structures of tryptophan and tyrosine.

> **Note:** (a) Prepare buffers fresh or from frozen stocks and use the highest reagent grade available. (b) Check the data sheets provided by the reagent's manufacturers and take appropriate health and safety precautions. (c) This method of measuring concentration is quick and non-destructive but can be subject to interference from nucleic acids, which also absorb light at this wavelength. (Use the correction factor: Protein (mg ml^{-1}) = 1.55 A_{280nm} −0.76 A_{260nm}.) (d) The majority of proteins have a percentage absorptivity coefficient in the range of 4.0–24.0. In general an absorbance reading of 1.0 approximates to a protein concentration of 1.0 mg ml^{-1} (i.e., $\varepsilon^{1\%}$ 280 nm = 10.0) (specific values BSA $\varepsilon^{1\%}$ 280 nm = 6.67 and **immunoglobulins** $\varepsilon^{1\%}$ 280 nm = 13–15 (use 14). (e) Small M_r metabolites such as the amino acids (tryptophan and tyrosine), peptides (containing tryptophan and tyrosine) and nucleotides will also contribute to the absorbance of light at 280 nm. The extract can be dialysed (see Protocol 4.9), subjected to ammonium sulphate precipitation (see Protocol 4.7) or SEC (see Section 7.6) to reduce the contamination from these components. (f) Crude extracts are sometimes cloudy due to **particulate** matter. This will contribute to the reading by scattering the light (**attenuance**). Clarifying the extract by centrifugation at 13,000 × g for 20 min (see Section 4.9) prior to reading the absorbance will help reduce this problem. (g) Warm the extract to room temperature prior to taking the reading to prevent moisture condensing on the surface of the **cuvette**.

Equipment

- Spectrophotometer that can generate and measure light in the UV wavelengths (200–340 nm).
- Quartz or disposable UV grade plastic cuvettes (1.0 or 3.0 ml volumes).

Method

- Switch on the spectrophotometer and set the wavelength to 280 nm.
- Allow the machine to stabilise (times vary with each machine).
- Fill the cuvette with buffer the sample is dissolved in and set absorbance to zero (blank).
- Replace the buffer with the protein sample and measure the absorbance of the sample.

Protocol 4.2 Bicinchoninic acid (BCA) protein assay (0–1.0 mg ml^{-1})

Note: (a) Prepare buffers fresh or from frozen stocks and use the highest reagent grade available. (b) Check the data sheets provided by the reagent's manufacturers and take appropriate health and safety precautions. (c) Read the samples within 10 min of each other (the BCA reaction with proteins is not a true endpoint reaction and the colour will continue to develop after the 30 min incubation, but this increase in colour is minimal at room temperature).

The reagents can be prepared as detailed below or a kit can be purchased (Sigma or Pierce) for very little difference in overall price.

Reagents A and B are can be stored at room temperature.

Reagent A: Dissolve 5.0 g BCA, 10.0 g sodium carbonate, 0.8 g sodium tartrate, 2.0 g sodium hydroxide and 4.75 g sodium bicarbonate in 400 ml of distilled and deionised water. Adjust the pH to 11.25 with concentrated sodium hydroxide and make up to 500 ml.

Reagent B: Dissolve 4 g copper sulphate (CuSO$_4$ pentahydrate).

Standard working reagent (SWR): Prepare enough for the assay by mixing 100 volumes of reagent A with 2 volumes of reagent B (apple-green colour).

Standard protein: 1.0 mg ml^{-1} Bovine serum albumin ε$^{1\%}$ 280 nm = 6.67).

(a) Microfuge tube	Sample buffer	1.0 mg ml^{-1} BSA	SWR	Protein concentration mg ml^{-1}
1	50.0 µl	0.00 µl	1.0 ml	0.0
2,3,4	45.0 µl	5.00 µl	1.0 ml	0.1
4,5,6	40.0 µl	10.0 µl	1.0 ml	0.2
7,8,9	30.0 µl	20.0 µl	1.0 ml	0.4
10,11,12	20.0 µl	30.0 µl	1.0 ml	0.6
13,14,15,	10.0 µl	40.0 µl	1.0 ml	0.8
16,17,18	0.00 µl	50.0 µl	1.0 ml	1.0

(b) Microplate (96 well)	Sample buffer	1.0 mg ml^{-1} BSA	SWR	Protein concentration mg ml^{-1}
A1, B1 and C1	20.0 µl	0.00 µl	0.2 ml	0.0
A2, B2 and C2	19.0 µl	1.0 µl	0.2 ml	0.05
A3, B3 and C3	18.0 µl	2.0 µl	0.2 ml	0.1
A4, B4 and C4	16.0 µl	4.0 µl	0.2 ml	0.2
A5, B5 and C5	12.0 µl	8.0 µl	0.2 ml	0.4
A6, B6 and C6	8.0 µl	12.0 µl	0.2 ml	0.6
A7, B7 and C7	4.0 µl	16.0 µl	0.2 ml	0.8
A8, B8 and C8	0.00 µl	20.0 µl	0.2 ml	1.0

- Incubate either microfuge tubes or 96 well microplate at 37°C for 30 min and measure the absorbance at 562 nm. Use the data to prepare a calibration graph of protein concentration (x-axis) mg ml^{-1} against absorbance (y-axis) at 562 nm.
- *Preparation of samples for a protein assay*: Prepare dilutions of the sample by adding (a) 50 μl of sample to 950 μl of sample buffer (1:20 dilution) and 100 μl of sample to 900 μl of sample buffer (1:10 dilution). Vortex mix the dilutions, before adding 3 × 50 μl to 3 microfuge tubes for the microfuge tube assay (a) or add 3 × 20 μl to three wells on a microplate. The samples can now be treated exactly as the standards (i.e., add the appropriate volume of SWR, incubate at 37°C for 30 min and read at 562 nm).
- Read the absorbance at 562 nm and, using the protein standard calibration graph (see above), convert the sample absorbance readings into protein concentration values.
- In practice the standards and samples can be prepared, incubated and read at the same time.
- Remember to multiply by the dilution factor to obtain the protein concentration of the samples.
- Avoid touching the bottom of the wells in a 96 well plate. Fingerprints on the wells can lead to erroneous absorbance readings.

Protocol 4.3 Bicinchoninic acid (BCA) protein assay (0.5–10 μg ml^{-1})

Note: (a) Prepare buffers fresh or from frozen stocks and use the highest reagent grade available. (b) Check the data sheets provided by the reagent's manufacturers and take appropriate health and safety precautions. (c) Read the samples within 10 min of each other (the BCA reaction with proteins is not a true endpoint reaction and the colour will continue to develop after the 30 min incubation, but this increase in colour is minimal at room temperature).

Reagent A: Dissolve 8 g sodium carbonate, 1.6 g sodium hydroxide, 1.5 g sodium tartrate in 50 ml of distilled water. Add solid sodium bicarbonate to adjust the pH to 11.25 and make up to 100 ml.

Reagent B: Dissolve 4 g BCA in 100 ml of distilled water.

Reagent C: Dissolve 4 g copper sulphate ($CuSO_4$ pentahydrate) in 100 ml of distilled water.

Reagents A, B and C are stable at room temperature.

Before use, prepare *Reagent D:* Mix 4 volumes of reagent C with 100 volumes of reagent B.

Standard working reagent: Mix 1 volume of reagent D with 1 volume of reagent A.

Standard protein: 1.0 mg ml^{-1} Bovine serum albumin ($\varepsilon^{1\%}$ 280 nm = 6.67)

Method

- Prepare bovine serum albumin (BSA) standards (0–10.0 μg ml^{-1}) in the same buffer as the sample in triplicate.
- Add 0.5 volume of standard working reagent to 0.5 ml of standards (or sample) in a microfuge tube.
- Mix and incubate at 60°C for 60 min.
- Cool to room temperature and measure absorbance at 562 nm.
- Use the readings from the standards to prepare a calibration graph.
- Convert the reading from the samples into protein concentration using the calibration graph.
- Remember to multiply by any dilution factor to obtain the final protein concentration.

Protocol 4.4 Coomassie blue dye binding protein assay

Note: (a) Prepare buffers fresh or from frozen stocks and use the highest reagent grade available. (b) Check the data sheets provided by the reagent's manufacturers and take appropriate health and safety precautions.

Reagent A: Dissolve 500 mg of Coomassie brilliant blue G-250 in 250 ml of 95% (v/v) ethanol, and then add 500 ml of 85% (v/v) phosphoric acid and store at room temperature.

Standard working reagent: Dilute reagent A (1:4) with distilled water and filter before use.

Standard protein: 1.0 mg ml^{-1} Bovine serum albumin ($\varepsilon^{1\%}$ 280 nm = 6.67)

Microfuge tube	Sample buffer	Standard protein	Standard working reagent	Protein concentration (mg ml^{-1})
1	20 μl	0 μl	1.0 ml	0.0
2,3,4	18 μl	2 μl	1.0 ml	0.1
4,5,6	16 μl	4 μl	1.0 ml	0.2
7,8,9	14 μl	6 μl	1.0 ml	0.3
10,11,12	12 μl	8 μl	1.0 ml	0.4
13,14,15	10 μl	10 μl	1.0 ml	0.5
16,17,18	5 μl	15 μl	1.0 ml	0.75
19,20,21	0 μl	20 μl	1.0 ml	1.0

- Prepare the standards as outlined above in the same buffer as the sample.
- Vortex mix the tubes, incubate for 5 min at room temperature and then measure the **absorbance** at 595 nm. Use the information to prepare a calibration graph of protein concentration mg ml^{-1} against absorbance at 562 nm.
- Add 1.0 ml of the standard working reagent to 20 μl of the undiluted sample and to 20 μl of two dilutions of the sample (e.g., 1/10 and 1/50) in triplicate. Vortex mix, incubate for 5 min at room temperature and measure the absorbance at 595 nm (the colour is usually stable for 60 min). Using the calibration graph, convert the sample absorbance readings into protein concentration values.
- Remember to multiply by the dilution factor to obtain the sample's protein concentration.

Protocol 4.5 Azocasein assay to determine the peptidase profile in crude extracts

Azocasein is an orange-coloured protein substrate for proteolytic enzymes. When the peptidase enzyme cleaves the azocasein, the orange polypeptide fragments are released into solution. After a period of incubation (5 min–24 hr), the reaction is stopped by the addition of cold acid trichloroacetic acid (TCA), which precipitates proteins and protein fragments (above approximately M_r 3000), leaving the azopeptide (orange-coloured) fragments from peptidase hydrolysis in solution. The colour produced can be read directly but is enhanced by the addition of alkali.

($\varepsilon^{1\%}$ at 440 nm in 0.1 M NaOH = 32–38.)

Reagent A: Dissolve 2.0 g of azocasein and 0.05 g of sodium azide in 100 ml distilled and deionised water.

- Add 0.25 ml of reagent A and 0.25 ml of buffer (extraction buffer) to a 1.5 ml microfuge tube and initiate the reaction by adding 0.25 ml of sample (an incubation with no enzyme should be initiated with 0.25 ml buffer instead of the sample).
- Incubate at 37°C (the time of incubation should be determined experimentally by incubation at different time points up to 16 hours. For long incubations the assay components should be sterile-filtered and the sample should be centrifuged at 13,000 × g for 30 min to remove bacterial contamination).
- The reaction is terminated by the addition of 0.25 ml of 20% (w/v) TCA.
- Leave on ice for 15 min (encourages the formation of precipitate) and then centrifuge at 10,000 × g for 10 min.
- Set the spectrophotometer to 440 nm.
- Mix 0.5 ml of the supernatant from the incubation with no enzyme with 0.5 ml of 2M NaOH, and use this to zero the spectrophotometer.
- Mix 0.5 ml of the enzyme incubation supernatant with 0.5 ml of 2M NaOH blank and read the absorbance at 440 nm.
- Take care to avoid any floating particles of precipitated azocasein.

When a suitable incubation time has been established, the assay can be repeated in the presence of a variety of proteolytic enzyme inhibitors (see Table 2.2) at different concentrations to establish the concentration required to prevent proteolysis of the target protein.

Protocol 4.6 Extraction of plant tissue material using a blender and concentration using ammonium sulphate

Note: (a) Prepare buffers fresh or from frozen stocks and use the highest reagent grade available. (b) Check the data sheets provided by the reagent's manufacturers and take appropriate health and safety precautions (c) The buffer components will depend on the requirements of the target protein. As an example, the details provided here are for the extraction of transglutaminase (E.C. 2.3.2.13) from 14-day-old *Pisum sativum* tissue.

Extraction buffer: 100 mM Tris/HCl pH 8.0 containing 10 mM 2-ME (add fresh), 250 mM sucrose, 3 mM ascorbic acid and 3 mM EDTA.

Membrane washing buffer: 5 mM Tris/HCl pH 7.2 containing 1mM DTT (add fresh), 250 mM sucrose and 1.0 M potassium chloride.

Membrane resuspension buffer: 5 mM Tris/Mes pH 7.2 containing 1 mM DTT (add fresh) and 250 mM sucrose.

Method

- Solid PVPP was added to the extraction buffer at a concentration of 5% (w/v) and left overnight at 4°C.
- Leaf tissue was harvested after 14 days and homogenised in ice cold extraction buffer in a ratio of 1:2 (w/v) with a blender, using 15 seconds bursts of blending followed by 30 seconds of cooling until the tissue was completely homogenised. After the first 15 second burst, proteolytic inhibitors (1 mM **PMSF**, 10 µM leupeptin, 1 µM pepstatin and 10 µM **E64**) and phenol oxidase inhibitors (1 mM **DIECA**) were added to the final concentrations indicated.
- The homogenate was strained through two layers of muslin and the pH re-adjusted to 7.4 using solid Tris.
- The extract was then centrifuged at 13000 × g for 20 min at 4°C using a centrifuge fitted with an 8 × 50.0 ml pre-chilled angle rotor (see Section 4.9).
- The pellet was discarded and the supernatant was further clarified by centrifugation at 80,000 × g for 45 min at 4°C to sediment the mixed membrane fraction using an ultra centrifuge fitted with a pre-chilled rotor.
- The protein in the supernatant was precipitated by the gradual addition of solid ammonium sulphate to 90% saturation at 4°C (0.6 g ammonium sulphate per ml of supernatant; see Section 4.11). After stirring for 20 min at 4°C the precipitated protein was collected by centrifugation (13000 × g for 20 min at 4°C) using a centrifuge fitted with an 8 × 50.0 ml pre-chilled angle rotor. The pellet was resuspended in 50 mM Tris/HCl buffer pH 7.4 containing 1 mM EDTA and 1 mM DTT and dialysed (see Protocol 4.9) against 5.0 L of the same buffer (changed twice).
- The dialysed extracted protein was clarified by centrifugation (13,000 × g for 20 min at 4°C) before storage at −25°C.
- The membrane pellet from the 80,000 g centrifugation was removed with a spatula and placed into a 5 ml Potter–Elvehjem homogeniser (see Section 4.6). The membrane fraction was resuspended in the membrane washing buffer before being centrifuged at 80,000 × g for 45 min.
- The supernatant was discarded and the membrane was resuspended as above in membrane resuspension buffer before being **aliquoted** and stored at −25°C.

Protocol 4.7 Extraction of animal tissue material using a Potter–Elvehjem homogeniser

Note: (a) Prepare buffers fresh or from frozen stocks and use the highest reagent grade available. (b) Check the data sheets provided by the reagent's manufacturers and take appropriate health and safety precautions. (c) The buffer components will depend on the requirements of the target protein. As an example, the details provided here are for the extraction of Type II (tissue) transglutaminase (E.C. 2.3.2.13) from guinea pig liver.

Extraction buffer: 100 mM Tris/HCl pH 7.4 containing 5 mM DTT and 3mM EDTA.

Method

- The liver tissue should be trimmed of fat and blood vessels and then cut into small pieces using a scalpel.
- The tissue was place into the pre-chilled mortar of a Potter–Elvehjem homogeniser (see Section 4.6) and homogenised in ice-cold extraction buffer in a ratio of 1:2 (w/v) using a handheld Teflon pestle. After several strokes with the pestle (on the down stroke rotate and grind the pestle; on the up stroke only rotate the pestle), the mortar was chilled on ice and proteolytic inhibitors were added (1 mM PMSF, 10 µM leupeptin and 1 µM pepstatin) to the final concentrations indicated. The homogenisation process was then repeated until the tissue was completely fragmented.
- The pH was adjusted to 7.4 using solid Tris.
- The extract was then centrifuged at $13,000 \times g$ for 20 min at 4°C using a centrifuge fitted with an 8×50.0 ml pre-chilled angle rotor (see Section 2.12).
- The pellet was discarded and the supernatant was further clarified by centrifugation at $80,000 \times g$ for 45 min at 4°C to sediment the mixed membrane fraction using an ultra centrifuge fitted with a pre-chilled rotor.
- The volume of the supernatant was measured and an **aliquot** of the crude homogenate kept for enzyme and protein assays. The remaining extract had a fraction of the protein precipitated by the gradual addition of solid ammonium sulphate to 30% saturation at 4°C (see Section 4.9). After stirring for 20 min at 4°C the precipitated protein was collected by centrifugation (13,000 g for 20 min at 4°C) using a centrifuge fitted with an 8×50.0 ml pre-chilled angle rotor.
- The supernatant's volume was measured and solid ammonium sulphate was gradually added to bring the % saturation to 70%. The mixture was left stirring at 4°C for 20 min and the pellet was collected by centrifugation ($13,000 \times g$ for 20 min at 4°C).
- The supernatant's volume was measured and solid ammonium sulphate was gradually added to bring the % saturation to 100%. The mixture was left stirring at 4°C for 30 min and the pellet was collected by centrifugation ($13,000 \times g$ for 20 min at 4°C).

- The three ammonium sulphate pellets were resuspended in 50 mM Tris/HCl buffer pH 7.8 containing 0.1 mM EDTA and 1 mM DTT and separately dialysed (see Protocol 4.9) against 5.0 L of the same buffer (changed twice).
- After dialysis the extracted protein was clarified by centrifugation (13,000 × g for 20 min at 4°C) and the volume of each fraction was measured.
- A protein and enzyme assay was performed on the crude homogenate and the three ammonium sulphate fractions to determine the fraction enriched in transglutaminase (see Chapter 8). The ammonium sulphate fraction enriched in transglutaminase was then stored at −70°C.

Protocol 4.8 The total (a) and fractional (b) precipitation of protein by ammonium sulphate

Note: (a) Prepare buffers fresh or from frozen stocks and use the highest reagent grade available. (b) Check the data sheets provided by the reagent's manufacturers and take appropriate health and safety precautions. (c) Ammonium sulphate concentration is usually quoted as percent saturation, assuming that the extract will dissolve the same amount of ammonium sulphate as pure water (the amount of ammonium sulphate to add to a given volume of extract can be acquired from Table 4.9; see Section 4.11, which provides the basis of protein precipitation using ammonium sulphate).

(a) Total protein (0–100% sat)

Place the protein solution in a beaker in a cold room (or on ice) on a magnetic stirrer. While stirring to every 100 ml of clarified extract slowly add 70.0 g of ammonium sulphate over a 5–10 min period (check the pH and adjust if necessary) and leave stirring for 20 min until the salt dissolves. The precipitate can be collected by centrifugation 13,000 × g for 20 min at 4°C (see Section 4.9) and again dissolved in buffer. If required, the concentration of ammonium ions can be reduced by dialysis (see Protocol 4.9) or by group size exclusion chromatography (SEC) (see Chapter 7).

(b) Fractional approach (0–40% sat, 40–70% sat, 70–100% sat)

- Place the protein solution in a beaker in a cold room (or on ice) on a magnetic stirrer. While stirring to every 100 ml of clarified extract slowly add 22.6 g of ammonium sulphate over a 5–10 min period (check the pH and adjust if necessary) and leave stirring for 20 min until the salt dissolves.

- The precipitate (P1) can be separated from the supernatant by centrifugation at 13,000 × g for 20 min at 4°C. The supernatant's volume should be measured and for every 100 ml slowly add 18.7 g of ammonium sulphate.

- When the salt has dissolved the precipitate (P2) can be separated from the supernatant by centrifugation at 13,000 × g for 20 min at 4°C. The volume of the supernatant should be measured and to every 100 ml of extract add 20.9 g of ammonium sulphate. When the salt has dissolved the precipitate (P3) can be separated from the supernatant by centrifugation at 13,000 × g for 20 min at 4°C and redissolved in buffer.

The precipitates P1, P2 and P3 can be dialysed (see Protocol 4.9) or desalted using SEC (see Chapter 7). Then the volume, protein concentration and the activity for the protein of interest can be measured (see Chapter 8). If the target protein is split between fractions, in subsequent experiments, the fractional additions of ammonium sulphate can be adjusted to capture all the target protein into one precipitate.

Protocol 4.9 Preparation of dialysis tubing

Dialysis (Visking) tubing is a semi-permeable membrane that allows movement of molecules below the M_r cutoff into and out of the dialysis bag. The tubing comes in a variety of sizes, usually with a M_r cutoff of approximately 12,000 but tubing with smaller and larger pore sizes can be obtained (Perbio, Pierce Ltd).

> **Note:** (a) Prepare buffers fresh or from frozen stocks and use the highest reagent grade available. (b) Check the data sheets provided by the reagent's manufacturers and take appropriate health and safety precautions. (c) Dialysis will result in an increase in the sample volume, so always leave some room in the tubing for expansion. (d) In dialysis "little and often" is best (i.e., multiple changes of smaller volumes of buffer are more efficient than large volumes changed infrequently).

Preparation

- Place a length of dialysis tubing in a glass beaker and boil in 2% (w/v) sodium bicarbonate and 0.05% (w/v) EDTA for 5 min to remove heavy metal ions.
- Rinse in distilled water.
- Boil in distilled water for 5 min.
- Rinse in distilled water and then store at 4°C in 20% (v/v) ethanol or 0.05% (w/v) sodium azide until required.

Sample Dialysis

- Cut a length of prepared dialysis tubing and tie a double knot at one end (alternatively, bag sealer can be purchased (e.g., Thermo Fisher Ltd).
- Rinse the inside of the tube with distilled water and check for leaks.
- Using a funnel, carefully add the sample.
- Expel the air from the tubing and tie another double knot at the end to seal the tubing. Remember to leave some room for the liquid to expand into.
- Place the dialysis bag with the sample in a large beaker containing buffer (the start buffer for the next chromatographic step?) at 4°C and stir (arrange the dialysis bag so that it does not touch the stirring mechanism) for 3–4 hr to allow the concentration of salt to reach equilibrium. Several changes of buffer may be necessary to lower the salt concentration to the desired level.

Protocol 4.10 Precipitation of protein from a small volume (0.1–5.0 ml) using acetone

Acetone is a clear, volatile, flammable solvent. Appropriate safety precautions should be instigated when working with this solvent (e.g., a fume cupboard and a freezerrated suitable for solvents).

Preparation

- Place the required volume of acetone in a −25°C freezer to cool to the required temperature.
- HPLC/GC glass sample vials with gastight seals are useful for the method.
- If glass sample vials are not available, please make sure that the containers are compatible with acetone.

Method for a 1.0 ml Sample

- Aliquot 100 µl of the sample into ten glass sample vials.
- Add 900 µl of ice cold acetone to each glass vial.
- Vortex mix and store overnight in the freezer (−25°C).
- The following morning transfer the contents of one sample vial into a microfuge tube and centrifuge at $12,000 \times g$ for 15 min.
- Place the microfuge tube in the micro centrifuge rotor with the hinge of the lid facing away from centre of the rotor (see Figure 4.17A). Even if a precipitate is not visible, the protein will gather at the bottom of the microfuge tube beneath the lid hinge (r_{max}; see Figure 4.4).
- After centrifugation open the lid and carefully remove the microfuge tube (try to hold the tube at the angle it was contained in the rotor). Transfer the solvent from the tube by pipetting from the opposite side to the hinge (see Figure 4.17B).
- Allow the tube to dry in the air.
- Add 50 µl of 0.5% (w/v) SDS in 0.1M NaOH and vortex mix.
- Assay for the protein concentration using the BCA protein assay (see Protocols 4.2 or 4.3 depending the amount of protein present).
- Knowing the amount of protein present in each tube will allow the operator to select the required number of tubes for further analysis (e.g., 1D- or 2D-PAGE).

RECOMMENDED READING

Research papers

Albertson, P. (1974) Separation of cells and cell organelles by partition in aqueous polymer two-phase systems. *Methods in Enzymology* 171:532-549.

Arakawa, T., Prestrelski, S.J. Kenney, W.C. and Carpenter, J.F. (2001) Factors affecting short-term and long-term stabilities of proteins. *Advanced Drug Delivery Reviews* 46:307-326.

Asenjo, J.A. and Andrews B.A. (2012) Aqueous two-phase systems for protein separation: phase separation and applications. *Journal of Chromatography (A)* 1238:1-10.

Bradford, M.M. (1976) A rapid and sensitive for the quantitation of microgram quantities of protein utilizing the principle of protein-dye binding. *Analytical Biochemistry* 72:248-254.

Brown, R.E., Jarvis, K.L. and Hyland, K.J. (1989) Protein measurement using bicinchoninic acid: Elimination of interfering substances. *Analytical Biochemistry* 180:136-139.

Burns, J.A., Butler, J.C., Moran, J. and Whitesides, G.M. (1991) Selective reduction of disulphides by Tris(2-carboxyethyl) phosphine. *Journal of Organic Chemistry* 56:2648-2650.

Dixon, M.A. (1953) A nomogram for ammonium sulphate solutions. *Biochemistry Journal* 54:457-458.

Ganong, B.R. and Delmore, J.P. (1991) Phase separation temperatures of mixtures of Triton X-114 and Triton X-45: Application to protein separation. *Analytical Biochemistry* 193:35-37.

Gornall, A.G., Bardawill, C.S. and David, M.M. (1949) Determination of serum proteins by means of the Biuret reaction. *J Biol Chem* 177:751-766.

Harrington C (1989) Lowry protein assay containing sodium dodecyl sulphate in microtiter plates for protein determinations on fractions from brain tissue. *Analytical Biochemistry* 186:285-287.

Huddleston, J., Albelaira, J.C., Wang, R. and Lyddiatt, A. (1996) Protein partition between the different phases comprising poly(ethylene glycol)-salt aqueous two-phase systems, hydrophobic interaction chromatography and precipitation: A generic description in terms of salting-out effects. *J. Chromatography (B) Biomedical Applications* 680:31-41.

Kasper, J.C., Winter, G. and Friess, W. (2013) Recent advances and further challenges in lyophilisation. *European Journal of Pharmaceutics and Biopharmaceutics* 85:162-169.

Krishan, K.N., Barry, D.T., Rees, R.C., Dodi, I.A., McArdle, S.E.B., Creaser, C.S. and Bonner, P.L.R. (2009) Estimation of peptide concentration by a modified bicinchoninic acid assay. *Analytical Biochemistry* 393:138-140.

Lopes, A.M., Magalhaes, P.O., Mazzola, P.G., Penna, T.C., Pessoa, A., and Rangel-Yagui, C. (2007) Methods of endotoxin removal from biological preparations: A Review. *J Pharm Pharmaceut Sci* 10:388-404.

Lowry, D., Rosebrough, N.J., Farr, A.R. and Randall, R.J. (1951) Protein measurement with Folin phenol reagent. *J Biol Chem* 193:265-275.

Majekodunmi, S. O. (2015) A review on centrifugation in the pharmaceutical industry. *American Journal of Biomedical Engineering* 5:67-78.

Raghupathi, R. N. and Diwan, A. M. (1994) A Protocol for protein estimation that gives a nearly constant colour yield with simple proteins and nullifies the effects of four known interfering agents: Micro estimation of peptide groups. *Analytical Biochemistry* 219:356-359.

Reid, E. and Williamson, R. (1974) Centrifugation. *Methods in Enzymology* 31:713-733.

Rodríguez-Vico, F., Martínez-Cayuela, M., García-Peregrín, E and Ramírez, H. (1989) A procedure for eliminating interferences in the Lowry method of protein determination. *Analytical Biochemistry* 183:275-278.

Shu-Sheng, Z. and Lundahl, P. (2000) A Micro-Bradford membrane protein assay. *Analytical Biochemistry* 284:162-164.

Smith, P.K., Krohn, R.I., Hermanson, G.T., Mallia, A.K., Gartner, F.H.,

Provenzano, M.D., Fujimoto, E.K., Goeke, N.M., Olson, R.J. and Klenk, D.C. (1985) Measurement of protein using bicinchoninic acid. *Analytical Biochemistry* 150:76-85.

Stevens, R., Stevens, L. and Price, N.C. (1983) The stabilities of various thiol compounds used in protein purification. *Biochemical Education* 11:70.

Warburg, O. and Christian, W. (1941) Isolation and crystallisation of enolase. *Biochem Z* 310:384-421.

Books

Beynon, R.J. and Easterby, J.S. (1996) *Buffer Solutions.* Biosis Sci Publishing Ltd., Oxford, UK.

Bonner, P.L.R. and Hargreaves, A.J. (2011) *Basic Bioscience Laboratory Techniques.* Wiley Blackwell, UK.

Cutler, P (Ed.) (2004) *Protein Purification Protocols.* 2nd ed. Humana Press, New Jersey, USA.

Deutscher, M.P (Ed.) (1990) *Guide to Protein Purification Methods in Enzymology,* 182. Academic Press, London, UK.

Patel, D. (2001) *Separating Cells.* Biosis Sci Publishing Ltd, Oxford, UK.

Roe, S. (Ed.) (2001) *Protein Purification: Methods.* 2nd ed. Oxford University Press, Oxford, UK.

Rosenberg, I.M. (2005) *Protein Analysis and Purification.* 2nd ed. Birkhauser, Boston, Massachusetts, USA.

Non-Affinity Absorption Techniques Used to Purify Proteins

5

5.1   INTRODUCTION

Effectively only four out of the five physical properties that biological polymers possess can be utilised to effect a purification (see Section 2.7).

1) Surface charge (positive, neutral or negative)
2) Polarity (from hydrophilic to hydrophobic)
3) Molecular size (metabolites, which are relatively small, through proteins, to nucleic acids which are relatively large)
4) Biospecificity (biological molecules are synthesised for a reason and their unique character can be exploited to select a molecule from a complex mixture). Post-translational modifications can be included in this section.

The exception:

5) Volatility (only a small range of biological molecules can easily enter the gas phase. Some (e.g., amino and fatty acids) can be chemically modified (derivatised) so that they will enter the gas phase. Large biological polymers (e.g., glycogen, proteins and nucleic acids) are very unlikely to enter the gas phase due to their size.

Fortunately, within each group (1–4, above) there is sufficient variety to provide a basis for protein purification procedures. For example, because proteins are derived from different genes, the extent of their surface charge will vary with the content of amino acids with weak acid functional groups (lysine, arginine, histidine, aspartic and glutamic acid) in their structure. Among different proteins there will be subtly different topographical locations of the charge, which may influence their interaction with different chromatography resins. The charges on the surface of proteins are described as weak acids (see Section 1.6), so the pH of the local environment in which proteins are dissolved will influence the surface charge.

Finally, the diversity of a protein's surface charge can be broadened with post-translational modifications. Some post-translational modifications will alter the extent and location of a recipient protein's surface charge (e.g., deamidation, phosphorylation or sulphation). The addition of the charged post-translational modification will result in some conformational change to the protein's structure, which in turn may alter the extent and accessibility of a protein's surface charge.

The nature, extent and location of these surface charges will influence a protein's interaction with a chromatographic resin and can be exploited to effect a successful purification procedure.

5.2   ION EXCHANGE (IEX) CHROMATOGRAPHY

Ion exchange (IEX) chromatography is a versatile technique that can be used for the purification of biological molecules with charged functional groups, including proteins, peptides, amino acids, nucleotides, nucleic acids and charged metabolites. The resins used in IEX are relatively inexpensive and they can be easily washed, sanitised ready for a repeat run using simple procedures. Ion exchange resins have a high capacity for the biological material applied; during elution they demonstrate good recovery of biological activity (non-denaturing) and show excellent resolution of complex protein mixtures.

Amino acids are zwitterionic molecules containing an amino group (basic) and a carboxyl group (acidic) (see Section 2.2). These groups are weak acids, showing pH-dependent ionisation (see Figure 3.1). At pK_{a1} 50% of the carboxyl group is in the ionised form, and at pK_{a2} 50% of the amino group is in the ionised form. The **isoelectric point (pI)** is the point on the pH scale where the positive charge is balanced by the negative charge and the overall charge on the molecule is zero.

Every protein has a free amino group at the first amino acid and a free carboxyl group at the terminal amino acid; these will be ionised in solution and the charge will be pH-dependent. In addition, some amino acids with charged functional groups (see Table 5.1) will point out from the protein's surface, interacting with water and keeping the protein in solution (see Section 2.4). The presence of these weak acid surface charges means that the overall charge on a protein will depend on the pH of the environment in which the protein is dissolved. At low pH the overall charge on the surface of a protein will be positive, and at a high pH the overall charge on the surface of a protein will be negative. There is a point on the pH scale when the protein's positive surface charges are balanced out by the negative surface charges, resulting in a net zero surface charge. This is the protein's pI. It is important to remember that at a protein's pI, there will be both positive and negative charges associated with the weak acid residues within their structure. It is just that these charges have cancelled each other out. At a pH value 0.5–1.0 units above a protein's pI, the overall charge on the protein will begin to be negative, and at 0.5–1.0 pH units

Table 5.1 The charges on amino acid functional groups at pH 5.0 and 7.0.				
Amino acid	Functional group	pK_a	Charge at pH 7.0	Charge at pH 5.0
Primary amino acid	$-NH_3^+ \leftrightarrow -NH_2 + H^+$	9.5	+ve	+ve
Terminal carboxyl group	$-COOH \leftrightarrow -COO^- + H^+$	2.5	−ve	−ve
Lysine (K)	$-NH_3^+ \leftrightarrow -NH_2 + H^+$	10.5	+ve	+ve
Arginine (R)	$-NH_3^+ \leftrightarrow -NH_2 + H^+$	12.5	+ve	+ve
Histidine (H)	$= NH^+ \leftrightarrow NH + H^+$	6.0	negligible	+ve
Aspartate (D)	$-COOH \leftrightarrow -COO^- + H^+$	3.9	−ve	−ve
Glutamate (Q)	$-COOH \leftrightarrow -COO^- + H^+$	4.3	−ve	−ve

below the pI of a protein, the overall charge will begin to be positive. At these pH values above and below a protein's pI (pI ±1.0), the protein will have sufficient charge to bind to a particle with an opposite charge (IEX; see Section 5.2.1) or move to an oppositely charged electrode under the influence of an electrical field (see Section 8.4).

At a physiological pH (7.0), the functional groups from the amino acids aspartate and glutamate contribute the negative charge on a protein's surface (see Table 5.1) and the functional groups from the amino acids arginine and lysine contribute the positive charge. In the lysosomes and vacuoles of eukaryotic cells (animal and plant, respectively), the pH is more acidic (pH 5.0–5.5) than in the cytoplasm (pH 7.0–7.4). At these pH values, the amino acid histidine's functional group will also contribute some positive charge on a lysosomal/vacuolar protein's surface charge.

Most proteins exhibit solubility problems as they approach their pI and as a result most proteins do not have a pI between pH 7.0–7.4. An analysis of the distributions of isoelectric points in prokaryotic and eukaryotic **proteomes** has shown that there is a trimodal distribution of proteins' isoelectric points, with two large distributions around pH 5.8 and pH 9.0 and a smaller grouping around pH 7.8. In one study of eukaryotic proteomes, the distribution of the proteins' pI's appeared to correlate with their intracellular location. The cytoplasmic proteins predominantly had acidic pI's, nuclear proteins had pI's at neutral pH values and membrane proteins predominantly had pI values in the basic pH range. In another study the multimodality was found to be a function of the pK_a of the amino acids side chains.

5.2.1   Ion exchange resins

There are two groups of ion exchange resins (see Table 5.2): anionic exchange resins, which are positively charged and attract negatively charged molecules (anions), and cation exchange resins, which are negatively charged and attract positively charged molecules (cations). Both groups of ion exchange resins can also be divided into strong and weak ion exchangers; this does not reflect the strength with which oppositely

Table 5.2 Functional groups on cation and anion exchange resins.

IEX matrix functional group	Functional group abbreviation	Strong/ Weak	Working pH range	Charge in the working pH range
Diethylaminoethyl	DEAE	Weak anion	2.0–9.0	+ve
Quaternary ammonium	Q	Strong anion	2.0–12.0	+ve
Quaternary aminoethyl	QAE	Strong anion	2.0–12.0	+ve
Carboxymethyl	CM	Weak cation	6.0–10.0	−ve
Methyl sulphonate	S	Strong cation	4.0–13.0	−ve
Sulphopropyl	SP	Strong cation	4.0–13.0	−ve

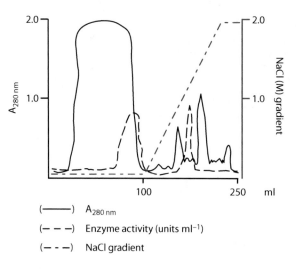

Figure 5.1 An ion exchange experiment exhibiting that the column's capacity to bind the target protein has been exceeded as demonstrated by the presence of the target protein in the later fraction of the unbound protein.

(———) $A_{280\,nm}$

(— — —) Enzyme activity (units ml^{-1})

(— · —) NaCl gradient

charged molecules bind but refers to their ionisation range (similar to the definition of strong and weak acids; see Section 1.6). Strong ion exchange resins ionise over a wider pH range than do weak ion exchange resins.

A variety of support matrices are available for IEX, including cellulose (Sober and Peterson, 1958), dextrans and agarose, all of which are suitable for low-pressure IEX. There are also more robust resins (cross-linked mixtures of dextrans/acrylamide, polyacrylate, ceramic, polystyrene and silica), strengthened to withstand compression by elevated pressures, that are suitable for use in medium- and high-pressure chromatography (see Section 3.7). The capacity of the resin to bind charged molecules is given by the number of functional groups present per gram of dried resin (mEq g^{-1}) or per volume of hydrated resin (mEq ml^{-1}). Often, the maximum capacity of an IEX resin is compromised by the steric hindrance caused by the proteins bound to its surface. The manufacturers often quote the capacity to bind a standard protein such as bovine serum albumin (BSA) in mg protein g^{-1} (or ml^{-1}) of resin (typically 10–100 mg BSA ml^{-1} resin). It may be argued that BSA is not a typical protein. However, it does provide a guide as to the amount/volume of resin required for an IEX experiment. One ml of IEX resin for every 25–50 mg of protein in the extract is a good starting point when deciding how much resin to use in a chromatography run. This can be adjusted in later experiments if the unbound material starts to show the presence of the target protein (see Figure 5.1).

In addition, it is possible to avoid resins and columns and use IEX functional groups bound to membranes as the stationary phase. The mobile phase can be pumped or centrifuged through membrane discs, and the sample is usually eluted isocratically using buffers with a fixed concentration of salt (see Figure 3.9). The low volume occupied by the membranes and the improved flow characteristics of the filters mean that these IEX membranes can be utilised to concentrate large volumes of dilute protein solutions, and thus are particularly of interest to the biotechnology industry.

5.2.2   Binding and elution of protein to IEX resins

Ion exchange chromatography relies on the association between a charged molecule in the mobile phase and an oppositely charged group bonded to the stationary phase. The functional groups on the stationary phase's surface are neutralized by oppositely charged counter ions in the mobile phase (e.g., Na^+ for cation IEX and Cl^- for anion IEX). When the protein sample is introduced into the column, it will diffuse to the stationary phase surface, displacing the counter ion. The displaced counter ion will flow through the column and be eluted with the mobile phase.

Short fat columns are used for IEX because binding to an ion exchange column is charge-dependent not concentration-dependent. This means that large volumes of dilute sample can be applied to an IEX resin and then eluted in a smaller volume, effectively concentrating the sample.

Prior to starting ion exchange column chromatography, the approximate binding and elution conditions for IEX can be elucidated using small scale experiments (see Protocol 5.1). Alternatively, a literature/web search may provide a short cut to the appropriate starting conditions. To facilitate the binding of proteins to an ion exchange resin, a buffer of between 10–25 mM is required, set to a pH approximately 1.0 pH unit above the pI of the target protein in anion IEX and 1.0 pH unit below the pI in cation IEX (see Table 5.3). The buffer ion should be of the same charge as the resin to avoid the buffer ion binding to the resin and taking up some of the resin's protein-binding capacity. The pH of the buffer should be adjusted after being equilibrated at the temperature at which the chromatographic run will occur, because some buffers (e.g., Tris) have different pH values at different temperatures (see Appendix 8).

The sample should ideally be in a buffer with the same composition (correct pH and low salt) as the starting buffer. This can be achieved by dialysis (see Protocol 4.9) or size exclusion chromatography (see Protocol 7.1). Alternatively, the sample can be diluted (1:5–1:10) with the starting buffer to prepare the sample for chromatography. These three techniques will increase the starting volume of the sample, but this is not a problem because sample binding using ion exchange chromatography is charge-dependent, not concentration-dependent, and the ion exchange resin will have a concentrating effect on dilute and salt-free samples. The sample should always be clarified before application to any chromatography column; this can be achieved by either filtration through a 0.2 μm membrane or centrifugation at $12,000 \times g$ for 15–20 min. This will remove any bacteria and protein aggregates that could block the pores in the resin, eventually resulting in an increase in the back pressure during the chromatography run.

Table 5.3 Examples of buffers that can be used for IEX.

	Buffer	Counter ion	pH range
Cation IEX	Lactate	Na^+	3.6–4.3
Cation IEX	Acetate	Na^+	4.8–5.2
Cation IEX	MES	Na^+	5.5–6.7
Cation IEX	Phosphate	Na^+	6.7–7.6
Anion IEX	Piperazine	Cl^-	5.0–6.0
Anion IEX	bis-Tris propane	Cl^-	6.4–7.3
Anion IEX	Tris	Cl^-	7.5–8.0
Anion IEX	Diethanolamine	Cl^-	8.4–9.4

The binding to the ion exchange resin is based upon the competition between the charged groups on the surface of the protein and the charge on the counter ions. The greater the overall charge on the protein, the more tightly it will bind to the IEX resin and the harder it will be to dislodge (see Figure 5.2). The bound protein will be dislodged when the counter ion concentration is sufficient to overcome the attraction between the protein and the IEX resin (see Figure 5.3). The concentration of the counter ion in the eluting buffer can be increased gradually using a gradient former over 10–25 column volumes (see Figure 3.9), or isocratically (see Figure 3.9) by running separate buffers (minimum of two column volumes each) through the resin at set (but increasing) concentrations of salt. The bound proteins will elute in order of their increasing surface charge.

A protein will only bind to an IEX resin when there is sufficient charge on the protein's surface above (anion IEX) or below (cation IEX) the protein's pI. Another method of eluting bound proteins from an IEX resin is to alter the pH of the eluting buffer, which will in turn alter the magnitude of the weak acid charges on the surface of the protein. To elute proteins bound to a cation exchange resin, a gradual increase in pH from the starting conditions is required. The opposite (i.e., a gradual decrease in pH from the starting conditions) is required to elute proteins bound to an anion exchange resin.

A change in the pH flowing through the ion exchange resin can be achieved using either a gradient chamber and a peristaltic pump (see Section 3.6.6). A descending pH gradient (in the case of anion exchange chromatography; ascending pH for cation exchange chromatography) can be formed with the high pH buffer placed in the mixing chamber and a lower pH buffer placed in the other chamber. The (high pH) solution leaving the mixing chamber and flowing to the column is replaced in the mixing chamber of the gradient former by an equal volume of the lower

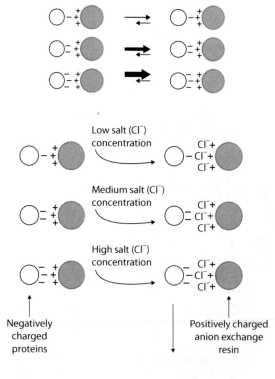

Figure 5.2 A schematic representation of protein binding to anion IEX.

Figure 5.3 A schematic representation of protein eluting from anion IEX.

pH buffer. This results in a gradual decrease in the pH of the buffer being pumped onto the column. A similar effect can be achieved using a dual buffer computer-controlled medium- or high-pressure gradient system (see Section 3.7). The linearity of the gradient generated can be checked by running a blank gradient through the system and measuring the pH in the fractions collected. Modern medium-pressure protein purification systems may have an inline pH detection probe at the column exit prior to the flow entering the UV detector. The proteins are eluted as the descending/ascending pH approaches their pI.

In practice, pH gradients generated by these methods are rarely linear and most proteins become irreversibly denatured as they approach their pI, making this procedure of academic value only. Almost-linear pH gradients with IEX resins can be obtained using the technique of chromatofocusing (see Section 5.3 below). The preferred method of elution from an IEX resin uses a gradient with an increasing/decreasing salt concentration.

If the pI of a target protein is not known, then binding to an anion exchange resin at pH 8.0 and elution of the bound protein using a gradient of 0–2.0 M NaCl over 10–15 column volumes is a reasonable set of starting conditions. If the target protein is unbound, then reapply the sample to clean and equilibrated IEX resin at a higher pH value. If the target protein has bound to the column but elutes late in the gradient profile at a relatively high salt concentration, this means that the starting pH is more than 1.0 pH unit above the protein's pI, imparting a large negative surface charge. Figure 5.4 outlines a flowchart for a typical anion IEX run for a protein with unknown charge characteristics. The approach is empirical at all stages; ideally, the binding conditions should be chosen so that the target protein elutes relatively early in the gradient profile and the salt gradient is sufficient to give the required resolution. At the early stages of purification, a five- to tenfold increase in the specific activity with >90% recovery of activity can be readily achieved with IEX.

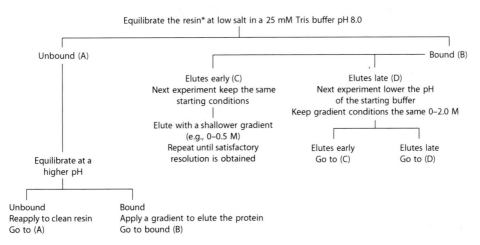

*In general the choice of resin depends on the pH stability of the sample; at pH 8.0 both strong and weak anion IEX resins (see Table 5.2) can be used. Different resins used at the same pH may produce some advantageous selectivity of the target molecule.

In the case of stages A, B, C and D, the resin and sample must be equilibrated in the new starting buffer before another chromatographic run. This may require fresh sample, or dialysis/desalting (see Protocols 4.9 and 7.1) of a collected sample.

Figure 5.4 A flow diagram of the events in a typical anion exchange chromatography experiment.

5.2.3   Regeneration and storage of IEX resins

After each IEX run, the resin should be washed prior to the next run. A wash of 4.0 M NaCl will remove most tightly bound proteins that do not elute during the chromatographic run. But to ensure complete removal of tightly bound proteins, a wash of 0.5–1.0 M NaOH will clean and sanitise the resin. The sodium hydroxide-treated IEX resin should be washed extensively with distilled water and then re-equilibrated with starting buffer before another run. If another run is not imminent, then the resin can be stored in a bactericide (either 0.05% (w/v) sodium azide or 20% (v/v) ethanol, depending on the manufacturer's recommendations).

5.3   CHROMATOFOCUSING

Chromatofocusing is a chromatographic technique that combines anion exchange chromatography with isoelectric focusing (IEF), separating proteins according to their pI. The anion exchange resin and the proteins to be separated are equilibrated in a low ionic strength buffer at a set pH. Those proteins with a pI below the starting pH of the column will have an overall positive charge and will not bind to the column. Proteins with a pI above the preset pH will bind to the anion exchange resin. The bound proteins are eluted with approximately 12.5 column volumes of an amphoteric buffer (GE Healthcare or Bio-Rad) set at a pH below the starting pH of the experiment. The eluting buffer has an even buffering capacity over the set pH range and establishes a pH gradient that is lower at the top of the column than at the bottom of the column. (The pH gradient is generated *in situ*, in contrast to pH elution in IEX, in which two buffers and a gradient mixer are used to generate a pH gradient; see Section 5.2.2.)

At the start of the elution, when the pH falls below the starting pH, bound proteins (with a pI between the starting and finishing pH) will become positively charged. The bound proteins will be repelled from the resin and start to migrate down the column, where they will encounter increasing pH values. At a point on the pH scale just beyond the protein's pI, it will again be negatively charged and will be retained by the resin. As the pH gradient is developed within the column, proteins will dissociate and bind to the resin, gradually becoming focused and eluting at a pH near their pI. Proteins with the highest pI elute first and proteins with the lowest pI elute last. If the target protein elutes in the unbound fraction, a gradient of lower pH is required, and if the protein remains bound to the resin, a gradient of higher pH is required. Any protein that does not elute during the pH gradient can be removed from the resin within the column by washing with two column volumes each of 2.0 M NaCl and 1.0 M NaOH.

During chromatography the pH values of each fraction should be measured immediately (with a pH probe or an in line pH detector) to avoid interference by atmospheric CO_2, which will dissolve in the fractions, acidifying the solution and altering the apparent pH. A plot of pH against the volume collected from the column can be prepared to enable an estimation of the target protein's pI (see Figure 5.5). After the pH has been measured, the pH in each fraction can be elevated by the addition of a small volume of concentrated buffer (e.g., Tris). This is will prevent the target protein from remaining at a pH value close to its pI, as proteins have a tendency to precipitate as they approach their pI. If the precipitation is observed during a chromatofocusing run, an increase in the concentration of the amphoteric buffers or inclusion of a low concentration of

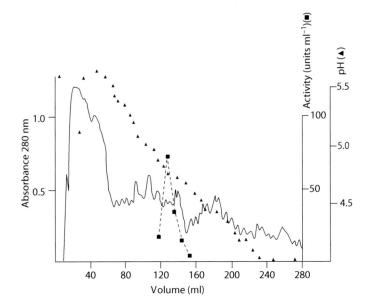

Figure 5.5 Chromatofocusing of a peptidase isolated from germinating *Vicia faba* cotyledons on a narrow pH gradient.

NaCl may alleviate this problem. The collected fractions can be assayed for the target protein's activity and pooled for the next chromatography step. When the approximate pI of the target protein has been established using a wide pH gradient (e.g., pH 7.0–4.0), the target protein can be reapplied to the chromatofocusing column and eluted over a narrower pH gradient, thus improving the resolution of the chromatofocusing chromatographic run (see Figure 5.5).

The amphoteric buffers used in chromatofocusing will interfere with protein assays based upon the biuret reaction (see Table 4.1; and Protocols 4.2 and 4.3), but they are compatible with the reagents in the Bradford protein assay (see Protocol 4.4). Salt precipitation (see Section 4.14.1 and Protocol 4.8), dialysis (see Protocol 4.9), size exclusion chromatography (see Section 7.1 and Protocol 7.1), affinity chromatography (see Section 6.1) and hydrophobic interaction chromatography (see Section 5.5) can be used to remove the amphoteric buffers from the sample.

5.4   HYDROXYAPATITE (HA) CHROMATOGRAPHY

Hydroxyapaptite is the crystalline form of calcium phosphate ($Ca_{10}(PO_4)_6(OH)_2$) prepared by mixing solutions of calcium chloride and sodium phosphate at neutral pH. The precipitate is collected and then boiled with either sodium or ammonium hydroxide to produce the crystalline form. These crystals can be used for chromatography but require careful handling as they are easily fragmented, generating "fines." These are small particulates that will block the pores in a chromatography resin, resulting in poor flow rates due to high back pressure. Hydroxyapatite encapsulated in agarose (HA Ultrogel; Pall Ltd) or coated to a solid ceramic support (CHT; Bio-Rad, Ltd) can be purchased and are easier to use.

The structure of hydroxyapatite has a surface comprised of pairs of positively charged of calcium ions, triplet clusters of negatively charged

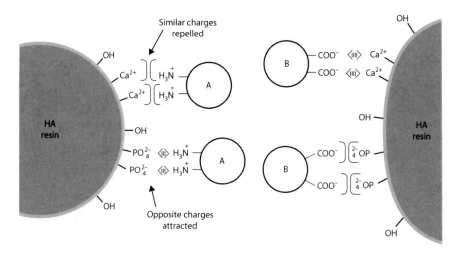

Figure 5.6 Protein binding to hydroxyapaptite (A is a basic protein and B is an acidic protein).

phosphates, and hydroxyl groups. When protein is added to hydroxyapatite, the positively charged amino groups on the surface of the protein are attracted to the phosphate groups and repelled by the positively charged calcium ions. The carboxyl groups on a protein's surface are repelled by the phosphate groups and attracted to the positively charged calcium ions (see Figure 5.6). The interaction between the carboxyl groups and the calcium ions is greater than mere electrostatic attraction and involves the formation of co-ordinate covalent (sometimes referred to as dative interactions) complexes (see Section 6.11). Phosphate groups on proteins will also co-ordinate with the calcium ions. The varied nature of these interactions makes it difficult to predict the outcome of a hydroxyapatite chromatographic run.

A typical chromatographic run with hydroxyapatite involves loading a sample in a low ionic strength buffer (1–10 mM phosphate pH 7.0) and eluting the bound acidic proteins with a phosphate gradient (100–400 mM). Alternative elution patterns after binding can involve sequential washing with (a) 5 mM $MgCl_2$ to elute bound basic proteins, followed by (b) a gradient of NaCl to elute proteins with a pI around 7.0 and then (c) a gradient of phosphate (100–400 mM) to elute the acidic proteins. Ceramic fluoroapatite ($Ca_{10}(PO_4)_6(F_2)$) (Bio-Rad, Ltd) can also be used for the separation of acidic proteins. The composite fluoroapatite and hydroxyapatite material has increased tensile strength and chemical stability in the low pH (5.0) range required to separate acidic proteins.

Hydroxyapatite can be a useful technique to use in any purification schedule because the interaction between the protein and the resin is not based solely on ionic interactions. It does require careful investigation of the binding and elution conditions and may have merit when used late in a purification schedule (after IEX and HIC) to resolve components that are difficult to remove by other chromatographic procedures.

5.5   HYDROPHOBIC INTERACTION CHROMATOGRAPHY (HIC)

Proteins have different quantities and content of the twenty different amino acids that make up protein structure. Included in these are the amino acids with hydrophobic functional groups (see Table 2.1), which avoid contact with water. These include the amino acids with aliphatic functional groups [isoleucine (I), leucine (L), valine (V), alanine (A), methionine (M) and those with aromatic functional groups (phenylalanine (F) tyrosine (Y) and tryptophan (W)]. To avoid contact with water in an aqueous environment, many of these residues are buried in the core of the protein's tertiary structure (see Section 2.4). Those that cannot be accommodated in the protein's core remain as hydrophobic patches near the surface of a protein's structure. To minimise their contact with water, the surface hydrophobic residues may be surrounded or masked by neighbouring polar and more hydrophilic amino acid functional groups. These hydrophobic surface patches may be involved in the biological role of a protein. For example, when the protein calmodulin binds calcium ions, it changes conformation, exposing hydrophobic patches that are subsequently involved in the interaction with calmodulin's target proteins.

The addition of increasing amounts of ammonium sulphate to a protein solution will alter a protein's solubility (see Section 4.11.2) by stripping away the protein's solvation shell, resulting in the exposure of hydrophobic patches on the surface of the protein. These hydrophobic patches will now come into contact with water molecules, generating clathrate (caged) water molecules, a situation that is thermodynamically unfavourable (see Appendix 1). To liberate the clathrate water molecules, hydrophobic patches on the surface of one protein will spontaneously interact with the hydrophobic patches on the surface of a neighbouring protein. This will liberate the clathrate water, increasing the entropy of the system and making it a thermodynamically favourable event. Different proteins interact and form a complex that eventually becomes too large to be maintained in solution and starts to form a precipitate.

If the ammonium sulphate is added to a concentration below the concentration required to form a precipitate, the hydrophobic patches on proteins will not interact with other but will be available to interact with a hydrophobic ligand attached to a chromatographic resin (see Figure 5.7). Binding of the hydrophobic patches on the surface of the protein to the hydrophobic ligand on the column in the presence of high salt is thermodynamically favourable, because it also releases clathrate water molecules (i.e., increases the entropy) and it occurs spontaneously. The protein will remain bound until the elution conditions are applied.

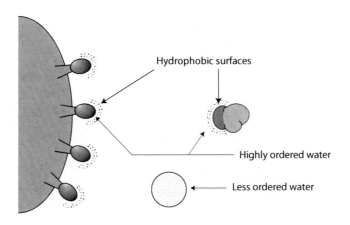

Hydrophobic surfaces

Highly ordered water

Less ordered water

Figure 5.7 Hydrophobic interaction chromatography involves displacement of clathrate water molecules from exposed hydrophobic pockets on the surface of the protein and those surrounding the ligand on the HIC resin.

5.5.1   The binding and elution conditions for HIC

Hydrophobic interaction chromatography has some similarities with reversed-phase chromatography (RPC) (see Sections 3.3 and 8.8). They both involve interaction of hydrophobic patches on a protein with hydrophobic ligands (aliphatic or aromatic) attached to a support resin. The support resins for HIC are usually cross-linked dextrans, agarose or acrylamides. The resins for RPC are usually silica or polymeric, and they have many more ligands bonded to the resin than the HIC resins. The result of this increase in ligand density is that proteins bind strongly to RPC resins. The consequence is that proteins bound to an RPC resin require stronger elution conditions, necessitating the use of organic solvents (e.g., methanol or acetonitrile). The use of these organic solvents results in the elution of protein from the reversed-phase column, but biological functionality is rarely retained. The lower ligand density on HIC resins does not compromise the resin's protein-binding capacity (typically 10–30 mg protein ml^{-1} resin), but it does allow milder binding and elution conditions that promote good recovery of biological activity.

Because HIC requires high salt concentrations at the start of the chromatographic run, it is a convenient technique to use after ammonium sulphate fractionation (see Section 4.11.2 and Protocol 4.8). The precipitate can be dissolved in a bufferand applied directly to a HIC resin that has been equilibrated in a buffer with a salt concentration just below where the target protein would start to precipitate (see Figure 5.8). If the chromatographic procedure is to be used later in a purification schedule, a salt (usually ammonium sulphate) is added to the target protein solution, again to a concentration just below where the target protein would normally start to precipitate (Figure 5.9 shows a flow diagram for a typical HIC experiment). To prevent fouling the HIC resin with low levels of precipitated protein (which would increase the back pressure during the chromatography run), the sample solution should be clarified by centrifugation at $12,000 \times g$ for 20 min at 4°C.

Binding to HIC resins is temperature-dependent and for most applications room temperature is used for binding and elution. There is little or no binding or elution at 4°C. If binding to a HIC resin is problematic, adjust the pH of the starting buffer such that it is close to the pI of the target protein, where binding is maximised. Ammonium sulphate can acidify a buffer solution, so always check the pH of the starting and elution conditions buffer for HIC before application of the sample and adjust the pH if necessary. Alternatively, the molarity of the starting buffer can be increased (50–100 mM).

Eluting the protein that has bound to an HIC resin is achieved by decreasing the salt concentration in the eluting buffer using a gradient or isocratic

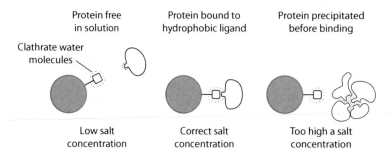

Protein free   Protein bound to   Protein precipitated
in solution   hydrophobic ligand   before binding

Clathrate water
molecules

Low salt   Correct salt   Too high a salt
concentration   concentration   concentration

Figure 5.8 The effect of increasing the salt concentration on protein binding to HIC.

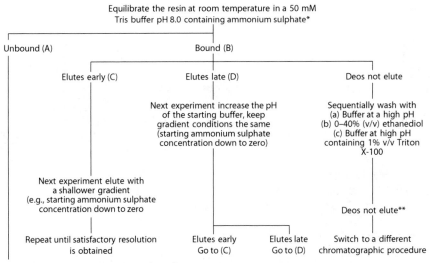

Equilibrate the resin at room temperature in a 50 mM
Tris buffer pH 8.0 containing ammonium sulphate*

Unbound (A)   Bound (B)

Elutes early (C)   Elutes late (D)   Deos not elute

Next experiment increase the pH
of the starting buffer, keep
gradient conditions the same
(starting ammonium sulphate
concentration down to zero)

Sequentially wash with
(a) Buffer at a high pH
(b) 0–40% (v/v) ethanediol
(c) Buffer at high pH
containing 1% v/v Triton
X-100

Next experiment elute with
a shallower gradient
(e.g., starting ammonium sulphate
concentration down to zero

Deos not elute**

Repeat until satisfactory resolution
is obtained

Elutes early
Go to (C)

Elutes late
Go to (D)

Switch to a different
chromatographic procedure

(i) Equilibrate at a lower pH and reapply to the same resin
(ii) Reapply to a more hydrophobic resin (e.g., octyl or butyl)

*It is best to start with a phenyl HIC resin (the least hydrophobic ligand). The ammonium sulphate concentration at the start of the experiment should be just below the concentration which brings about the 'salting out' of the target protein.

In the case of stages A, B, C and D, the resin and sample must be equilibrated in the new starting buffer before another chromatographic run. This may require fresh sample, or dialysis/desalting (see Protocols 4.9 and 7.1) of a collected sample.

**Wash the resin sequentially in 1.0 M NaOH (five column volumes), water (two column volumes), 30% (v/v) isopropanol (10 column volumes and water (two column volumes). The resin can then be equilibrated in starting buffer for the next experiment or stored in 20% (v/v) ethanol.

Figure 5.9 A flow diagram of the events in a typical HIC experiment.

elution (see Section 3.6.7 and Figure 5.10). When the eluting salt concentration decreases from a concentration that encourages ligand and hydrophobic patch interaction, the protein will start to regain its solvation shell and refold into its original conformation, hiding the hydrophobic patches with more polar amino acid functional groups. The protein will disengage from the ligand and it will be eluted in a lower ammonium sulphate salt concentration. After elution, it may be necessary to remove or reduce the ammonium sulphate concentration by desalting using group size exclusion chromatography (see Section 7.1 and Protocol 7.1) or dialysis (see Protocol 4.9) before undertaking a protein assay (see Protocols 4.1–4.4)

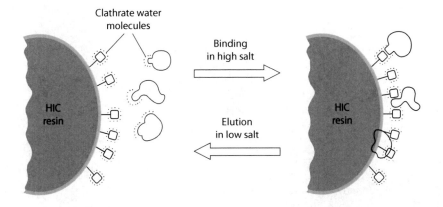

Clathrate water
molecules

Binding
in high salt

HIC
resin

HIC
resin

Elution
in low salt

Figure 5.10 Binding and elution from HIC is dependent on the salt concentration (high salt for binding and low salt for elution).

or before application to another chromatographic procedure. The starting conditions for IEX (see Protocol 5.1) require a low salt concentration and will work with large volumes of dilute feedstock, making it an ideal procedure to follow HIC.

Proteins that show a strong interaction with the HIC ligand and do not elute at zero ammonium sulphate concentration may be eluted with a buffer set at a pH higher than the protein's pI, because bound proteins will gain charge and become more hydrophilic at higher pH values. If this fails to elute the bound target protein, a gradient of 0–40% (v/v) ethanediol or a wash with a 1% (v/v) solution of a non-ionic detergent (e.g., Tween or Triton) in a high pH buffer can be used, and if this elutes the target protein it will usually remain active. Should the target protein elute in ethanediol or detergent, an alternative HIC ligand that shows reduced hydrophobicity should be considered in future HIC experiments. It is better to start with the least hydrophobic ligand (phenyl) before progressing onto the more hydrophobic octyl (C_8) and butyl (C_5) ligands.

5.5.2   The regeneration and storage of HIC resins

To elute precipitated proteins, lipoproteins and lipids that show a very strong interaction with the HIC ligand, the HIC resin can then be washed with five column volumes of 1.0 M NaOH, followed by two column volumes of water and then ten column volumes of 30% (v/v) isopropanol. Alternatively, two column volume washes of a 0.5% (v/v) solution of a non-ionic detergent such as Triton X-100, followed by five column volumes of 70% (v/v) ethanol and five column volumes of water. The resin can then be stored in 20% (v/v) ethanol or a bactericide such as 0.05% (w/v) sodium azide (see manufacturer's recommendations).

5.6   HYDROPHOBIC CHARGE INDUCTION CHROMATOGRAPHY (HCIC)

In traditional HIC, protein binding to the HIC ligand is controlled by the concentration of lyotropic salts (see Figure 4.10). In hydrophobic charge induction chromatography (HCIC), the binding of proteins to the hydrophobic ligand is controlled by the pH.

A modified cellulose resin has 4-mercapto-ethyl-pyridine (4-MEP) (Pall Ltd) (see Figure 5.11) as the ligand and has been designed as an alternative to protein A or **protein G** (see Protocol 6.1) for the purification of immunoglobulins from culture media, ascites fluid or blood serum. The interaction between the MEP ligands on the chromatography media and the antibodies (typically 30.0 mg IgG ml^{-1} resin) has been described as involving both a "pseudoaffinity" molecular interaction with the Fc region on the antibody and hydrophobic interactions at neutral pH. The aliphatic spacer arm that connects the ligand to the cellulose resin also contributes to the hydrophobic interactions with the immunoglobulins.

The buffer solution containing the target antibody is passed through the column at neutral pH and the unbound protein is washed through the column. The bound antibody typically elutes from the resin at approximately pH 5.0. When the pH is lowered from the binding conditions at neutral pH to pH 4.0 (independent of the salt concentration), both the resin and the antibody gradually gather positive charge, repelling each other

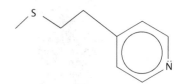

4-Mercaptoethylpyridine (4-MEP)
pK$_a$ = 4.8

Figure 5.11 The structure of the MEP ligand head group.

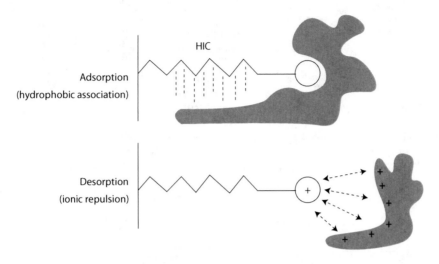

Figure 5.12 Binding of IgG in HCIC involves weak hydrophobic interactions and elution involves charge repulsion.

(see Figure 5.12). This is achieved by washing the resin isocratically (see Figure 3.9) with two column volumes of a 50 mM sodium acetate or citrate buffer at gradually decreasing pH values (e.g., pH 6.0, 5.5, 5.0, 4.5, 4.0 and 3.0). The exact elution conditions for an antibody may vary depending on the source of the antibody, but by careful adjustment of the elution conditions it is possible to elute the antibody substantially free from contaminating proteins (e.g., albumin). The resin can then be washed sequentially with two column volumes of 0.1 M acetic acid and 1.0 M NaOH before a final wash with five column volumes of distilled water and storage in 20% (v/v) ethanol.

The binding and elution of an antibody to HCIC is independent of salt concentration (although low-salt binding conditions would help reduce non-specific interactions with other hydrophobic proteins), which makes it an ideal resin to use with large volumes of dilute antibody solutions. After elution, the low-salt conditions mean that the eluted protein can be submitted to another chromatographic procedure such as IEX (see Section 5.1). Although HCIC has been designed for the purification of immunoglobulins, the resin could be used as an alternative HIC resin for the purification of other proteins. The binding and elution conditions would have to be determined empirically.

5.7   INTRODUCTION TO MIXED MODE (MULTIMODAL) CHROMATOGRAPHY (MMC)

Mixed mode chromatography is the name given to chromatographic techniques that separate molecules based on more than one chromatographic principle (e.g., GE Healthcare's Capto MMC media, Pall's MBI media and Bio-Rad's Nuvia™ cPrime™ media). The ligands associated with these mixed modal resins are designed to provide separation media that can provide an alternative separation route, particularly in process scale chromatography. The label "mixed or multimodal chromatography" can be misleading, as it implies that only these resins provide a separation process with more than one interaction between the stationary phase (ligand attached to the resin) and the proteins applied to the mobile phase entering the column. In truth, most chromatographic methods engage more than one of the separation processes (charge, polarity, size and biospecificity; not volatility) that can be used to separate proteins or metabolites (see Sections 3.3, 3.4 and 5.1). Small differences in the construction of the chromatographic media by different manufacturers can influence the result of the separation process. The applied proteins may interact with the primary separation ligand attached to the resin and then form secondary interactions with either the spacer arm used to distance the ligand from the surface of the resin or with the surface of the resin itself. For example, size exclusion resins can be constructed with cross-linked dextrans, so the primary mode of separation is based on the size and shape of the molecules applied (**hydrodynamic** volume; see Section 7.1). However, the dextrans used to form the porous network retain some surface charge, which can also exert ion exchange effects on the proteins introduced to the mobile phase. In this example, we could suggest that the use of dextrans in SEC is multimodal separation with size and shape as the dominant separation process but also with some secondary effects of IEX (which can be overcome by including 150 mM NaCl in the mobile phase buffer).

5.7.1   Capto™ MMC (GE Healthcare)

Capto™ Multimodal chromatography is a novel multimodal cation exchange resin that offers the capability to bind proteins in high or low ionic strength buffers. The resin also offers high flow rates and high binding capacity, coupled with the traditional good recovery (associated with IEX) of biologically active material. In addition, the structure of the cation exchange ligand (see Figure 5.13) bonded to the resin can provide different selectivity than conventional cation IEX, allowing the binding of proteins in high-salt starting conditions (0–300 mM). However, the ideal starting pH (typically 0.5–2.5 units below the eluting pH) and salt concentration (conductivity) would need to be determined empirically. The elution conditions are typically 0.0–2.0 M NaCl at a pH 0.5–2.0 units above the binding pH. The exact binding and elution conditions would need to be determined empirically using a suitable automated chromatography system (with method scouting programmes), small volume chromatography columns (e.g., small volume GE Healthcare HiTrap™ columns used with a syringe) or scale experimentation (see Protocol 5.1).

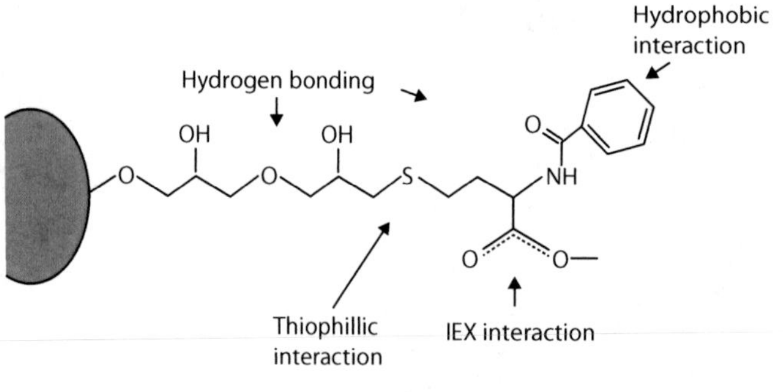

Figure 5.13 Structure of Capto MMC.

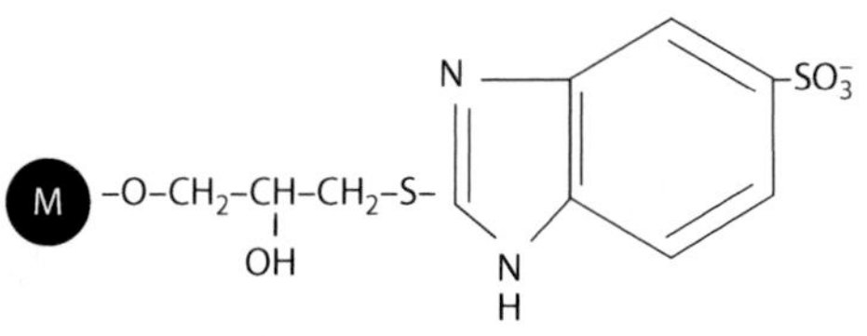

Figure 5.14 The structure of the MBI ligand.

5.7.2   Mercapto-benzimidazole sulfonic acid (MBI)

Mercapto-benzimidazole sulfonic acid (MBI; Pall Ltd) is a zwitterionic ligand bonded to modified cellulose resin that interacts with immunoglobulins in a "mixed function" mode. There is interaction with the Fc region of the immunoglobulins ("pseudoaffinity") and electrostatic interaction between the ligand and the immunoglobulin (the ligand remains negatively charged throughout the procedure). At the binding conditions (the capacity of the resin is typically 30.0 mg IgG ml^{-1} resin) of 50 mM sodium acetate pH 5.0–5.5 in the presence of 0.15 M NaCl, the resin carries a negatively charged sulphonate group (see Figure 5.14) that interacts with the positively charged IgG molecules. At this pH the negatively charged albumin should not interact with the resin. Elution of the bound antibody is achieved by increasing the pH to pH 9.0, which increases the negative charge on the antibody. These elution conditions are mild compared to the elution conditions when purifying immunoglobulins using protein A or protein G chromatography (see Protocol 6.1) where the elution conditions are low pH buffers (pH 2.0).

The column can be regenerated by washing with two column volumes 1.0 M NaOH followed by five column volumes of distilled water prior to equilibration with the starting conditions buffer for another chromatographic run, or two column volumes of 20% (v/v) ethanol if the resin is to be stored at 4°C.

Other MMC resins from Pall Ltd, include hexylamine (HEA) and phenylpropylamine (PPA), which offer different selectivity to conventional resins and can be used to resolve proteins with similar pI values. This is a separation that cannot be easily achieved using conventional IEX.

5.7.3   Nuvia cPrime (Bio-Rad)

The Nuvia cPrime resin from Bio-Rad is a cation exchange resin with hydrophobic interaction properties and is primarily aimed at process scale chromatography users. Proteins that bind may also develop secondary hydrogen bonding interactions with the ligand's structural elements (see Figure 5.15).

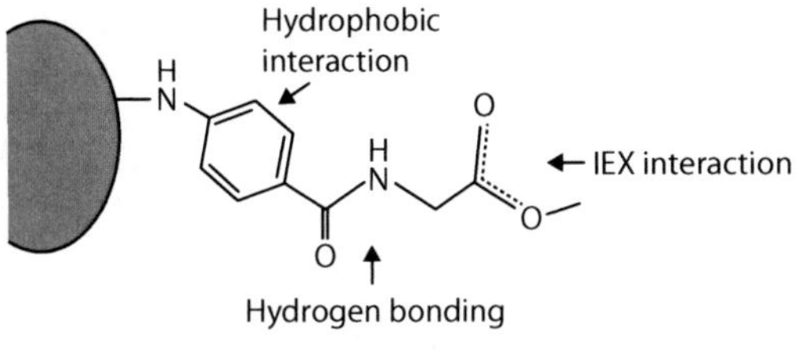

Figure 5.15 The structure of the Nuvia cPrime ligand.

The binding and elution conditions should be determined empirically. This resin may provide a means to purify proteins that have proved troublesome to purify with conventional IEX or HIC.

5.8   SUMMARY

The non-affinity absorption techniques described in this chapter provide the operator with methods that are benign, offer good resolution and excellent recovery of biologically active material. For example, the charge on a protein's surface is provided the zwitterionic amino acids with weak acid charges as their functional groups (see Chapter 2). The negative charges on a protein's surface are contributed by the functional groups of aspartate and glutamate and the positive charges by the functional groups of lysine and arginine. These charges effectively make protein zwitterionic molecules with an isoelectric point (pI) and variable charge depending on the pH of the environment they are located in. Exploiting the charge on a protein's surface is an appropriate and effective principle to start a purification schedule. The procedure of ion exchange chromatography (IEX) provides the operator with a technique that has good capacity, admirable resolution and excellent recovery of biologically active material. In addition, because binding is based upon charge not concentration, IEX can also function to concentrate dilute solution of starting material. Hydrophobic interaction chromatography (HIC) and a variety of resins described as mixed modal provide the operator with additional techniques with excellent capacity, resolution and recovery but different selectivity. These adsorption techniques function to provide the operator with an ideal staring point in a purification schedule.

PROTOCOLS FOR CHAPTER 5

Protocol 5.1 Small-scale screening experiments to establish the appropriate binding and elution conditions for chromatographic resins

This protocol describes a small-scale screening with an anion exchange resin, but the principle can be applied to other chromatographic resins (e.g., cation exchange chromatography or hydrophobic interaction chromatography). The starting and eluting buffers may change for other resins.

> **Note:** (a) Prepare buffers fresh or from frozen stocks and use the highest reagent grade available. (b) Check the data sheets provided by the reagent's manufacturers and take appropriate health and safety precautions. (c) Use the highest quality water available to make the buffers and filter through 0.2 μm membrane before use. (d) Conduct the experiment at the temperature at which the chromatographic run is to be conducted; this will depend on the thermal stability of the target protein. (e) Check and adjust the pH of the buffers at the working temperature, as some buffers (e.g., Tris) show alterations in the pH with temperature.

Equipment

- 10 ml of washed anion exchange resin (after the preservative has been removed) suspended in an equal volume of distilled and deionised water.
- A micro centrifuge and 1.5–2.0 ml microfuge tubes.
- 200–1000 μl pipette and appropriate pipette tips.
- 10 ml each of 25 mM bis Tris propane/HCl buffer with the pH adjusted to pH 6.5 and pH 7.0; also 10 ml each of the buffers at the set pH value containing 0.5 M, 1.0 M and 2.0 M NaCl.
- 10 ml each of 25 mM Tris/HCl buffer with the pH adjusted to pH 7.5, 8.0, 8.5 and 9.0; also 10 ml each of the buffers at the set pH value containing 0.5 M, 1.0 M and 2.0 M NaCl.
- 10 ml of homogenate clarified by centrifugation at $12,000 \times g$ for 20 min (see Protocol 4.8 if ammonium sulphate precipitation is required to concentrate the protein in the extract). The extract should be essentially salt-free before ion exchange chromatography (IEX) and should be either dialysed (see Protocol 4.9) against 10 mM Tris buffer pH 7.5 or subjected to group size exclusion chromatography (see Protocol 7.1) using either Sephadex G25/G50 or Biogel P6/P10 equilibrated in 10 mM Tris buffer pH 7.5.

Method

- Slurry the resin by gently swirling the resin in the distilled water. Allow the bulk of the resin to settle and remove any floating particles ("fines"). Repeat this two or three times until the liquid above the settled resin looks clear.
- Cut the bottom 5 mm from the end of 1.0 ml pipette tip.
- Dispense 1.0 ml of the resin slurry into six microfuge tubes using the 200–1000 μl pipette and the pipette tip with the bottom 5 mm removed.
- Centrifuge the tubes in the bench top **microfuge** at $2000 \times g$ for 1 min.

- Pipette off the liquid and add 1.0 ml of the buffers at different pH values to each tube (remember to label the tubes). Vortex mix the resin in the buffer and then centrifuge the tubes in the microfuge at $2000 \times g$ for 1 min. Remove the liquid and repeat three times.
- In a separate microfuge tube add 0.5 ml of the appropriate buffer to 0.5 ml of the extract. Centrifuge at $12,000 \times g$ for 5 min to clarify the liquid and remove any precipitation.
- Add 0.5 ml of the extract at different pH values to the IEX resins in the microfuge tubes equilibrated at that pH value, retaining 0.5 ml for a protein and activity assay (B).
- Gently mix the resin and buffered extract for 1 min by inverting the tube.
- Centrifuge the tubes in the bench top microfuge at $2000 \times g$ for 1 min.
- Remove the supernatant liquid and place this in a separate labelled microfuge tube (C).
- Add 0.5 ml of the appropriate buffer containing 0.5 M NaCl to the microfuge.
- Gently mix the resin, centrifuge and remove the liquid into a labelled microfuge as described above (D).
- Repeat this for the buffers containing 1.0 M and 2.0 M NaCl (E and F).

Analysing the Results

- Measure the volume of the retained liquid (A–F) the protein concentration (see Protocols 4.1–4.4) and the biological activity of the target protein.
- Determine the specific activity, total activity, fold purity and % recovery (see Section 8.3 and Exercise 8.1) for each fraction.
- For IEX the ideal starting conditions will give 100% binding (at and above the pH, which is 0.5–1.0 pH values above the target protein's pI) with 100% recovery (at the salt concentration at which the target protein elutes from the IEX resin), coupled with a five- to tenfold increase in the fold purity (the binding, recovery and increases in the purity will depend on the target protein and the resin being used).
- After analysis these screening experiments can be repeated to fine-tune the starting and elution conditions before starting the scaled-up chromatographic procedures.
- For a protein to bind to an anion exchange resin, the pH of the buffer has to be approximately >0.5–1.0 above the isoelectric point (pI) of the protein. The minimum pH for binding to the anion IEX resin will give an indication of the pI value for the target protein.

Protocol 5.2 The purification of calcium-dependent proteins using hydrophobic interaction chromatography (HIC)

This procedure was based upon a publication by Brockhart et al. (1983). Normally, proteins bind to HIC resins in the presence of high salt. However, at low salt some calcium-activated proteins can expose hydrophobic pockets near to their surfaces in the presence of calcium ions. The low salt conditions ensure that the vast majority of proteins in an extract will pass through the HIC column without binding whereas the calcium activated proteins will bind. The calcium dependent binding of the target protein can be reversed either by a wash in calcium free buffer or by the inclusion of calcium chelating agents (e.g., EDTA) or EGTA in a buffer (see Figure 5.16).

<u>Starting and initial wash buffer</u>: 50 mM Tris pH 8.5 containing 5 mM $CaCl_2$

<u>Zero calcium wash buffer</u>: 50 mM Tris pH 8.5

<u>EDTA wash buffer</u>: 50 mM Tris pH 8.5 containing 5 mM EDTA

Method

- A column of Phenyl-Sepharose 6FF (or another suitable HIC resin) was equilibrated with two column volumes of 50 mM Tris pH 8.5 containing 5 mM $CaCl_2$.
- The absorbance at 280 nm was set to zero.
- The sample is applied and the fractions collected.
- The column is washed with 50 mM Tris pH 8.5 containing 5 mM $CaCl_2$ until the absorbance at 280 nm reaches <0.1.
- The column is then washed with a zero-calcium buffer (e.g., 50 mM Tris pH 8.5) until the absorbance at 280 nm reaches <0.1.
- To elute the majority of calcium bound proteins the column is washed with 50 mM Tris pH 8.5 containing 5 mM EDTA until the absorbance at 280 nm reaches <0.1.
- To wash the HIC resin of proteins which have bound but not yet eluted the column is washed with water until the absorbance at 280 nm reaches <0.1.

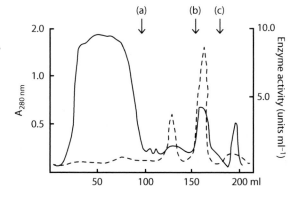

(a) Remove $CaCl_2$ from the elution buffer
(b) Added EDTA to the elution buffer
(c) Wash the column with water to elute protein that have bound to the column with a non-specific interaction

Figure 5.16 Hydrophobic interaction chromatography (10 ml phenyl sepharose) showing the calcium dependant elution of an enzyme extracted from *Vicia faba* cotyledons.

If the wash with water fails to restore the baseline zero over twenty column volumes, a more stringent wash procedure could be instigated.

If the column has been packed into an empty glass column, first remove the resin from the column and slurry the resin in a beaker in distilled and deionised water. Pour the slurred resin into a glass funnel with a sintered glass floor.

The water can be removed under vacuum.

Stop the vacuum before the resin dries out (do not let the resin dry completely).

In the filter add five column volumes of 0.1 M NaOH (to dissolve any precipitated proteins) and suspend the chromatography resin in the NaOH.

Leave for 5 min and then reapply the vacuum.

Wash with distilled water until the pH of the exit liquid has returned to <pH 8.0.

The HIC chromatography resin can then be stored in 20% (v/v) ethanol at 4°C.

To remove lipids/lipoproteins it may be necessary to wash with 30% (v/v) isopropanol or 30% (v/v) acetonitrile, followed by copious amounts of water and then storage in 20% (v/v) ethanol at 4°C.

If the HIC column is a pre-packed proprietary column, please remember to release the pressure on the resin in the column by backing off the top inlet adaptor by a 2–5 mm.

Then flow the washing liquids (outlined above) in the reverse direction by inverting the column before reattaching the column to the chromatography system in the conventional flow direction.

In a chromatography system these steps can be performed efficiently. Do not let the 0.1 M NaOH reside in the column or the system for a prolonged period of time.

Protocol 5.3 The affinity elution (displacement) of enzymes from an ion exchange column

This method of elution from an IEX resin is based upon a method described by Maruyama et al. (1985).

If the target protein is known (or suspected) to exhibit conformational changes on binding to substrates, inhibitors or cofactors, this protocol may be a useful variant of the normal IEX procedures.

The procedure requires a <u>two</u>-stage ion exchange process. The chromatography in this protocol is ideally conducted with a protein purification chromatography system with a controlled gradient, an inline conductivity monitor, a fraction collector and a computer-based data analysis (see Section 3.7). This procedure describes the use of a proprietary anion exchange resin in a 1.0 ml column, but the principle can be applied to other chromatographic resins or different volumes of resin (the starting and eluting buffers may change for different resins and column volumes).

> **Note:** (a) Prepare buffers fresh or from frozen stocks and use the highest reagent grade available. (b) Check the data sheets provided by the reagent's manufacturers and take appropriate health and safety precautions. (c) Use the highest quality water available to make the buffers and filter through 0.2 μm membrane before use. (d) Conduct the experiment at the appropriate temperature to maintain the thermal stability of the target protein. (e) Check and adjust the pH of the buffers at the working temperature as some buffers (e.g., Tris) show alterations in the pH with temperature.

Equipment

- 10 ml of washed anion exchange resin (after the preservative has been removed—see Section 5.2) in an equal volume of distilled and deionised water.
- A protein purification chromatography system (e.g., GE Healthcare AKTA).
- Buffer A: 100 ml of 25 mM Tris/HCl buffer pH 8.0.
- Buffer B: 100 ml of 25 mM Tris/HCl buffer pH 8.0 containing 0.5 M NaCl.
- 10 ml of 500 mM $CaCl_2$.
- The solution of sample should be essentially salt-free before ion exchange chromatography (IEX). If it does contain some salt, the sample can be either dialysed (see Protocol 4.9) against 10 mM Tris buffer pH 8.5 or subjected to group size exclusion chromatography (see Protocol 7.1) using either Sephadex G25/G50 or Biogel P6/P10 equilibrated in 10 mM Tris buffer pH 8.5.
- Prior to applying the sample to the chromatography resin, the sample should be clarified by centrifugation at $12,000 \times g$ for 20 min (see Section 4.10.1) or filtered through 0.2 μm membrane filter.

First Ion Exchange Method

- Set the flow rate at 0.5 ml min^{-1} and equilibrate the anion exchange resin in the 1.0ml with 10.0 ml of buffer A.
- Set the absorbance at 280 nm to zero.
- Load the 1.0 ml of sample onto the column using the injection loop (see Figure 3.8) and wash through with 10.0 ml of buffer A.

- Start collecting 0.5 ml fractions.
- Elute the target protein with a gradient (0–100% buffer B) over twenty column volumes and collect the fractions.
- At the end of the gradient wash 5.0 ml of buffer B through the column followed by 10.0 ml of buffer A to put the column back into the starting conditions.
- Take the fractions collected and assay for the activity of the target protein.
- Record the volume where the peak activity elutes and using the graphical output, determine the precise salt concentration that elutes the target protein. (Remember that the fraction number at which the target protein has been collected **will not** be at the exact point of elution. This is because the fraction volume at which the target protein has been collected includes the volume of the column and the volume from the end of the column to the outlet of the fraction collector. You will need to project back from the apparent elution conditions to the exact elution conditions [see Figure 5.17A].)

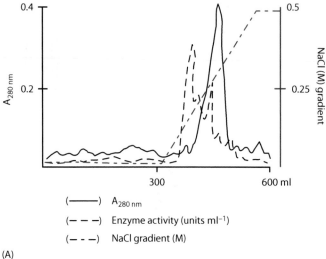

(———) A$_{280\,nm}$

(— — —) Enzyme activity (units ml^{-1})

(— · — ·) NaCl gradient (M)

(A)

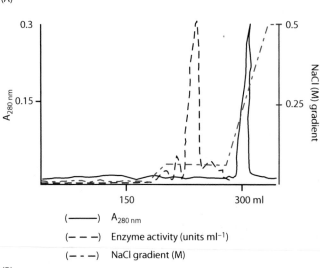

(———) A$_{280\,nm}$

(— — —) Enzyme activity (units ml^{-1})

(— · — ·) NaCl gradient (M)

(B)

Figure 5.17 (A) Ion excahnge chromatography (10 ml Q10 anion exchange Bio-Rad) of the enzyme activity eluted from HIC (see Figure 5.16) using NaCl gradient. (B) Calcium affinity elution of the enzyme extracted from *Vicia faba* cotyledons after (i) Figure 5.16 and (ii) Figure 5.17A. The active fractions from Figure 5.17A were diluted and reapplied to 10 ml Q10 anion exchange (Bio-Rad) as described in Protocol 5.3.

Second Ion Exchange (Affinity Elution)

When the exact elution concentration of salt has been determined, prepare buffer A1 (see above) with the salt concentration that is 5 mM below the salt concentration that elutes the target protein. For example, if the concentration of salt that eluted the target protein was 45 mM NaCl, then prepare buffer A1 as follows: 25 mM Tris/HCl pH 8.5 containing 40 mM NaCl (see Figure 5.17A).

Prepare buffer A2 to include the NaCl concentration of buffer A1 and an appropriate concentration of the affinity eluent (e.g., 25 mM Tris/HCl pH 8.5 containing 40 mM NaCl and 5 mM $CaCl_2$).

- Take the pooled active sample and add an equal volume of buffer A1.
- Wash 5.0 ml of buffer A1 through the column and set the absorbance at 280 nm to zero.
- Reapply the sample to the IEX column and start to collect fractions.
- Wash through two column volumes with buffer A1.
- When the absorbance at 280 nm reaches zero, apply 5.0 ml of buffer A2.
- Collect 0.5 ml fractions.
- An increase in the absorbance at 280 nm will indicate protein has been released from the ion exchange column.
- Confirm the presence of the target protein by assaying all the fractions.

An alternative affinity elution procedure could be performed by sequentially applying injections of NaCl containing gradually increasing concentrations of $CaCl_2$. If, for example, the target protein eluted from the first ion exchange experiment at 45 mM, the following injections may be appropriate: 40 mM NaCl plus 1 mM $CaCl_2$, 42 mM NaCl plus 2 mM $CaCl_2$, 45 mM NaCl plus 5 mM $CaCl_2$.

> **Note:** This protocol is open to many different variations (e.g., inhibitors, activators, and cofactors). A suitable affinity elution would need to be tailored to the target protein and the procedure modified through empirical experimentation.

RECOMMENDED READING

Research papers

Brookhart, P.P., McMahon, P.L. and Takahasi, M. (1983) Purification of guinea pig liver transglutaminase using a phenylalanine-Sepharose 4B affinity column. *Anal Biochem* 128:202-205.

Huddleston, J., Albelaira, J.C., Wang, R. and Lyddiatt, A. (1996) Protein partition between the different phases comprising poly(ethylene glycol)-salt aqueous two-phase systems, hydrophobic interaction chromatography and precipitation: A generic description in terms of salting-out effects. *J Chromatogr B Biomed Appl* 680:31-41.

Maruyama, K., Ebisawa, K. and Nonomura, Y. (1985) Purification of vitamin D-dependent 28 000-M_r calcium-binding protein from bovine cerebellum and kidney by calcium dependent elution from DEAE-Cellulose DE-52 column chromatography. *Anal Biochem* 151:1-6.

Nandi, S., Mehra, N., Lynn, A.M., and Bhattacharya, A. (2005) Comparison of theoretical proteomes: Identification of COGs with conserved and variable pI within the multimodal pI distribution. *BMC Genomics* 6:116.

Sober, H.A. and Peterson E.A. (1958) Protein chromatography on ion exchange cellulose. *Fred Proc* 17:1116-1126.

Wolfe, L.S., Barringer, C.P., Mostafa, S.S. and Shukla, A.A. (2014) Mixed-mode chromatography in pharmaceutical and biopharmaceutical applications. *J Chromatogr A* 340:151-156.

Wu, S., Wan, P., Li, J., Li, D., Zhu, Y. and He, F. (2006) Multi-modality of pI distribution in whole proteome. *Proteomics* 6:449-455.

Zang, K. and Lui, X. (2016) Mixed-mode chromatography in pharmaceutical and biopharmaceutical applications. *J Pharm Biomed Appl* 128:73-88.

Books

Cutler, P. (Ed.) (2004) *Protein Purification Protocols*. 2nd ed. Humana Press, New Jersey, USA.

Deutscher, M.P. (Ed.) (1990) "Guide to protein purification." *Methods in Enzymology* 182. Academic Press, London, UK.

Roe, S. (Ed.) (2001) *Protein Purification: Methods*. 2nd ed. Oxford University Press, Oxford, UK.

Rosenberg, I.M. (2005) *Protein Analysis and Purification*. 2nd ed. Birkhauser, Boston, USA.

Yamamoto, S., Nakanishi, K. and Matsuno, R. (1988) *Ion Exchange Chromatography of Proteins*. Marcel Dekker, New York, USA.

Affinity-Based Procedures Used to Purify Proteins

6

6.1 INTRODUCTION TO AFFINITY CHROMATOGRAPHY

Proteins are synthesised from the information contained within genes; as a result they each have a different content and total number of amino acids. All proteins possess these physical properties and the differences in these parameters can be exploited to purify proteins. Proteins are synthesised for a unique cellular role and this property can also be exploited to purify a protein from a complex mixture.

Affinity chromatography does not exploit the physical differences between proteins. Instead, it relies upon a target protein's unique biospecificity to resolve the target protein from a complex protein mixture. It still involves an interaction between two immiscible phases because it involves a reversible interaction between a ligand (a small molecule such as an enzyme substrate or a macromolecule such as an antibody [e.g., IgG]) immobilised onto a resin (stationary phase) and a target protein contained within a **solute** (mobile phase). The technique was originally developed as a means of purifying enzymes, but it has expanded to cover a wide variety of interactions, including: the interaction of nucleic acids and proteins, antibodies with antigens (immunoaffinity chromatography), receptors with agonists, glycoproteins with lectins (sugar-binding proteins) and ligands with intact cells or cell membranes.

For example, enzymes will bind with a high affinity to their substrates because their active sites become stereospecific upon binding to the substrate. Therefore, an enzyme's substrate (ligand) immobilised onto a resin can be used to bind a target enzyme to the exclusion of all the other proteins present in the mixture (see Figure 6.1). Other enzymes will not bind to the ligand because their active sites do not match the three dimentional shape of the ligand molecule; they will percolate through the resin and elute in the unbound fraction. The enzyme bound to the ligand can be eluted from the resin in a highly purified format. In theory, affinity chromatography provides the means to purify and concentrate a target protein from a complex mixture in one chromatographic step. However, in practise, successful one-step purifications are rare and affinity chromatography is usually used in conjunction with other chromatographic procedures (e.g., ion exchange chromatography, hydrophobic interaction chromatography or size exclusion chromatography; see Chapters 5 and 7) to successfully purify a protein of interest to homogeneity.

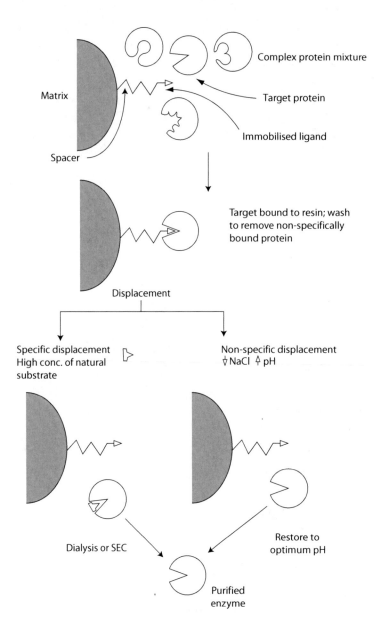

Figure 6.1 The basis of affinity chromatography.

6.2   THE RESINS USED IN AFFINITY CHROMATOGRAPHY

There is a wide choice of support resins available for affinity chromatography, including agarose, Sephadex, polyacrylamide and silica. If the resin is porous (agarose or Sepharose), a large pore size (particle size 50–400 μm) will help minimise any size exclusion effects of the resin. In addition, the resin should be chemically stable during ligand coupling and during the chromatography of the target protein. The stability of the coupling and leakage of the ligand from the resin is particularly important if the target protein is to be used therapeutically.

6.3   THE AFFINITY LIGAND

Prior knowledge about the protein of interest (substrate specificity, cofactor requirements, inhibitor/activator profile) will help determine the choice of a good ligand for affinity chromatography.

$$\underset{\text{Protein+Ligand}}{\underline{P+L}} \quad \leftrightarrow \quad \underset{\text{protein ligand complex}}{\underline{PL}}$$

The equilibrium/dissociation (affinity) constant (K_a) for the interaction between a protein and a ligand is given by

$$K_a = \frac{[PL]}{[P][L]}$$

where [PL] is the concentration of the protein ligand complex, [P] is the concentration of the protein and [L] is the concentration of free ligand. A value for K_a can be determined using equilibrium dialysis (kits are available from ThermoFisher Scientific Ltd) and values ranging between 10^{-5}–10^{-11} M are usually required for a good affinity ligand. It is important to remember that when a ligand is bound to a resin, it no longer has completely free movement about every atom. Particularly, the atom used to attach the ligand to the resin will have restricted movement compared to the free ligand. This will affect the interaction between the ligand and the target protein. Consequently, the value for K_a between a protein and a ligand can be up to a thousandfold less when the ligand is bound to a resin.

Successful affinity chromatography depends upon the reversible binding of the target molecule to a ligand attached to a support resin. Ideally, the interaction between the target protein and the ligand should have sufficient strength and specificity to retain the target protein, thus allowing all the unwanted proteins to percolate through the resin in the unbound fraction. However, the interaction should also be weak enough to allow gentle elution conditions to be applied (typically a rise in the concentration of free ligand or a rise in the salt concentration) that will sever the protein ligand interaction, resulting in both high yield and fold purity of the target protein (see Chapter 8). These ideal affinity chromatography conditions are very rarely encountered; often it is relatively easy to prepare an affinity resin for an enzyme that shows specific binding of the target protein, but the strength of the interaction between the target protein and the ligand often means harsh elution conditions (typically low pH or the use of chaotrophic salts) are needed to release the target protein from the ligand bound to the resin. The interaction between the protein and the ligand is altered because the ligand does not have complete freedom of movement. The binding can occur, but the necessary molecular movements required to release the target ligand (e.g., substrate for an enzyme) are prevented from taking place. The subsequent harsh conditions employed to release the target protein will result in the majority of the target protein eluting in denatured conformations, which impacts the recovery of biologically active material. If a strong interaction between the ligand and the target protein is observed, it may be possible to alter the chemistry of the ligand to reduce the strength of the binding. Alternatively, it may be possible to attach the ligand via a different functional group (see Table 6.1), retaining the binding but also allowing gentler elution conditions. These alternatives would have to be determined empirically.

Table 6.1 Commercially available activated matrices for coupling ligands.

Name	Coupling groups	Comments	Supplier*
Affi 10 (coupling proteins PL >6.5) and Affi 15 (coupling protein PL<6.5)	Proteins with available -NH$_2$	N-hydroxysuccinimide esters	Bio-Rad
Epoxy activated sepharose	Coupling of free **thiols**, hydroxyls and amino groups	Conditions pH 9–13 for 16–72 hr. Useful for small ligands	GE Healthcare
Affi gel Hz	Coupling of glycoproteins via oxidised aldehyde in a carbohydrate residue		Bio-Rad
Thiopropyl Sepharose	Coupling via thiols		GE Healthcare
Cyanogen activated Sepharose 4B	Proteins with available -NH$_2$	Conditions pH 7–9 16 hr. No spacer arm	GE Healthcare
EAH Sepharose	Coupling of ligands with free carboxyl groups	Use water-soluble N-ethyl-N'-(3-dimethylaminopropyl) carbodiimide HCl (EDC)	GE Healthcare
EAH Sepharose	Coupling of ligands with free amino groups	Use EDC	GE Healthcare
AminoLink (gel and kit format)	Coupling through a primary amino group	Lysine and the terminal amino group	ThermoFisher Scientific
MicroLink peptide kit	Coupling through sulphydryl groups	Sulphydryl containing peptides and proteins	ThermoFisher Scientific
Reacti-Gel CDI supports	Coupling through a free amino group at pH 9–11.0	(a) Three different matrices (b) Stable imidazolyl carbamate attachment	ThermoFisher Scientific

When small ligands are attached to an affinity resin, they will be physically close to the resin's surface, which may impact the ability of a target protein to approach and successfully interact with the ligand. To overcome this impasse, small ligands may require the presence of a spacer arm to present the ligand away from the surface of the resin, thus allowing a successful interaction between the ligand and the target protein moving through the mobile phase. The spacer arm is usually 6–10 carbons atoms (or equivalent) in length (e.g., 1, 6, diaminohexane or 6-aminohexanoic acid). The structure of the spacer arm (predominantly hydrophobic) and the nature of the support resin can be important additional factors in determining a successful interaction (see Section 5.7). This is through promoting H-bonding, hydrophobic, ionic or dipole interactions between the spacer arm and the protein that binds to the resin. Many of the commercially available affinity resins have pre-set spacer arms attached for ligand binding (see Table 6.1). The reaction scheme for two popular activated resins are shown in Figures 6.2 and 6.3.

Large ligands (e.g., proteins) can be attached directly to an affinity resin and still retain their attractiveness to the target molecule. A protein will typically be attached to an affinity resin via the ε-amino group of lysine residues. It should be remembered that proteins will contain many ε-amino groups and thus multiple attachment sites of the protein to the affinity resin. This will impact the orientation of the ligand protein, resulting in

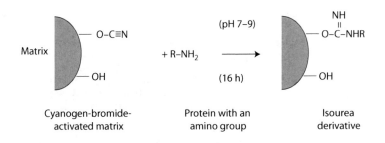

Figure 6.2 The coupling of proteins with a free amino group to a cyanogen bromide-activated Sepharose (GE Healthcare).

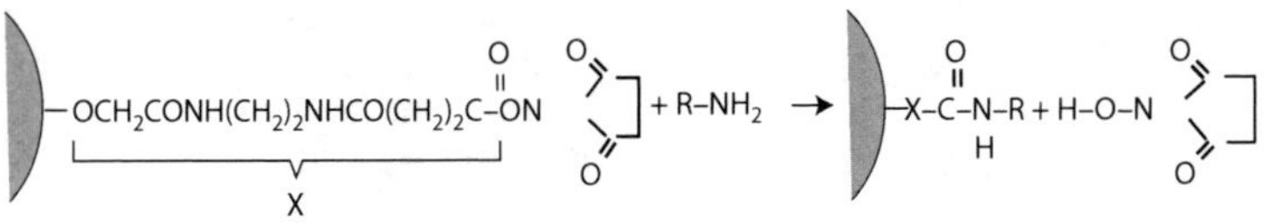

Cyanogen-bromide-activated matrix

Protein with an amino group

Isourea derivative

Figure 6.3 The coupling of proteins with a free amino group to Affi gel 10 (Bio-Rad).

many redundant attachments, as only a limited number of the protein molecules will be in the correct orientation to interact with the target molecule in the mobile phase. This problem is difficult to overcome, and the operator may need to factor this in by producing a larger (e.g., five- to tenfold) volume of the affinity resin to produce an affinity ligand with sufficient ligand protein molecules in the correct conformation. Whether the ligand attached to the affinity resin is large or small, they should ideally not leak from the support during the course of the affinity process. Minor contaminating pieces of the affinity ligand can be a major headache in the purification and use of therapeutic proteins.

6.4 THE BINDING AND ELUTION CONDITIONS FOR AFFINITY CHROMATOGRAPHY

The ideal binding and elution conditions for affinity chromatography must be determined experimentally and can initially be determined on a small scale (adapting the method described in Protocol 5.1). Binding should be conducted in a buffer (containing cofactors [e.g., metal ions]) set at a pH that encourages an interaction between the target protein and the ligand. This could be ±1.0 about the pH optimum of an enzyme. Bear in mind that the ligand attached to the affinity resin will have some restriction in movement, and this may also impact the pH optimum for binding and elution. If the affinity interaction involves any hydrophobic forces, the inclusion of 0.1–0.5 M NaCl may help promote binding and also help overcome any non-specific ion exchange interactions between the proteins in the sample and the affinity resin. Due to the specificity of the interactions in affinity chromatography, columns with smaller volumes (<20.0 ml) that are run at slow flow rates (e.g., 10 cm h^{-1}) can help promote the affinity interactions by promoting mass transfer between the target protein in the mobile phase and the ligand on the stationary phase (see Section 3.3.2). If the target protein is perceived to be present at a low concentration in the sample, the flow through the column can be recycled (see Figure 6.4A) for many hours at a slow flow rate before the column washing and elution steps. Alternatively, the affinity resin can be mixed with the sample in an "end-over-end" mixer (see Figure 6.4B) for a period of time before the mixture of resin and sample is loaded into a column, washed to remove

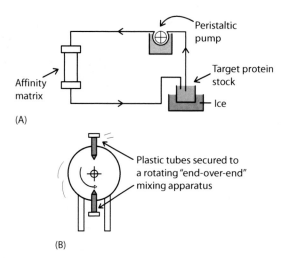

(A)

(B)

Figure 6.4 Recycled stock setups which can be used in affinity chromatography. (A) Recycled stock affinity setup. The peristaltic pump moves the target protein stock solution at a slow rate (e.g., <0.2 ml min⁻¹) overnight at 4°C. After 16 hours the bound protein is eluted from the affinity matrix. (B) The target protein stock is mixed with the affinity matrix to form a slurry that is placed into sealable plastic tubes. After overnight mixing the matrix is poured into a column for washing and elution.

the unbound material and then subjected to the elution conditions. However, the adsorption efficiency of this technique is generally poorer than using a column with the same volume of resin (see Section 4.12.2). A flow diagram of a typical affinity chromatography experiment is shown in Figure 6.5.

Depending on the degree of interaction between the target protein in the mobile phase and the ligand bound to the stationary phase, there could

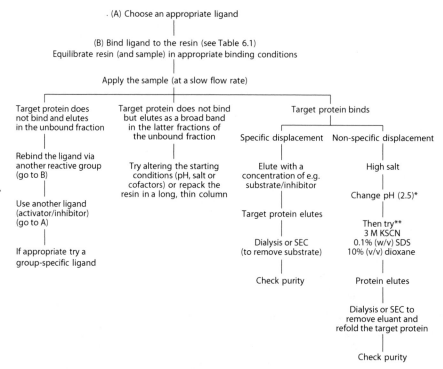

*Put an aliquot of high pH buffer into the tubes of the fraction collector to quickly restore ideal conditions for the target protein.
**Use of these conditions may compromise the recovery of biologically active material. But it may still be suitable for the production of antibodies.

Figure 6.5 A flow diagram of the events in a typical affinity chromatography experiment.

be a number of outcomes. Ideally, if the ligand concentration is high and there is a strong association between the target protein and ligand, the free protein will be immediately captured by free ligand, resulting in a concentrated band of target protein at or near the top of the resin in the column. The elution conditions will move the equilibrium in favour of free protein in the mobile phase, resulting in the target protein eluting in a single sharp peak. To avoid dilution of the eluted target protein as it moves from the top of the column to the exit, the elution conditions can be applied in the reverse direction to the application. This simple procedure will gather the target protein in a small concentrated volume (see Figure 6.6).

If the interaction between the target protein and the bound ligand is weak, the protein may move onto and off the ligand bound to the resin. Its progress down the column will be retarded and it will elute later in the elution profile of the unbound proteins. If this is the case, it does not mean that the affinity column has proven ineffective, but it does require a different approach. The sample should be applied to the affinity resin packed into a long thin column, using a slow flow rate at a temperature lower than room temperature. This will help maximise the interaction between the target protein and the affinity ligand, delaying the target protein's progress down the column such that it elutes (probably in a broad peak) after the unbound and unwanted protein has eluted. The target protein can then be concentrated by a variety of methods (see Section 4.11).

Displacement of the target protein bound to the ligand on the resin may be achieved by using a high concentration of the target enzyme's substrate. Alternatively, an inhibitor (or activator) in the eluting buffer can be used to induce conformational changes in the bound protein to specifically displace ligand-bound enzymes. If the enzyme requires a cofactor such as metal ions, the inclusion of EDTA or other chelating reagents (see Table 4.3) in the eluting buffer may induce displacement of the bound protein from the ligand. Often, specific displacement will not remove the target protein from the affinity ligand and non-specific displacement conditions have to be employed. Increasing the salt concentration to >1.0 M NaCl or decreasing the pH to 2.0 are non-specific elution procedures that can be applied. If a dramatic change in pH is selected for elution

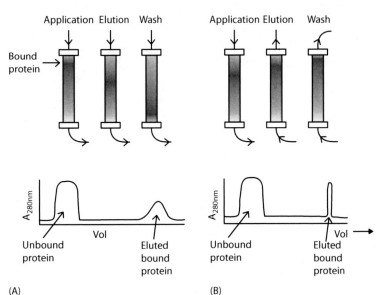

Figure 6.6 Elution profiles from affinity columns eluted in (A) the direction of flow and (B) against the flow.

(e.g., immunoaffinity chromatography; see Section 6.4), care must be taken to quickly return the eluted fractions to the ideal storage pH for the target protein (see Section 4.14). Denaturation of the eluted protein can be minimised by (a) reducing the length of the tubing between the column outlet and the fraction collector (dead volume) and (b) including a small volume of concentrated buffer in the bottom of the fraction collector tubes (e.g., 1.0 M Tris pH 8.5). This will minimise the time the target protein spends in a low pH environment.

Non-specific displacement conditions can provide good recovery of the target protein (as judged by SDS-PAGE and Western blot analysis; see Sections 8.3 and 8.4), but in most cases the experience of a low pH environment will result in poor recovery of biological activity. This is the contrast between the physical recovery of protein, as judged by electrophoresis, and biologically active protein, as judged by biological activity (see Section 8.2). The loss of biological activity will be due to the failure of the majority of the target protein to correctly refold into its active conformation when the pH is adjusted back to the proteins ideal conditions. The inclusion of substrates, reversible inhibitors, metal ion cofactors, and reducing agents in the high pH buffer present in the fraction collection tubes may aid the recovery of more active target protein. These additional molecules may provide a template for part of the protein structure to latch onto, so that the rest of the protein structure can be encouraged into an active conformation. The high concentration of buffer and additions can be removed by dialysis (see Protocol 4.9) or by size exclusion chromatography (see Protocol 7.1). Size exclusion chromatography is a technique that is routinely used at the end of a purification procedure to remove trace aggregates and contaminating proteins (see Section 7.5.2). If a target protein is very tightly bound to an affinity resin, an elution with a buffer containing either 3.0 M KSCN, 2.0 M potassium iodide, 4.0 M $MgCl_2$, 8.0 M urea, 6.0 M guanidine/HCl, or 10% (v/v) dioxane can be tried to remove the protein. After these harsh elution conditions, dialysis (see Protocol 4.9) or size exclusion chromatography (see Protocol 7.1) can be used to separate the target enzyme from contaminating low molecular mass components.

The preceding information has been directed towards binding and eluting a protein from its interaction with a small molecule attached to a resin. If the molecule attached to the affinity resin is a protein, care must be taken to ensure the integrity of the protein on the affinity ligand during the binding and elution of the target molecule in the applied sample. The use of non-specific elution conditions (see above) may compromise the integrity of the protein being used as an affinity ligand, effectively resulting in a "one use" affinity matrix.

Affinity chromatography can be a highly resolving technique, but some of the non-specific elution conditions can result in poor yields (see Section 8.1) due to denaturation and incorrect refolding of the target protein. The loss of activity and three-dimensional structure may be a problem if the eluted protein is to be used for kinetic analysis or for the growth of crystals but may not be a problem if the eluted protein is to be used to generate antibodies.

6.5   THE REGENERATION AND STORAGE OF AFFINITY RESINS

Cleaning the affinity resin will depend on the nature of the ligand. Resins coupled to low M_r substrates can be washed with low pH (e.g., 1.0 M

Ligand	Target proteins
Protein A or Protein G	Immunoglobulins
Melon gel	Immunoglobulins (ThermoFisher Scientific)
Benzamidine	Serine proteases
Calmodulin	Calmodulin-binding proteins
Lectin(s)	Glycoproteins (see Section 6.10 and Table 6.3)
Cibacron Blue	Dehydrogenases, kinases and albumin
5'AMP, ATP	Dehydrogenases
NAD^+, $NADP^+$	Dehydrogenases
Heparin	Lipoproteins, coagulation factors (DNA and RNA)
Lysine	Plasminogen (rRNA and dsDNA)

Table 6.2 Some examples of commercially available group-specific ligands.

CH_3COOH) and high pH (1.0 M NaOH) buffers, followed by ten columns volumes of water, before storage in 20% (v/v) ethanol. Resins that have a protein ligand can be washed in high salt (4.0 M NaCl) before storage in 0.05% (w/v) sodium azide. (Lectin protein affinity ligands may require storage in the presence of metal ions; please check the manufacturer's recommendations; see Section 6.10.)

6.6 GROUP-SPECIFIC LIGANDS

Designing a specific affinity ligand for a protein can be difficult and expensive, so it may be possible to exploit a general property of a target protein to purify all the proteins in a complex mixture with the same general property (e.g., the use of lectin affinity chromatography to purify a group of glycoproteins; see Section 6.10). After elution, other chromatographic techniques can be used to isolate the target protein from the group-specific mixture. There are many commercially available affinity resins with group-specific ligands pre-attached (see Table 6.2); these resins are available for low- and high-pressure chromatography systems.

6.7 COVALENT CHROMATOGRAPHY

6.7.1 Introduction to covalent chromatography

If a protein has been synthesised to be exported from the cell, its tertiary and/or quaternary structure may be stabilised by the presence of covalent disulphide bridges formed by the oxidation of two cysteine residues. These proteins destined for export from the cell are synthesised on ribosomes attached to the endoplasmic reticulum ("rough" ER). They are then processed through the ER before being exported to the Golgi bodies and then journeying to the plasma membrane for export. This means that proteins with disulphide bridges will also be present in the endomembrane system of the cell. These disulphide double bonds confer additional structural strength upon the exported proteins, contributing to their extracellular

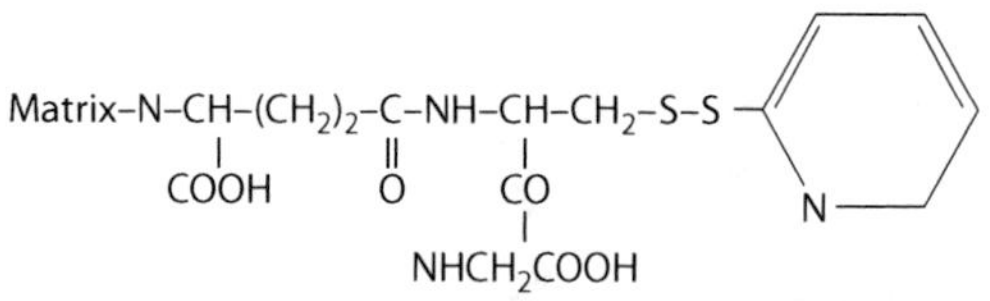

Matrix–N–CH–(CH$_2$)$_2$–C–NH–CH–CH$_2$–S–S

COOH   O   CO

NHCH$_2$COOH

Figure 6.7 The partial structure of activated thiol Sepharose 4B.

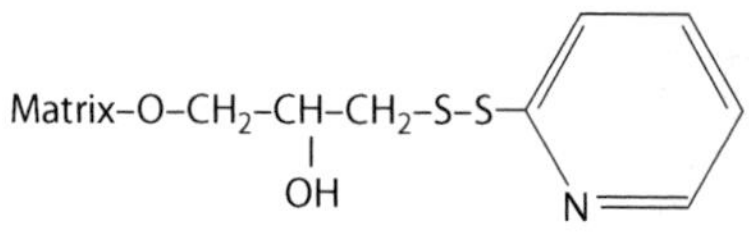

Matrix–O–CH$_2$–CH–CH$_2$–S–S

OH

Figure 6.8 The partial structure of thiopropyl Sepharose 6B.

longevity. Cytoplasmic proteins contain cysteine amino acids, and in the reducing atmosphere of the cytoplasm there will be reduced cysteine residues present on the surface of proteins or at the active site of enzymes that do not form disulphide bridges. A ligand containing a **thiol** residue attached to a resin (stationary phase) can be reacted with these surface and/or active site sulphydryl groups to form a covalent mixed disulphide complex, covalently attaching the protein to the affinity resin.

Covalent chromatography is a separation technique developed to isolate thiol containing proteins and peptides. Activated thiol Sepharose (see Figure 6.7), a low capacity resin (1 mmol 2-pyridyl sulphide groups ml^{-1} resin), and thiopropyl Sepharose (see Figure 6.8), a high capacity resin (20 mmol 2-pyridyl sulphide groups ml^{-1} resin), are commercially available (GE Healthcare, UK).

6.7.2   The binding and elution conditions for covalent chromatography

The covalent chromatography resin of choice should be equilibrated in a starting buffer (which should be degassed before use to help prevent oxidation of the free thiols) that is compatible with the target protein (e.g., 0.1 M Tris/HCl pH 7.5 containing 0.5 M NaCl and 1 mM EDTA to chelate heavy metals, which react irreversibly with thiols). The column size will depend on the sample size, and typically low flow rates (5–10 cm h^{-1}) are used during the run. The reaction scheme for covalent chromatography is shown in Figure 6.9 and involves displacement of pyridine 2-thione by the thiol groups present on the protein. The pyridine 2-thione absorbs light at 343 nm and can be used to check that protein has bound to the column.

After washing to remove non-specifically bound protein, the covalently bound protein can be eluted with a buffer at pH 8.0 containing either 5–25 mM L-cysteine, 20–50 mM 2-mercaptoethanol (useful because 2-ME can be removed by freeze drying) or 20–50 mM dithiothreitol (DTT). Different thiol-containing proteins may be separated by a gradient or sequential isocratic elution with these reducing agents (see Section 3.6.7). Unreacted pyridine 2-thione will also elute with the protein but can easily be removed by dialysis (see Protocol 4.9) or size exclusion chromatography (see Protocol 7.1). Alternatively, prior to eluting the bound protein, the column should be washed with 50 mM sodium acetate buffer pH 4.0 containing 4 mM 2-ME or DTT, which will displace the unreactive pyridine 2-thione. The column can then be re-equilibrated with a buffer at pH 8.0 before applying the conditions that will elute the covalently bound protein (as above).

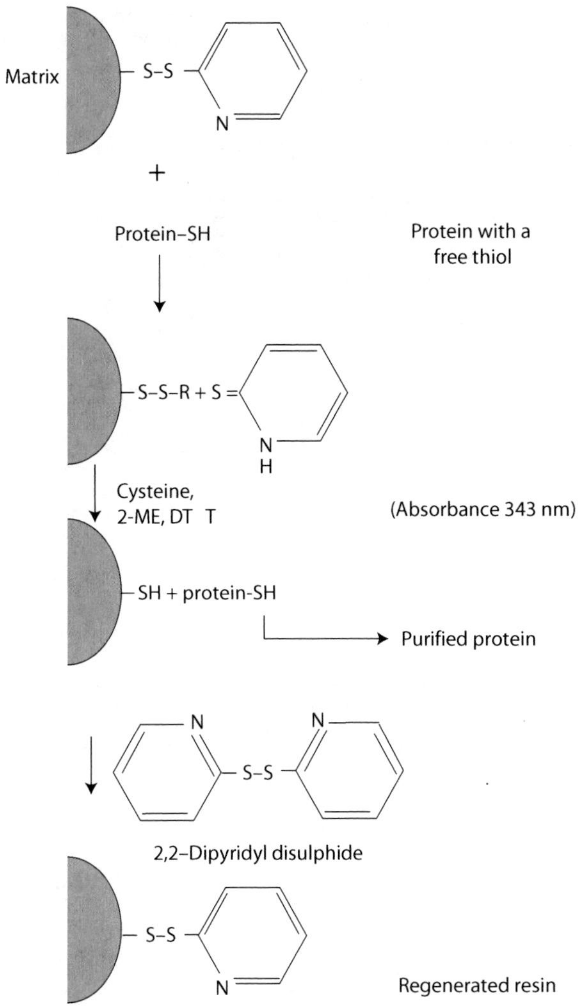

Figure 6.9 The reaction scheme for covalent chromatography on activated thiol Sepharose.

6.7.3 The regeneration and storage of covalent chromatography resins

The column can be regenerated by passing two column volumes of saturated 2,2′-dipyridyl disulphide (stir 40 mg of dipyridyl disulphide in 50 ml buffer at room temperature for a few hours); remove the insoluble material by centrifugation (12,000 × g for 20 min) and adjust to pH 8.0 Equilbrate the column with two column volumes of the pH 8.0 buffer containing the dipyridyl sulphide. The column can then be washed with a buffer pH 8.0 containing 0.05% (w/v) sodium azide and stored at 4°C.

6.8 DYE LIGAND AFFINITY CHROMATOGRAPHY

Aromatic triazine dyes bound to a support matrix (Sepharose or agarose) have been shown to selectively bind proteins. The affinity process was originally identified using size exclusion chromatography in the presence of blue dye (used to determine the void volume [V_0] of a size exclusion column; see Section 7.5.1). This resulted in the elution volumes of certain

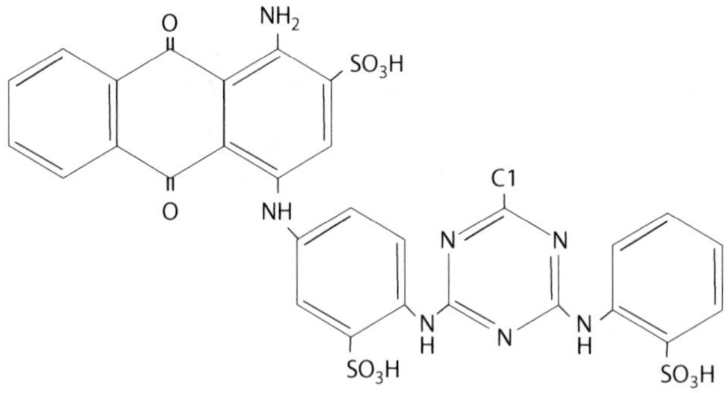

Figure 6.10 The structure of Cibacron blue FG-3A triazine dye.

proteins being smaller than predicted. The proteins had bound to the Cibacron blue FG-3A dye on the blue Dextran used to measure the void volume (V_0) of the column, eluting in the void volume and appearing as if they had a large molecular mass. It has been suggested that the structure of the dyes (see Figure 6.10) resembles the structure of metabolic nucleotide cofactors (e.g., NAD^+). Indeed, dehydrogenases and other proteins can be competively eluted from dye ligand resins using substrates or cofactors. However, other proteins (e.g., endonucleases and albumin) bind to dyes without a nucleotide cofactor requirement. The use of dye ligand chromatography has been used to partially separate antibodies from contaminating albumins. The interaction between a protein and the dye bound to a resin appears to involve both hydrophobic and ionic interactions, making predictions about binding and elution difficult (mixed modal chromatography; see Section 5.7).

A range of different triazine dyes attached to resins in small volume columns are commercially available for screening the binding and elution of a target protein on a small scale (see Protocol 5.1), allowing the operator to establish the best conditions before purchasing a larger volume of resin for the purification process. Alternatively, once the appropriate dye has been established in these small-scale experiments, the dye can be purchased and attached to an activated resin (see Table 6.1) via the reactive chloro-group.

The correct pH for binding usually lies between pH 7.0 and 8.5, and the elution of bound protein is usually achieved by increasing the salt concentration up to 1.0 M NaCl or by inclusion of an affinity displacement agent. The gel can be regenerated by washing in 2.0 M NaCl, 1.0 M NaOH or 6.0 M guanidine/HCl. If the gel is to be stored, a further two column volume wash with a buffer containing a preservative (e.g., 0.05% [w/v] sodium azide or 20% [v/v] ethanol) is required.

6.9 IMMUNOAFFINITY CHROMATOGRAPHY

6.9.1 Introduction to immunoaffinity chromatography

Immunoglobulin G (IgG) is the major class of antibody circulating in blood and lymph fluid. An antigen circulating in the blood, on binding to a B-cell surface antigen receptor with the presence of helper T-cells, initiates the B-cell to differentiate, multiply and produce antibodies to the antigen. These freshly produced circulating antibodies will coat the antigen target with antibodies, preventing the antigen from contacting any cell surfaces. They will also activate other cells to phagocytose and break down the antibody/antigen complex, as well as activating the complement system. The IgG proteins (M_r 150,000) have two identical heavy chains (M_r 50,000) and two identical light chains (M_r 25,000). The IgG "Y"-shaped conformation has two identical antigen recognition sites with the structure strengthened by covalent disulphide bonds (see Figure 6.11). An important co-translational modification on immunoglobulins is *N*-glycosylation in the endoplasmic reticulum. These sugar residues have been shown to confer pro- and anti-inflammatory properties, depending on the presence or absence of specific sugar residues.

A variety of immunoglobulins are now being produced by biotechnology companies for therapeutic, diagnostic and academic uses. Following immunisation, the antibodies raised against the antigen can be extracted from animal blood and will contain a range of IgG antibodies (polyclonal) directed against different sites on the target antigen. Alternatively, monoclonal antibodies (Mab) can be produced that interact specifically with one epitope on the antigen. The monoclonal hybridomas can be cultured indefinitely to produce the monoclonal IgG directed specifically at one epitope on the target antigen.

The purification of IgG from exsanguinated blood taken from an immunised animal or from the monoclonal cell culture supernatant can be achieved using a number of different chromatography techniques. In both cases, the specific antibody of interest will be present as a low percentage of the total protein. It has been estimated that 1 ml of monoclonal antibody culture supernatant with a protein concentration >10.0 mg ml^{-1} protein will contain only 1–10 µg ml^{-1} of the desired monoclonal antibody. The most abundant proteins in the monoclonal culture supernatant will be the albumins (up to 60% of the total protein in the culture supernatant) from the fetal calf serum (FCS) required to keep the monoclonal cell culture happy. This means that in the monoclonal cell culture supernatant, the required monoclonal antibody will be a small percentage of the total protein. The requirement to quickly concentrate and purify the target antibody will be imperative.

Antibodies produced from antisera, ascites fluid or from monoclonal cell culture supernatant can be enriched by either selecting positively for the antibody and excluding all the unwanted proteins or vice versa. Dye ligand affinity chromatography (e.g., Cibacron blue agarose; see Section 6.8) has been used to preferentially bind and remove albumins in the purification of antibodies. "Melon gel" is a proprietary resin sold by ThermoFisher

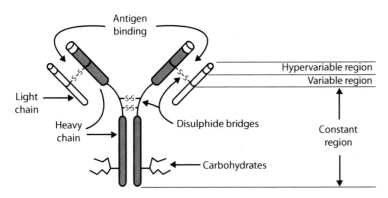

Figure 6.11 Structures of eukaryotic antibodies.

Scientific Ltd that facilitates the purification of antibodies by retaining all the non-IgG proteins (e.g., albumin and transferrin) and allowing the antibodies to flow through and be collected. The required antibodies can be purified using affinity chromatography with protein A or protein G bound to agarose or Sepharose (see Table 6.2 and Protocol 6.1). Alternatively, IgG can be purified using IEX (see Section 5.2 and Protocol 6.2) or hydrophobic charge induction chromatography (see Section 5.6).

Antibodies raised to an antigen can be species-specific for the target protein or it may show cross-reactivity with the same protein present in different species. In immunoaffinity (immunoadsorption) chromatography, the antibody, or fragment of the antibody, is bound to an activated resin (see Table 6.2) and used to select the target protein (antigen) from a complex protein mixture. Binding of the IgG via free amino groups using activated resins will randomly orient some of the antibody in a configuration that will not allow interaction with the target antigen, thus reducing the capacity of the column. Protein A (or protein G) does not bind to the IgG in the variable region, so by first binding IgG to protein A agarose (see Protocol 6.1) and then covalently cross-linking the IgG to the protein A, it is possible to construct an immunoaffinity column with all the bound IgG free to interact with the antigen in solution (IgG orientation kits from ThermoFisher Scientific Ltd). Alternatively, IgG (a glycoprotein) can be bound to an activated hydrazine resin (see Table 6.1) via its saccharide residues; this will also correctly orient the IgG to maximise the antigen-binding capacity of the immunoaffinity resin.

6.9.2   The binding and elution conditions for immunoaffinity resins

Binding conditions for immunoaffinity chromatography are usually at pH 7.0 in the presence of 0.5 M NaCl (to reduce the non-specific binding of unwanted proteins' ion exchange interactions), coupled with a slow flow rate (30 cm h^{-1}) to encourage the antibody and antigen interaction. Alternatively, the output from the column can be slowly recycled through the column input for a period of time (hrs) before washing the column to remove the unbound material (see Section 6.1.3). Low concentrations of detergents (0.05% [v/v] Tween 80 or Triton X100) can be included in the wash to improve the stringency of the wash and facilitate the removal of non-specifically bound proteins. This should be followed by extensive washing with a buffer without detergent prior to elution.

The specificity between an antibody and its antigen is high and this provides the means to extract and concentrate a target protein from a complex protein mixture. But because the specificity is high, harsh elution conditions may have to be employed to prise the target protein from the antibody complex. A low pH buffer (e.g., 0.1 M glycine/HCl, pH 2.8) is commonly used as a harsh eluent, and the target protein should elute in a sharp peak. Denaturation of the eluted protein due to the low pH can be minimised by reducing the dead volume between the column outlet and the fraction collector. The addition of a small volume of concentrated buffer (e.g., 1.0 M Tris pH 8.5) into the collection tubes will minimise the time the target protein spends in the low pH buffer. This harsh elution regime usually guarantees good recovery of protein but with reduced recovery of activity. After the bound target protein has been released from the column, the column itself should be quickly washed in a neutral pH

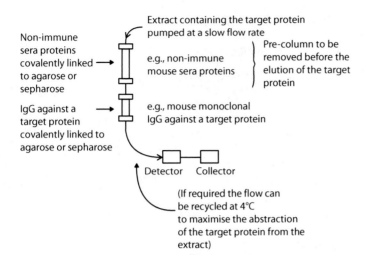

Extract containing the target protein
pumped at a slow flow rate

Non-immune
sera proteins
covalently linked
to agarose or
sepharose

e.g., non-immune
mouse sera proteins

Pre-column to be
removed before the
elution of the target
protein

IgG against a
target protein
covalently linked to
agarose or sepharose

e.g., mouse monoclonal
IgG against a target protein

Detector   Collector

(If required the flow can
be recycled at 4°C
to maximise the abstraction
of the target protein from the
extract)

Figure 6.12 The use of a non-immune serum pre-column to reduce non-specific binding to an immunoaffinity column.

buffer (to help prevent irreversible denaturation of the bound IgG) and then stored in a preservative (e.g., 0.05% [w/v] sodium azide) at 4°C.

Other methods of immunoaffinity elution that can be tried include: a high pH buffer (e.g., 1.0 M NH_4OH or 50 mM diethylamine pH 8.0–8.5); a high salt buffer (e.g., 0.1 M Tris/HCl containing 2.0 M NaCl) in the presence and absence of a detergent (e.g., 0.1–1% [w/v] SDS); a buffer containing chaotrophic salts (e.g., 0.1 M Tris/HCl containing 3.5 M $MgCl_2$, 3.0 M NaSCN or 3.0 M KSCN); denaturants (e.g., 6.0 M guanidine/HCl or 6.0 M urea); or organic solvents (e.g., 50% [v/v] ethanediol, 10% [v/v] dioxane, or 40–80% [v/v] acetonitrile). After being subjected to these elution conditions, the sample may have to be dialysed (see Protocol 4.9) or desalted (see Protocol 7.1) into an appropriate buffer to remove the components of the harsh affinity elution buffers. These harsh elution procedures will allow the target protein to be recovered and identified (SDS-PAGE and Western blotting; see Sections 8.3 and 8.5) using tryptic digestion and mass spectrometry. However, biological activity is unlikely to be recovered.

Immunoaffinity chromatography can be used early in a purification protocol because of the high specificity between the antibody and antigen. But in the early stages of a purification protocol, the peptidase enzyme activity present in a crude extract (see Section 4.4.5) may result in the hydrolysis of the ligand (antibody) bound to the resin. In addition, using the resin with crude extracts may result in an increase in the non-specific protein binding to the antibody on the resin. This can be reduced by increasing the salt concentration in the starting buffer or by passing the extract through an additional immunoaffinity column that has non-immune IgG attached to the resin prior to using the antigen-specific immunoaffinity column (see Figure 6.12).

6.9.3 Regeneration and storage of immunoaffinity resins

The resin should be washed with two column volumes of 0.1 M Tris/HCl pH 7.5 containing 2.0 M NaCl and 0.01% (v/v) Tween 80 (or Triton X100), followed by five-ten column volumes of 0.1 M Tris/HCl pH 7.5. The resin can be stored in 0.1 M Tris/HCl pH 7.5 containing 0.05% (w/v) sodium azide at 4°C.

6.10   LECTIN AFFINITY CHROMATOGRAPHY

6.10.1   Introduction to lectin affinity chromatography

Many eukaryotic proteins destined for the plasma membrane and those released from the cell into the extracellular matrix have oligosaccharides (glycoproteins) attached. The oligosaccharides may be attached co-translationally as the polypeptide is being synthesised on the rough ER (N-linked) and during the protein's progress through the endomembrane system (O-linked and GPI-linked). The oligosaccharides attached to the protein are complex branched structures built from many different saccharides.

Lectins are carbohydrate-binding proteins that were originally found in plant tissue but have subsequently been shown to be present throughout nature. They have an affinity for saccharides and will interact with the saccharide residues on the surface of glycoproteins, glycopeptides, membranes and cells. Lectins have quaternary structure (usually tetrameric) and if composed of different subunits they can bind more than one type of saccharide. There are commercial sources of lectin affinity resins (see Table 6.3) or the lectin proteins can be attached to activated affinity resins

Table 6.3 The common lectins used to fractionate glycoproteins.

Lectin	Specificity	Useful eluents	Uses
Concanavalin A from *Canavalia ensiformis* (Jack bean) (requires Mn^{2+} and Ca^{2+} for binding)	α-D-mannoside with free hydroxyl groups at C3, C4 and C6	(a) 0.01–0.5 M Methyl α-D-mannoside (b) D-mannose (c) D-glucose	Separation of glycoproteins. Binding efficiency is reduced in the presence of a detergent
Lens culinaris	Terminal-α-D-mannoside or α-D-glucoside	(a) Methyl α-D-glucoside (b) 0.15 M Methyl α-D-mannoside (c) 0.1 M sodium borate pH 6.5	Glycoproteins bind less strongly than Concanavalin A Binding takes place in the presence of 0.1% (w/v) sodium deoxycholate. Useful for the isolation of membrane glycoproteins
Tritium vulgaris	N-acetyl-D-glucosamine	0.1 M N-acetyl-D-glucosamine	Binding takes place in the presence of 0.1% (w/v) sodium deoxycholate. Purification of RNA polymerase transcription factors
Ricinus communis	α-D-galactoside	0.15 M D-galactose	
Jacalin from *Artocarpus integrifolia*	α-D-galactoside	(a) O-linked sugars 20 mM α-methyl-galactoside (b) 800 mM D-galactose	(a) Separation of O-linked sugars (b) IgA from IgG
Galanthus nivalis	Multiple α-(1-3) mannose residues	0.5 M methyl-α-D-mannoside	Mouse IgM
Mannan-binding protein Requires Ca^{2+} (part of mammalian collection family of lectins)	Terminal non-reducing sugar residues, mannose, N-acetyl-D-glucosamine GlcNAc, fucose and glucose	(a) 25 mM mannose (b) N-acetyl-D-glucosamine	Mouse IgM

Table 6.4 Protective saccharides used when coupling a lectin to a preactivated resin (see Table 6.1).

Lectin	Protective saccharide
Concanavalin A	Methyl-α-D-mannoside
L. culinaris	Methyl-α-D-mannoside
T. vulgaris	Chitin oligosaccharides
R. communis	Methyl-α-D-galactoside
Jacalin	D-galactoside

(see Table 6.1). If using an activated affinity resin, protection must be provided to the lectin's saccharide binding site on the protein by coupling the lectin to the resin in the presence of the appropriate saccharide (see Table 6.4).

6.10.2   The binding and elution conditions for lectin affinity chromatography

If the saccharide content of the target glycoprotein is not known, then a range of lectin affinity resins should be tested prior to packing the most effective resin into a column (adapt the method in Protocol 5.1). A long thin column can be used to resolve mixtures of glycoproteins and short fat columns can be used to remove unwanted glycoproteins from a protein mixture containing the target protein (non-glycoprotein). The binding of glycoproteins to lectin columns involves hydrophobic, not ionic, interactions, and this allows the sample to be applied using buffers (pH between pH 3–10) with high salt concentrations. If required, low concentrations of appropriate metal ions (see Table 6.3) should be included in the chromatographic buffers. Avoid the use of chelating agents (e.g., EDTA).

The sample can be applied at a slow flow rate and the column washed to remove the unbound proteins. Always check the later volumes of the unbound fraction, which may include glycoproteins that have had their progress down the column retarded because of a weak interaction with the resin. If this is the case, in subsequent experiments slow the flow rate and extend the column length, thus maximising the interaction between the glycoprotein and the lectin bound to the column.

Bound glycoproteins on the lectin column can be eluted isocratically or with a gradient (see Section 3.6.6.1) of the appropriate saccharide in a buffer (see Table 6.3). Altering the pH, switching to a borate buffer (which forms complexes with glycoproteins) or washing with 0–40% (v/v) ethanediol may result in the elution of active glycoproteins.

6.10.3   Regeneration and storage of lectin resins

After use, the lectin resin can be stored in a buffer (with appropriately low concentrations of metal ions, if required) in the presence of a bactericide (e.g., 0.05% [w/v] sodium azide).

Strongly bound glycoproteins can be removed using buffers containing detergents (e.g., 0–5% [w/v] SDS) in 6.0 M urea at elevated temperatures.

This will denature both the glycoprotein and the resin-bound lectin and render the lectin affinity resin to a one-use experimental material.

6.11   IMMOBILISED METAL (ION) AFFINITY CHROMATOGRAPHY (IMAC)

6.11.1   Introduction to immobilised metal affinity chromatography

In covalent bonding one atom shares an electron with another atom, satisfying both atoms' outer orbital electron requirements. In co-ordinate covalent (dative) bonding, one atom provides both electrons for another atom with a vacant orbital to share. Again, both atoms have satisfied the electron requirements for those atomic orbitals. At a physiological pH, some of the amino acids present in a protein's structure have electron-rich atoms, including: the imidazole group of histidine, the carboxylic acid residues in aspartic/glutamic acid, the thiol group of cysteine and the indole group of tryptophan. These electron-rich atoms can form co-ordinate covalent bonds with different metal ions. These metal ions include: the divalent transition metal ions Mn^{2+}, Fe^{2+}, Ni^{2+}, Co^{2+}, Cu^{2+}, Zn^{2+} Hg^{2+} and Cd^{2+}, the alkali earth metal ions Mg^{2+} and Ca^{2+} or the trivalent metal ions Fe^{3+}, Al^{3+} and Ga^{3+}. The common co-ordinate covalent valences for these metal ions are 2, 4 and 6. As shown in Figure 6.13A, the divalent metal ion (M) interacts with the tridentate iminodiacetate (IDA) attached to the resin with a co-ordinate covalent valency of 4. The same divalent metal ion (M) interacts with the quadridentate nitrilotriacetic acid (NTA) with a co-ordinate covalent valency of 6 (see Figure 6.13B).

Above pH 3.0 the carboxyl groups in the IDA or NTA are deprotonated and become electron-rich. When a metal ion is added to a buffer flowing through the IMAC resin, a co-ordinate covalent complex can form between the metal ion and the electron-rich nitrogen and carboxyl groups in the IDA and NTA attached to the resin. The metal ion is held in the complex by co-ordinate covalent bonding. Water molecules occupy the remaining co-ordinate valency sites in the complex, until they are displaced when electron-rich atoms present on the surface of a protein flow through the IMAC column.

At the physiological pH of 7.0, the nitrogen atom in position 1 of the imidazole group of histidine is electron-rich (see Table 2.1 and Table 5.1) and has the ability to form co-ordinate covalent bonds with metal ions immobilised on an IMAC resin. Other electron-rich atoms in cysteine

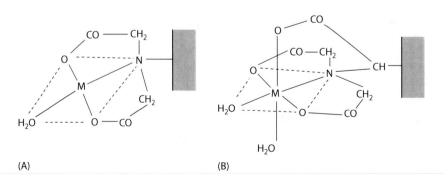

(A)   (B)

Figure 6.13 The partial structure of iminodiacetate and nitrilotriacetate bonded to a matrix.

and tryptophan can also complex with the immobilised metal ion, but histidine residues in proteins form the major complexes. Different proteins have different numbers of accessible histidine residues and these differences form the basis of IMAC chromatographic separation. At higher pH values (>9.0), selectivity is lost as the amino group on every protein's first amino acid starts to become deprotonated and electron-rich.

Examples of co-ordinate covalent bonding in biology include the retention of Fe^{2+}/Fe^{3+} ions at the centre of the porphyrin ring in haemoglobin and of Mg^{2+} ions by electron-rich nitrogen atoms in the chlorin ring of chlorophyll. Also, as many enzymes require Ca^{2+} ions for activity (described as calcium-dependent), Ca^{2+} ions are temporarily retained in discrete areas within the structure of the enzyme by the electron-rich oxygen atoms in the carboxylic acid residues from aspartic acid (e.g., the EF-hand motif see Section 2.5). In addition, the two final phosphates on nucleotide triphosphates such as ATP form a co-ordinate covalent interaction with Mg^{2+} ions (see Figure 6.14) in solution.

6.11.2   The binding and elution conditions for IMAC

After the bactericide has been removed, the IMAC resin should be washed in 5mM EDTA to remove any trace metal ions and then loaded with a solution of the metal ion of choice. Copper or nickel ions are popular choices for IMAC, with copper ions providing stronger binding (the most appropriate metal ion should be determined empirically). The metal ion binding capacity of the resin should be known (see the manufacturer's data sheet) and a concentration of metal ions should be applied to fill 75–80% of the column's metal ion binding capacity. For example: a 1.0 ml IMAC HiTrap column (GE Healthcare) has a metal ion binding capacity of 23 μmol. To achieve approximately 80% of the total capacity, apply 1.0 ml of an 18 mM solution of the chosen metal ion. This leaves the bottom 20% of the column free from metal ion and able to trap any metal ion released during the elution process. After the application of the metal ions, the column should be washed with three column volumes of distilled and deionised water, and then three column volumes of a starting buffer that is compatible with the metal ion on the column and with the target protein to be applied to the column.

As mentioned previously, protein interactions in IMAC are best achieved at neutral conditions in the absence of chelating agents. Phosphate buffers form insoluble salts at neutral pH with some metal ions and Tris buffers have chelating properties that can be used to reduce the strength of the interaction between the protein-bound histidine and the resin. All starting buffers should contain 0.5–1.0 M NaCl to reduce non-specific electrostatic interactions between the applied protein sample and the resin.

Elution is achieved by displacement at neutral pH with imidazole (0–250 mM), histidine, glycine or ammonium chloride. This can be applied as an isocratic wash or as a gradient (see Section 3.6.6.7). Alternatively, decreasing the pH (0.05–0.1 M sodium acetate buffer pH 6.0–4.0) below pH 5.6 will protonate the histidine residues on the target protein and release the histidines in the protein's structure from their interaction with the metal ion. Many proteins may denature and form precipitates as they approach their pI; for this reason elution by displacement (typically using imidazole) should be attempted first. Denaturing agents such as urea or guanidine/HCl can be included to help overcome the problem of protein precipitation. These additions can then be removed by dialysis (see Protocol 4.9) or size exclusion chromatography (see Protocol 7.1).

•Ammonium ions:

$$H_3N: \rightarrow H^+ \rightleftharpoons NH_4^+$$
$$\text{pKa } 9.24$$

•Magnesium ions (Mg^{2+} chelated by ATP):

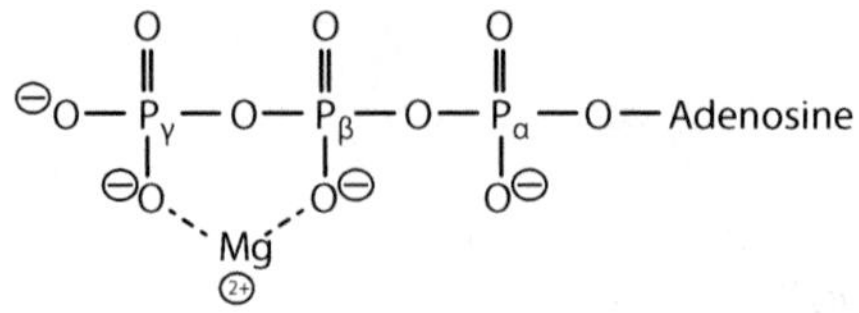

•Haem group in haemoglobin:
   (Fe^{2+})

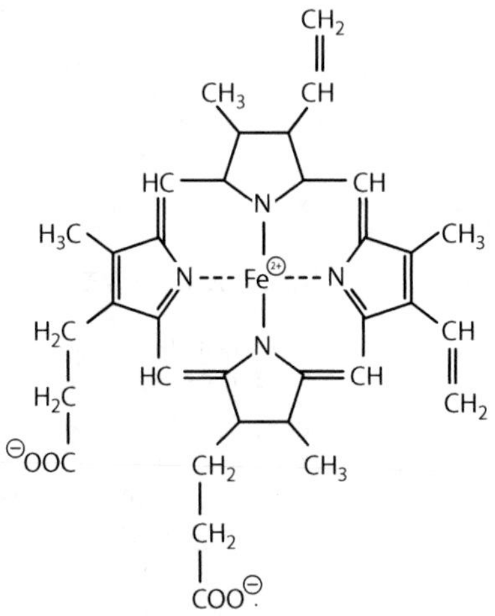

Chemical structure of the Fe(II)-protoporphyrin IX heme group in myoglobin and hemoglobin.

Magnesium ions in chlorophyll:

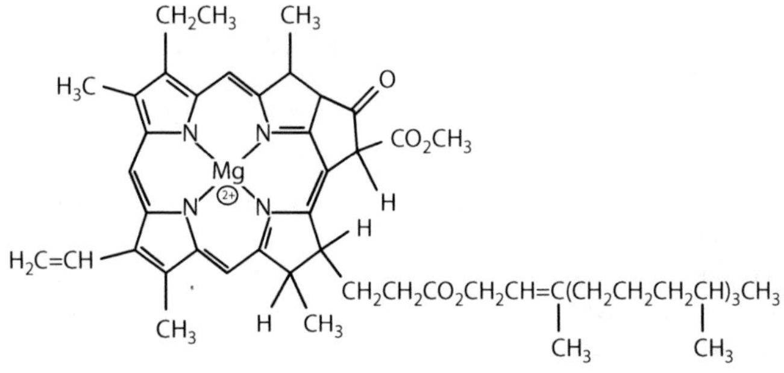

Figure 6.14 Examples of co-ordinate covalent bonding in biology.

6.11.3   The regeneration and storage of IMAC resins

After the elution of the target protein, the IMAC resin can be stripped of metal ions by a wash with 50 mM EDTA, and the resin can then be stored in 0.05% (w/v) sodium azide or 20% (v/v) ethanol.

6.12   THE PURIFICATION OF RECOMBINANT PROTEINS

6.12.1   Introduction to the purification of recombinant proteins

When affinity chromatography is used in a purification protocol with crude cell lysates, it has the necessary credentials to purify a target protein in a single chromatographic step. However, affinity chromatography resins can be expensive to design and make, and they are usually used after the target protein has been partially purified using salt precipitation (see Section 4.11.2) and IEX or HIC (see Sections 5.2 and 5.5). This is primarily because the target protein may be present at a fraction of a percent of the total protein. A partially purified preparation applied to an affinity chromatography resin would reduce non-specific interactions and be essentially free from proteolytic enzymes (important if the ligand used is a protein, e.g., IgG).

It may not be possible to purify the large amounts of protein from natural sources required for structural studies, kinetics analysis or for the production of therapeutic proteins. If the gene for the target protein is available, it is possible to incorporate it into an expression plasmid and overproduce the recombinant protein in an expression system—a prokaryotic (e.g., *Escherichia coli* [*E. coli*]), fungal (e.g., *Picchia*) or eukaryotic (e.g., yeast, insect and mammalian) cell line. The increase in total protein would in itself significantly help the purification process. But these expression systems also allow the addition of affinity components or signal sequences that greatly facilitate the target protein's purification.

The gene for the target protein can be placed into an expression vector under the control of an inducible operon (e.g., in *E. coli* the *lac* operon can be induced by isopropylthiogalactoside IPTG). In general, the N-terminus of a protein does not play a major functional role in most proteins and affinity/signal sequence additions at the N-terminus can range from a few amino acids to a complete protein (see Table 6.5). After plasmid induction and cell growth, the target protein can be recovered by cell lysis (see Sections 4.4–4.9). The target protein's N-terminal addition can be used to purify the protein by binding and elution from an affinity resin. The affinity label can then be removed to reveal a homogenous preparation of the target protein (see the examples below).

Expression of recombinant proteins in *E. coli* is popular, although the high levels of expression (up to 40% of the total cell protein) may result in the production of insoluble cytoplasmic aggregates of the target protein called **inclusion bodies**. After extraction, the inclusion bodies can be collected by centrifugation (12,000 × g for 20 min). The inclusion body aggregates will require solubilisation, purification and refolding of the protein, which will reduce the final yield. Another problem with the expression of eukaryotic proteins in a prokaryotic expression system is that the prokaryotes do not have the necessary enzymes to correctly add eukaryotic post-translational modifications (e.g., glycosylation). These post-translational modifications

Table 6.5 Examples of some fusion systems that can be used to purify recombinant proteins.

Purification Tag	M_r	Ligand	Elution
β-galactosidase	116,000	APTG (p-aminophenyl-β-D-thiogalactose)	Borate pH 10.0
Glutathione S-transferase	26,000	Glutathione	Glutathione
Chloramphenicol acetyltransferase	24,000	Chloramphenicol	Chloramphenicol
Protein A	31,000	IgG	pH 3.5
Maltose-binding protein	40,000	Amylose	Maltose
Flag peptide	Asp-Tyr-Lys-Asp-Asp-Asp-Asp-Lys	Anti-flag antibody	pH 3.5
Poly arg	$(Arginine)_5$	IEX	Salt gradient
6 His	$(Histidine)_6$	IMAC	(0-250 mM) Imidazole
Cys	$(Cysteine)_4$	Thiopropyl	2-ME or DTT

may be required for correct folding of the protein and achieving biological functionality. For post-translationally modified proteins, a eukaryotic expression system may be required.

6.12.2 The use of IMAC to purify recombinant proteins

Six consecutive histidine residues in a protein's sequence is unlikely to occur in the proteome of any cell. A sequence of six histidines placed at the N-terminus of a recombinant protein will result in it binding strongly to an IMAC resin loaded with either Cu^{2+} or Ni^{2+} ions (see Section 6.6).

Table 6.6 Cleavage peptides used in fusion proteins.

Peptide	Method	Product
N-Met-C (5)	Cyanogen bromide	N-Met and C
N-Asp-Pro-C (6)	Acid	N-Asp and Pro-C
N-Lys/Arg-C (7)	Trypsin	N-Lys/Arg and C
N-Glu/Asp-C (8)	V-8 peptidase	N-Glu/Asp and C
N-Lys-Arg-C (9)	Clostropain	N-Lys-Arg and C
N-(Lys)n/(Arg)n (10)	Carboxypeptidase B	n(Lys)/n(Arg) and N
N-Asp-Asp-Lys-C (11)	Enterokinase	N-Asp-Asp-Lys and C
Glu-Ala-Glu-C (12)	Aminopeptidase I	Glu-Ala-Glu and C
N-Ile-Glu-Gly-Arg-C (13)	Factor Xa	N-Ile-Glu-Gly-Arg and C
N-Pro-X-Gly-Pro-C (14)	Collagenase	N-Pro-X and Gly-Pro-C

The amino acid sequences above (where X indicates any amino acid) have been used infusion proteins to allow a specific hydrolysis reaction. Depending on the hydrolysis method, these cleavage peptides may be used with fusion polypeptides linked at either or both their amino and carboxy termini. These are indicated as N and C polypeptides, respectively.

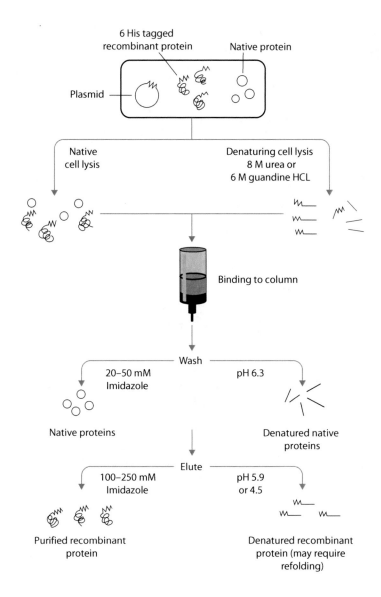

Figure 6.15 Purification of 6 His tag recombinant proteins in denaturing and non-denaturing conditions.

The presence of the 6 His tag (or His tag) may not interfere with the functionality of the target protein, but if it proves to be an issue it can be removed by the action of peptidases (Qiagen, Ltd, UK) or by the inclusion of a proteolytic cleavage sequence (see Table 6.6) after the 6 His sequence and prior to the N-terminal amino acid of the target protein. The peptide fragment can be removed from the target protein by dialysis (see Protocol 4.9) or size exclusion chromatography (see Protocol 7.1). One of the major advantages of using the 6 His affinity label to purify recombinant proteins is that the binding to IMAC can occur in the presence of detergents, which makes it a technique suitable for the purification of proteins from inclusion bodies (see above and Figure 6.15). However, trace levels of host proteins from the expression system or aggregates (dimers, etc.) can be a problem, and the use of other chromatographic techniques (IEX, HIC, RP, or SEC; see Chapters 5 and 7) may be required to drive purification to the levels required for the growth of crystals and therapeutic applications (see Section 5.5).

6.12.3   The use of fusion proteins to purify recombinant proteins

A popular method for the purification of recombinant proteins is to fuse the target protein to another protein (e.g., glutathione S-transferase, IgG or maltose binding protein) that is easy to purify by affinity chromatography. In addition, if the presence of the target protein is difficult to monitor, fusion to an enzyme (e.g., β-galactosidase; see Table 4.5) with an easy colourimetric assay can also provide a means to monitor the presence of the target protein as it is being purified. After cell lysis, the fusion protein can be purified by affinity chromatography e.g glutathione-agarose, followed by treatment with a proteolytic enzyme to cleave a sequence (see Table 6.6) spanning the protein fusion. The two proteins can then be separated

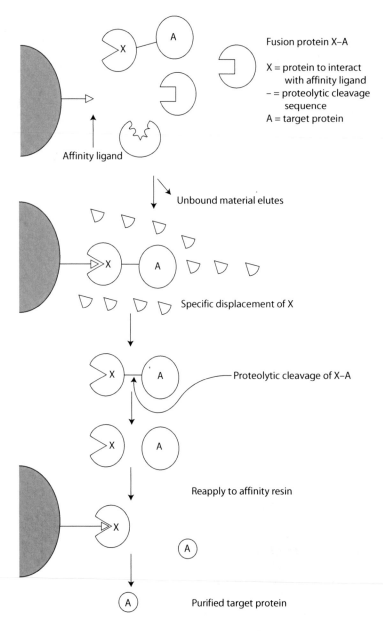

Fusion protein X–A

X = protein to interact
      with affinity ligand
– = proteolytic cleavage
      sequence
A = target protein

Affinity ligand

Unbound material elutes

Specific displacement of X

Proteolytic cleavage of X–A

Reapply to affinity resin

Purified target protein

Figure 6.16 The recovery of a target protein after production as a recombinant fusion protein.

by reapplication to the affinity resin used to isolate the fusion protein from the cell extract (see Figure 6.16).

6.13 AFFINITY PARTITIONING (PRECIPITATION)

Affinity chromatography is a separation usually conducted in a column, relying upon an interaction between a binding site on a protein and a ligand bound to a resin. The column format can have limitations, such as column fouling, when used with crude extracts, and sometimes there are slow association rates between the target protein and the resin-bound ligand due to diffusion limitations. A variation upon column-based affinity chromatography is affinity precipitation, in which the target protein binds to a ligand in free solution, resulting in the formation of a precipitate which can then be collected by centrifugation or membrane filtration.

The use of "bis" affinity ligands was developed for the purification of the tetrameric enzyme lactate dehydrogenase (LDH) using a bis-NAD^+ ligand (N_2,N'_1-adiposdihydrazido-bis-(N^6-carbonyl-methyl)-NAD^+ (see Figure 6.17). The NAD^+ molecules on the ends of the spacer arm can interact with two different LDH molecules, and the subunits on each of these molecules can be linked to other affinity ligands, forming a network that eventually becomes large enough to precipitate.

The target protein must have a quaternary structure to form a precipitable complex, and the length of the spacer arm used in the "bis" affinity ligand was found to be important in preventing **intramolecular** and encouraging **intermolecular** interactions. The specificity and strength of complex formation can be increased by the inclusion of substrate analogues of the target enzyme. The precipitate can be separated by centrifugation and the complex can be competitively displaced with high concentrations of the enzyme's substrate. These low molecular weight contaminants can then be removed by dialysis (see Protocol 4.9) or size exclusion chromatography (see Protocol 7.1).

The technique can also be used to isolate proteins that do not have a quaternary structure. In this form of affinity precipitation, multiple ligands are attached to a polymer whose solubility depends on a number of parameters. The interaction between the target protein and the ligand on the polymer does not result in precipitation. To facilitate precipitation of the protein polymer complex, the environment (e.g., pH or temperature) is altered and the precipitate can be collected by centrifugation. Examples of both techniques can be found in Table 6.7.

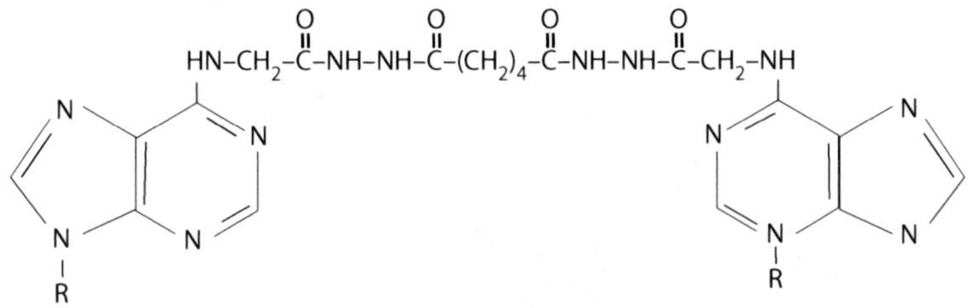

Figure 6.17 The structure of N2,N′1-adiposdihydrazido-bis-(N6-carbonyl-methyl)-NAD+.

Table 6.7 Examples of proteins purified using affinity precipitation with bis affinity ligands.

Affinity precipitatant	Protein purified
bis-Cibacron blue	LDH, albumin and chymosin
bis-ATP	Phosphofructokinase
bis-Borate	IgG
Biotin-phospholipid	Avidin and IgG
bis-Copper chelate	Human haemoglobin and galactose dehydrogenase
Copolymer of N-acryloyl-p-aminobenzoic acid and N-acryloyl-m-aminobenzamide	Trypsin (adjust the pH to below 4.0 to precipitate the complex)
Cibacron blue dextran	Lactate dehydrogenase (add Concanavalin A [see Table 4.3] to form a precipitable complex)
Protein A attached to Edragit S100 (copolymer of methyl methacrylate and methacrylic acid)	Monoclonal antibodies (adjust the pH below 4.5 to precipitate the complex)
Protein A attached to a copolymer of N-isoproplyl acrylamide and N-acryloxysuccimide	Monoclonal antibodies (adjust the temperature above 32°C to precipitate the complex)

6.14 SUMMARY

The chromatography of all components is governed by a limited number of properties (affinity, adsorption, charge, polarity, size and volatility). Unlike smaller molecules (e.g., alcohols), proteins are too big to enter the gas phase. The property of affinity has greater relevance in the chromatography of proteins because all proteins have a structure to fulfil a unique biological function. Proteins have three-dimensional biospecificity that can be exploited in chromatography to extract a target protein from a complex mixture. The design and use of affinity ligands in chromatography can be both beneficial and problematic. The advent of gene technology has allowed target proteins to be synthesised in recombinant protein systems. In addition, affinity tags can be introduced to aid the purification of the target proteins from the recombinant host proteins with an increase in yield and a decrease in the time the purification procedure requires. The resultant target protein may still contain either trace amounts of host proteins or oligomers of the target protein. This contamination can be addressed by recourse to a selection of other chromatographic or electrophoretic techniques.

PROTOCOLS FOR CHAPTER 6

Protocol 6.1 Purification of IgG using protein A agarose

There are a range of bacterial proteins (protein A, G and L) that bind selectively to different classes of mammalian immunoglobulins. They can be purchased (Thermo Fisher) in a number of different formats: native or recombinant, free or attached to agarose/acrylamide, coated on microplates or attached to magnetic beads. The bacterial proteins all bind almost entirely to IgG, but each has a slightly different selectivity for the different IgG subclasses and with the IgG from different animals. There is a recombinant protein (A/G fusion protein) that contains immuno-globulin binding sites for protein A and G, providing the best coverage for animal IgG purification. Protein L (*Peptostreptococcus magnus*) binds to the kappa light chains of immunoglobulins and can be used to purify a range of immunoglobulins (IgA, IgD, IgE, IgG and IgM) from different mammalian sources.

This protocol will also work with protein A, G or the hybrid A/G bound to a support resin (e.g., agarose or acrylamide). However, the exact conditions should be determined experimentally.

All the buffers should be prepared in ultrapure water and filtered through a 0.2 μm membrane. The sample should be centrifuged at $12,000 \times g$ for 20 mins or filtered through a 0.2 μm membrane prior to chromatography.

Required Equipment and Reagents

- Chromatographic columns and equipment
- Protein A agarose (self-made or purchased)

Method

- Remove the bactericide from the affinity resin by filtration or centrifugation.
- Suspend the protein A agarose in the start buffer 0.1 M Tris/HCl pH 8.0 containing 0.5 M NaCl (pH 5.0 for protein G and pH 7.0 for protein L).
- Add the resin to the column and wash with five column volumes of start buffer.
- Apply the sample at a relatively slow flow rate (e.g., 1.0 ml min^{-1}).
- Start to collect fractions. The unbound protein fraction should always be checked for the presence of IgG. This will confirm that the volume of protein A agarose is sufficient to bind all the IgG in the volume of sample applied to the column.
- After the sample has been applied, proceed to wash the protein A agarose with 5–10 column volumes of the start buffer or until the A_{280nm} is <0.1.
- Prior to elution, add 0.1 ml (for a 1.0 ml fraction) of 1.0M Tris/HCl pH 9.0 to the tubes in the fraction collector. This will minimise the time the eluted immunoglobulin protein spends in a low pH environment.
- Apply the eluting buffer (0.2 M glycine/HCl pH3.0) and collect fractions until the A_{280nm} reaches zero.
- Gather together the fractions containing affinity purified immunoglobulin, check that the pH is near neutral and measure the protein concentration (see Protocols 4.1–4.4) before aliquoting into suitable volumes for storage at –25°C or –80°C.

- Diluting the antibody before storage in a buffer containing 20–50% glycerol or ethanediol can help prevent damaging the immunoglobulins at low temperatures and extend their useful lifespan.
- Regenerate the column by washing with two column volumes of 1.0% (v/v) phosphoric acid pH 1.5 until the A_{280nm} reaches near zero. This will help remove unwanted protein in the sample that has bound to the protein A agarose.
- Wash the resin in the start buffer until the pH reaches 8.0.
- Wash the resin in the start buffer containing 3 M guanidine/HCl for two column volumes to help remove unwanted protein in the sample that has bound to the protein A agarose.
- Wash the resin in start buffer (5–10 column volumes) before storage in bactericide (0.05% [w/v] sodium azide or 0.1% [w/v] thiomersal) at 4°C.

Protocol 6.2 Purification of anti-transglutaminase 2 (TG2) monoclonal antibody ID10 (NTU) from a monoclonal cell culture supernatant using cation exchange chromatography

This method of purifying IgG antibodies from culture supernatant is relatively straightforward and uses SP Sepharose Fast Flow (GE Healthcare) cation exchange resin. The ion exchange resin concentrates the target immunoglobulin and the elution process is more benign than the low pH elution required for the antibodies in protein A affinity chromatography (see Protocol 6.1). The cation exchange resin has a high protein–binding capacity (>100 mg bovine serum albumin ml^{-1} of resin).

The method described was useful in the purification of Mab ID10 (NTU) and could be useful in the purification of other monoclonal antibodies with an adjustment of the pH of the starting conditions.

All the buffers should be prepared in ultrapure water and filtered through a 0.2 μm membrane. The sample should be centrifuged at 12,000 g for 20 min or filtered through a 0.2 μm membrane prior to chromatography.

Method

- Remove the 20% (v/v) ethanol preservative from the SP Sepharose cation exchange resin by filtration or centrifugation.
- Suspend the SP Sepharose resin in 0.1 M sodium acetate buffer pH 5.5 containing 0.5 M NaCl.
- Add the resin to the column and when packed wash with 5 column volumes of start buffer (0.1 M sodium acetate pH 5.5 containing 50 mM NaCl).
- The monoclonal antibody culture supernatant was diluted at least 1:4 with the start buffer prior to its application to the ion exchange resin. The sample at a flow rate of 5.0 ml min^{-1}.
- The unbound protein fractions were collected and checked for the presence of the target IgG. This will confirm that the volume of cation exchange resin is sufficient to bind all the target IgG in the diluted culture supernatant applied.
- After the sample has been applied, the column was washed with the start buffer. Fractions were collected until A$_{280nm}$ in the buffer leaving the column was <0.1.
- Apply the eluting buffer (0.1 M sodium acetate pH 5.5 containing 500 mM NaCl) and collect 1.0 ml fractions until the A$_{280nm}$ reaches zero.
- All the fractions were tested for the presence of Mab ID10 by using a 96 well micro plate coated with Guinea pig liver TG2 (gplTG2; Sigma, UK)
- The wells of the microplate were coated with 100 μl of phosphate buffered saline containing gplTG2 at 0.1 mg ml^{-1}. After 2 hr incubation at 37°C the gplTG2 was removed.
- The microplate was washed twice with phosphate buffered saline containing 0.05% (v/v) Tween-80 (PBS-Tween).
- Uncoated protein binding sites were blocked by adding 250 μl 3% (w/v) bovine serum albumin in PBS-Tween to each well. The plate was blocked at 37°C for 2 hr.
- The microplate was washed twice with phosphate buffered saline containing 0.05% (v/v) Tween-80 (PBS-Tween).
- 100 μl of each fraction from the ion exchange chromatography experiment in duplicate was added to the microplate wells, followed by 50 μl of PBS-Tween.
- The plate was incubated for 2 hr at 37°C.

- The fractions in the microplate were removed and the plate was washed twice in PBS-Tween.
- 100 μl of anti-mouse IgG secondary antibody horse radish peroxidase conjugate (2 μl in 10.0 ml of 1% [w/v] bovine serum albumin in PBS-Tween; Sigma, UK) was added to each well and the plate was incubated at 37°C for 2 hr.
- The fractions in the microplate were removed and the plate was washed twice in PBS-Tween.
- The developing solution of 0.1 M sodium acetate pH 6.0 containing 75 μl of 10 mg ml^{-1} 3,3',5,5'-Tetramethylbenzidine and 3.0 μl of hydrogen peroxide (30% [v/v] solution) was prepared.
- To each well was added 150 ml of the developing solution and the plate was incubated at room temperature for 15 min.
- The peroxidase reaction was stopped by the addition of 50 μl of 5 M H_2SO_4 and the yellow colour developed was recorded using a microplate reader set at 405$_{nm}$.
- The high salt fractions containing anti TG2 mab ID10 were pooled and the protein concentration was measured using the BCA protein assay (see Protocol 4.3) before being stored in aliquots at –25°C.
- Regenerate the column by washing with 2 column volumes of the start buffer containing 4.0 M NaCl, followed by 5 column volumes of distilled water and two column volumes of 20% (v/v) ethanol before storage at 4°C.

RECOMMENDED READING

Research papers

Arnold, F.H. (1991) Metal-affinity separations: A new dimension in protein processing. *Nat Biotechnol* 9:151-156.

Burnouf, T. and Radosevich, M. (2001) Affinity chromatography in the industrial purification of plasma proteins for therapeutic use. *J Biochem Biophys Methods* 49:575-586.

Burton, S.C. and Harding, D.R.K. (2001) Salt-independent adsorption chromatography: New broad-spectrum affinity methods for protein capture. *J Biochem Biophys Methods* 49:275-287.

Caron, M., Seve, A.P., Baldier, D. and Joubert-Caron, R. (1998) Glycoaffinity chromatography and biological recognition. *J Chromatogr B* 715:153-161.

Chaga, G.S. (2001) Twenty-five years of immobilised metal ion affinity chromatography: Past present and future. *J Biochem Biophys Methods* 49:313-334.

Firer, M.A. (2001). Efficient elution of functional proteins in affinity chromatography *J Biochem Biophys Methods* 49:433-442.

Gottschalk, I., Lagerquist, C., Zuo, S.S., Lundqvist, A. and Lundahl, P. (2002). Immobilised-biomembrane affinity chromatography for binding studies of membrane proteins. *J Chromatogr B* 768:31-40.

Hansen, S., Thiel, S., Willis, A., Holmskov, U. and Jensenius J.C. (2000). Purification and characterisation of two mannan-binding lectins from mouse serum. *J Immunol* 164:2610-2618.

Hilbrig, F. and Freitag, R. (2003). Protein purification by affinity precipitation. *J Chromatogr B* 790:79-90.

Huse, K., Bohme, H.J. and Scholz, G.H. (2002). Purification of antibodies by affinity chromatography. *J Biochem Biophys Methods* 51:217-231.

Imam-Sghiouar, N., Joubert-Caron, R. and Caron, M. (2005). Application of metal-chelate affinity chromatography to the study of the phosphoproteome. *Amino Acids* 28:105-109.

Muronetz, V.I. and Korpela, T. (2003). Isolation of antigens and antibodies by affinity chromatography. *J Chromatogr B* 790:53-66.

Raggiaschi, R., Gotto, S. and Terstappen, G.C. (2005). Phosphoproteome analysis. *Biosci Rep* 25:33-34.

Riggs, P. (2000). Expression and purification of recombinant proteins by fusion to maltose-binding protein. *Mol Biotechnol* 15:51-63.

Shen, S.Y., Lui, Y.C. and Chang, C.S. (2003). Exploiting immobilised metal affinity membranes for the isolation or purification of therapeutically relevant species. *J Chromatogr B* 797:305-315.

Zou, H., Lou, Q. and Zhou, D. (2001). Affinity membrane chromatography for the analysis and purification of proteins. *J Biochem Biophys Methods* 49:199-240.

Books

Clark, D.P. and Pazdernik, N.J. (2016). *Biotechnology.* 2nd ed. Elsevier, London, UK.

Cutler, P. (Ed.) (2004). *Protein Purification Protocols.* 2nd ed. Humana Press, New Jersey, USA.

Deutscher, M.P. (Ed.) (1990). "Guide to Protein Purification." *Methods in Enzymology*, 182. Academic Press, London, UK.

Janson J.C. and Ryden L. (Eds.) (1998). *Protein Purification.* 2nd ed. Wiley-VCH, New York, USA.

Roe, S. (Ed.) (2001). *Protein Purification: Methods.* 2nd ed. Oxford University Press, Oxford, UK.

Rosenberg I.M. (2005). *Protein Analysis and Purification.* 2nd ed. Birkhauser, Boston, Massachusetts, USA.

Non-Absorption Techniques for Purifying Proteins

7

7.1 INTRODUCTION TO SIZE EXCLUSION CHROMATOGRAPHY (SEC)

Size exclusion chromatography (SEC) is also known as gel permeation chromatography (GPC) and gel filtration chromatography (GFC). The term "GPC" is preferred for the size separation of chemical polymers in organic solvents and "SEC" or "GFC" is preferred for the separation of biological polymers (e.g., proteins and nucleic acids) in aqueous buffers, but in each case the principle of the separation process is identical. I prefer "SEC" for the separation of proteins because the term "size exclusion chromatography" includes the separation principle of the technique.

Lathe and Ruthven (1956) reported the first use of columns of starch in water to separate molecules based only on their size. Starch had the benefit of being an inert support material but included the inherent drawback of heterogeneity, which did not aid replication of the results. The starch and water columns were superseded by cross-linked dextrans, which provided an inert support with greater mechanical stability and reproducibility (Porath and Flodin 1959). Later the Swedish pharmaceutical firm Pharmacia produced "Sephadex" (**Se**paration **Pha**rmacia **Dex**tran), cross-linked dextrans suitable for the separation of peptides and proteins by SEC. The cross-linking of the dextrans could be controlled, which allowed the generation of a range of SEC resins with different pore sizes and fractionation ranges (see Table 7.1 and Figure 7.1).

Size exclusion chromatography involves the partition of molecules between two liquid volumes; the volume of the mobile phase and the accessible volume contained within the stationary porous bead (see Figure 7.1). The separation in SEC of a complex mixture of proteins is independent of the eluent used and does not involve any binding between the sample in the mobile phase and the porous stationary phase bead. The term "size" can be somewhat misleading, as it implies that the physical mass of the protein is the only factor of importance in SEC. However, we know that proteins vary in both size and shape (see Chapter 2), so a better way to view the separation process is to relate it to the hydrodynamic volume that the protein occupies. This takes into account the size and shape of the protein in relation to the volume in the porous bead that the protein can partition into as it travels down the SEC column.

Size exclusion chromatography can be used at any stage of a purification schedule because the proteins are separated in their native conformation, and there is good recovery of biological activity because there is no

Table 7.1 A selection of resins for SEC with the fractionation range for proteins.

Manufacturers/ Suppliers	Name	Material	Bead diameter μm	Protein fractionation range	pH stability
GE Healthcare	**Sephadex** range	Cross-linked dextran	20–300	1×10^2–7×10^4	2–13
GE Healthcare	**Sephacryl** range	Cross-linked dextrans and acrylamide	25–75	1×10^3–8×10^6	2–11
GE Healthcare	**Sepharose** range	Agarose	45–165	1×10^3–4×10^7	4–9
GE Healthcare	**Superdex** range	Dextran and cross-linked agarose	24–44	1×10^4–6×10^5	3–12
Bio-Rad	Bio-gel P100 fine	Acrylamide	45–90	2×10^2–1×10^5	2–10
Merk	Fractogels	Polymeric	45–90	5×10^3–1×10^5	1–14
Pall	Ultrogel	Acrylamide/agarose	60–140	1×10^3–1.2×10^6	3–10
Phenomenex	Biosep-SEC-S	Silica	5	2×10^3–3×10^6	3–7

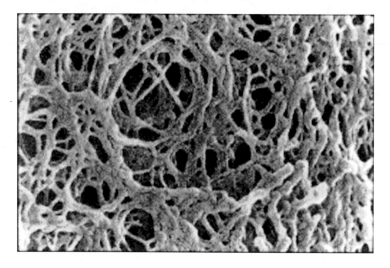

Figure 7.1 A scanning electron micrograph of a porous agarose gel.

interaction with the resin. It is the technique of choice in the biotechnology industry for rapid buffer exchanges (see Section 7.5.3). However, there are disadvantages with SEC; it will dilute the sample applied, it has low capacity for sample loading, and it shows at best moderate resolution. For these reasons SEC is usually used towards the end of a purification schedule as a technique that can gather all the desired target protein in a peak resolved from minor contamination.

7.2   THE THEORY OF SIZE EXCLUSION CHROMATOGRAPHY

The technique is described as size exclusion chromatography (SEC) because the pores within the material (see Figure 7.1) have a maximum pore size. Any component that is larger than the pore size will be excluded from entering the porous material and will travel down the column in the liquid volume surrounding the porous beads. Small molecules travel down the column in the liquid volume surrounding the porous beads as well, but they will also be able to diffuse into the volume within the porous beads. These smaller molecules can diffuse (partition) into a larger volume of the mobile phase. If a complex mixture of molecules is applied to a column containing size exclusion porous beads, they will be separated according to their size and shape (hydrodynamic volume). The larger molecules will elute first from the column and other molecules will elute in order of decreasing molecular mass.

When complex mixtures of protein molecules are applied to SEC columns (see Figure 7.2), they can effectively occupy three different volumes within the column. Depending on the fractionation range of the resin (see Table 7.1), large proteins may be totally excluded from the volume of the beads, and will elute first in the volume of liquid surrounding the beads called the void volume (V_0). If the protein molecules are small enough, they will occupy both the volume of liquid surrounding the beads (V_0) and the volume of liquid contained within the porous beads. The volume of the porous beads plus the void volume (V_0) is called the total column volume (V_t). Proteins that can occupy some (but not all) of the volume of the beads will elute in a volume (V_e = elution volume) between the two extremes of V_0 and V_t. Only the proteins eluting in a volume (V_e) between V_0 and V_t will be fractionated. This is because, depending on their mass, they will be able to occupy a lot of the volume of the beads (in which case they will elute towards V_t) or very little of the volume of the beads (in which case they will elute towards V_0) (see Figure 7.3).

An effective partition coefficient (K_{av}) can be determined for proteins fractionated using SEC.

$$K_{av} = \frac{V_e - V_0}{V_t - V_0}$$

where V_e is the elution volume of the sample of interest, V_0 is the void volume of the column, and V_t is the total volume column.

The partition coefficient K_{av} is an approximation of the true partition coefficient K_D (see Chapter 3) because ($V_t - V_0$) does not take into account the volume occupied by the cross-linked material that the porous bead is constructed from, only the volume contained within the resin. However, K_{av}

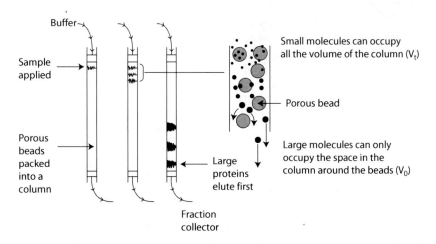

Figure 7.2 Schematic representation of size exclusion chromatography.

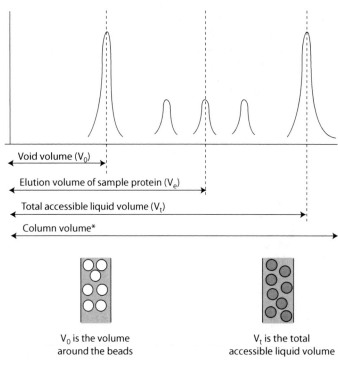

Figure 7.3 The three sample volumes that are accessible in SEC.

V_0 is the volume around the beads

V_t is the total accessible liquid volume

*Volume of the empty column. The difference between V_t and the column volume is the volume occupied by the polymers making up the beads.

is easy to measure and represents the fraction of the stationary gel volume that is available for the diffusion (partition) of a given solute species. It is a number between 0 (V_0) and 1.0 (V_t) and is effectively the percentage of the stationary gel volume occupied by the fractionated protein. The value of K_{av} is thus related to the volume the protein occupies (hydrodynamic volume), which is related to the protein's interaction with the mobile phase as well as the protein's size and shape (tertiary and/or quaternary structure; see Chapter 2). In SEC the effective partition coefficient (K_{av}) of a protein is inversely proportional to the log_{10} of the protein's relative molecular mass (M_r) (see Exercises 7.1 and 7.2).

Some proteins do not conform to the standard elution behaviour in SEC. Glycoproteins can have substantial carbohydrate additions to their protein core, and these "candelabra-like" carbohydrate structures physically impose restrictions on the available space within the porous beads into which the protein can diffuse. This means that glycoproteins will elute earlier than their amino acid sequence's M_r would suggest, giving an erroneously high M_r estimation. Performing SEC in the presence of chaotrophic salts (e.g., guanidine hydrochloride; see Chapter 2), which open up the tertiary structure of a protein and generate a random coil, leads to a more accurate determination of a protein's M_r.

If the M_r of the target protein is not known, then a resin with a broad fractionation range (e.g. Sephacryl S200) would be a good resin to choose for the first SEC experiment (see Table 7.1). If the column packing is acceptable, the column can be calibrated using proteins of known M_r or used directly for sample fractionation. A flow diagram for a typical SEC experiment is shown in Figure 7.4.

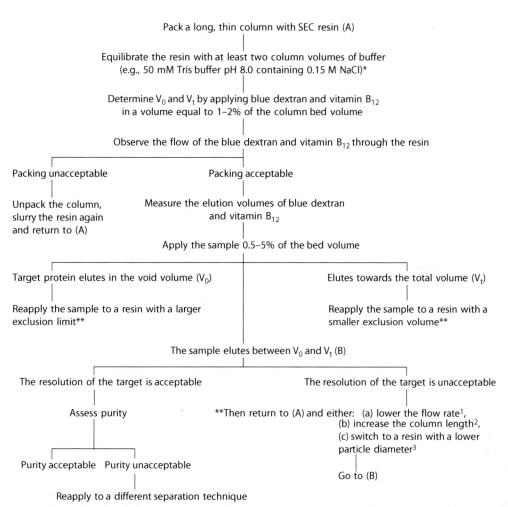

Pack a long, thin column with SEC resin (A)

Equilibrate the resin with at least two column volumes of buffer
(e.g., 50 mM Tris buffer pH 8.0 containing 0.15 M NaCl)*

Determine V_0 and V_t by applying blue dextran and vitamin B_{12}
in a volume equal to 1–2% of the column bed volume

Observe the flow of the blue dextran and vitamin B_{12} through the resin

Packing unacceptable   Packing acceptable

Unpack the column,   Measure the elution volumes of blue dextran
slurry the resin again   and vitamin B_{12}
and return to (A)

Apply the sample 0.5–5% of the bed volume

Target protein elutes in the void volume (V_0)   Elutes towards the total volume (V_t)

Reapply the sample to a resin with a larger   Reapply the sample to a resin with a
exclusion limit**   smaller exclusion volume**

The sample elutes between V_0 and V_t (B)

The resolution of the target is acceptable   The resolution of the target is unacceptable

Assess purity   **Then return to (A) and either: (a) lower the flow rate[1],
                                    (b) increase the column length[2],
                                    (c) switch to a resin with a lower
                                    particle diameter[3]

Purity acceptable   Purity unacceptable   Go to (B)

Reapply to a different separation technique

*In general the choice of resin depends on the estimated M_r of the sample. Table 5.1 provides the suppliers of different resins. A convenient starting resin might be Sephacryl S200. The choice of buffer, additives and the pH will depend on the stability of the sample. If agarose- or dextran-based resins are used a minimum of 0.15 M NaCl should be included in the equilibration buffer. If acrylamide-based resins are used the salt concentration should not be high enough to encourage hydrophobic interactions that may arise between the resin and the target protein.

**The sample may need concentrating (see Section 4.11) before (re)application to a new SEC resin.

[1]The flow rate needs to be a compromise between improved resolution and the stability of the sample.

[2]Use a longer column or connect two (or more) columns (filled with the same resin) in series. Remember that this will increase the dilution of your sample at the end of the SEC run.

[3]Before switching to a resin with a smaller bead size, check that there is a pumping system that can cope with the increased pressure requirements of smaller diameter beads.

Figure 7.4 A flowchart of the events in an SEC experiment.

7.3   FACTORS TO CONSIDER IN SIZE EXCLUSION CHROMATOGRAPHY

7.3.1   The resin

The resins used in SEC of proteins are constructed from essentially inert biocompatible material. There are many different resins to choose from with different fractionation ranges for separating complex protein samples (see Table 7.1). Try to match the fractionation range of the resin to the M_r of the target protein (if known). Many resins have been strengthened by chemical cross-linking, allowing higher flow rates without damaging the structure of the porous beads due to the increased pressure that higher flow rates generate. In addition, there are many SEC resins compatible with medium- to high-pressure pumping systems (see Chapter 3). The choice of resin depends on the application required and the budget available.

7.3.2   The bead size of the resin

In general, smaller diameter (3–15 μm) resin beads will improve the resolution (true for all chromatography). This is because as the diameter of the bead decreases, more beads can be packed into each column volume, which increases the volume available for proteins to partition into. The columns with smaller diameter beads need higher pressures to move the liquid through the column and require medium- to high-pressure pumping systems (see Section 3.7).

7.3.3   The flow rate

In SEC, long, thin columns packed with porous beads (see Table 7.1) should be used and operated at relatively slow flow rates. This will maximise the possible partition interactions between the sample in the mobile phase and the liquid in the porous beads. Flow rates are usually measured in ml min^{-1}, which is fine for individual experiments, but to compare runs of the same sample on different columns a linear flow rate is used: cm h^{-1} = ml h^{-1}/cross-sectional area of the column (cm^2). Fast flow rates in SEC may compromise the resolution of the protein mixture applied, because the sample will be quickly moved past the SEC beads, preventing any diffusion into the porous spaces of the beads (see Section 3.3.2). Too slow a flow rate, on the other hand, may result in peak broadening. Longer flow volumes improve the resolution and can be achieved by connecting smaller columns in series. Remember that the additional flow volume will increase the dilution of the eluted sample.

7.3.4   The size of the sample

The resolution in SEC depends upon the sample volume applied. A low sample volume to column volume ratio results in the best resolution. The ideal ratio needs to be determined experimentally, but in general a sample volume between 0.5–5.0% of the column bed volume should be used.

7.3.5   The sample viscosity

Sample viscosity increases as the concentration of protein increases. If the sample viscosity is higher than the viscosity of the mobile phase (more than twofold, which happens at approximately 70.0 mg ml^{-1} protein concentrations), the sample will have a reduced rate of diffusion into the accessible volume contained within the porous beads. This means that at the early stages of the chromatographic run, the sample will move past the size exclusion beads without partitioning into the volume contained within the beads. As the sample moves down the column it will be diluted in the mobile phase and the viscosity will decrease, allowing the sample proteins to move into the volume contained within the beads. This will underestimate the elution volume (V_e) for the proteins in the sample and result in erroneous estimations of the protein's relative molecular mass (M_r).

7.3.6   The composition of the buffer

All mobile phase buffers should be degassed and filtered through 0.2 µm membranes before being used in SEC. To overcome minor ion exchange interactions between the protein in the sample and the charged sulphate groups on agarose resins or charged carboxyl groups on dextrans, a minimum salt concentration of 0.15 M should be used in mobile phase buffers. The opposite may be the case when using acrylamide-based resins, as some proteins in the presence of high salt may show increased hydrophobic interactions (see Section 5.5). All eluting buffers should be set at a pH chosen to maintain the stability of the target protein and the integrity of the resin (see Table 7.1). After SEC, the protein sample can be concentrated by a number of different methods (see Section 4.11). If lyophilisation (freeze drying) is the chosen method, a volatile buffer (with no additional salt) should be used for the mobile phase (see Table 4.10).

7.4   SIZE EXCLUSION MEDIA PREPARATION AND STORAGE

Size exclusion media are supplied either pre-swollen in 20% (v/v) ethanol or as a dry powder. To use the pre-swollen resins, the preservative should be removed by filtration. The resin can then be resuspended in the desired buffer and degassed under vacuum before being packed into a column (see Chapter 3). The dry SEC powders will be swollen for use in an excess of buffer at room temperature overnight or heated in a water bath for three hours at 100°C. After allowing the gel to cool and settle, any floating material ("fines") should be poured off prior to packing into a column. If not removed, these "fines" (fragments of resin) will lodge in the pores of the beads and eventually cause problems with an increase in the back pressure.

When an SEC column has been packed and calibrated, the column can be left (with the inlet and outlet tubes blocked off) in a cold storage area after two column volumes of preservative (e.g., 20% [v/v] ethanol; see manufacturer's recommendations) have been pumped through the resin.

7.5   APPLICATIONS OF SIZE EXCLUSION CHROMATOGRAPHY

7.5.1   Analytical SEC

To determine the void (V_0) and total (V_t) volume of a packed SEC column and to assess the column packing efficiency, a solution of blue dextran (approximate M_r 2,000,000) and vitamin B_{12} (pink; M_r 1385) or potassium dichromate (yellow; M_r 294) can be used. The two coloured markers should be mixed and applied to the column in a small volume (<1% of the estimated column volume). The progress of the coloured compounds as they flow down the column can be monitored (see Figure 7.5). At the start of the calibration, the markers will visible as a dark coloured mixture at the interface

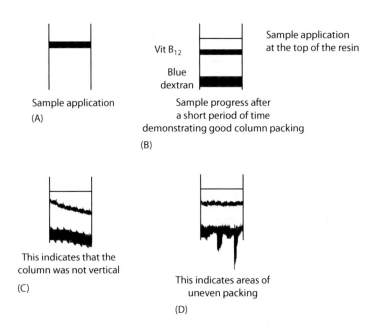

Sample application
(A)

Vit B$_{12}$

Blue
dextran

Sample application
at the top of the resin

Sample progress after
a short period of time
demonstrating good column packing
(B)

This indicates that the
column was not vertical
(C)

This indicates areas of
uneven packing
(D)

Figure 7.5 Determination of V$_0$ and V$_t$. In size exclusion chromatography at the start of the run, the sample should load as an even band (see A). When more mobile phase is added the components in the sample move down the column and separate into the quick moving larger molecules and the slower moving smaller molecules (see B). Observation of the bands as they progress down the column will provide information on the packing efficiency. Excellent packing (see B), poor alignment during packing (see C) and poor packing (see D).

between the top flow adaptor and the SEC resin (see Figure 7.5A). The flow should be set at the rate intended for the forthcoming separation of the components in the target sample, and the fraction collector should be initiated to collect the liquid flowing through the column. The coloured markers will begin to separate almost immediately, with the high molecular weight blue dextran seeming to race ahead of the low molecular weight pink vitamin B$_{12}$ (or yellow potassium dichromate). The two calibration reagents should flow down the column in level bands (see Figure 7.5B). As they progress down the column, the bands will become more diffuse (broader) because SEC will dilute any sample. Monitor the progress of the bands as they move down the column; if the bands deviate from a level band (see Figure 7.5C), the column was not vertical when the column was packed. Occasionally, you may notice fast-running areas of the band as it progresses down the column (see Figure 7.5D). This will indicate that the chromatography resin was not packed uniformly. Either of these packing errors will result in flow distortion of an applied sample, giving asymmetrical peaks as the sample elutes from the bottom of the column. To rectify these problems, the column can be repacked or, if the distortion is near the inlet (or outlet) of the column, the flow adaptor can be removed and the resin bed disturbed with a glass rod and additional buffer. The disturbed resin can be allowed to settle before reinserting the flow adaptor and running the column at the required flow rate. The determination of V$_0$ and V$_t$ using the coloured reagents should be repeated.

The elution volume of blue dextran and vitamin B$_{12}$ (or potassium dichromate) is from the midpoint of the sample volume application to the midpoint of the elution volume (see Figure 7.3). If the packing is judged to be workable, the column can then be calibrated by the application of a series of standard proteins of known M$_r$. The elution volumes (V$_e$) of these proteins can be measured, and their K$_{av}$'s can be determined and used to construct a calibration plot for the column (see Exercise 7.1). The K$_{av}$'s of the standard proteins will be plotted against their log$_{10}$ M$_r$. When a protein sample is applied to the same column, the elution volume (V$_e$) can be measured for the sample and the K$_{av}$ for the target protein can be determined. Using the K$_{av}$ for the sample protein and the calibration plot for the column, the target protein's

M_r can be estimated (see Exercises 7.1 and 7.2). It is important to remember that the sample protein will flow down the column in its native conformation and that the estimation of the sample's M_r will reflect this (see Exercise 7.1).

7.5.2   Separation of aggregates or removal of low amounts of contaminating material by size exclusion chromatography

After completing separations based upon a protein's surface charge (see Section 5.2), biospecificity (see Chapter 6) and hydrophobicity (see Section 5.5), there may be still low levels of contaminating protein present in the sample, as visualised by SDS-PAGE of the putative final sample of the target protein. These trace levels of contamination can arise from a number of sources. They may be trace amounts of genuine host proteins that have co-purified with the target protein (perhaps by "piggy backing" on the target protein), unfolded aggregates (either soluble or insoluble) of the target protein or a combination of both host and target protein aggregates.

Proteins in solution will be an equilibrium mixture of folded and partially unfolded structures, the extent of which will be determined by factors such as the protein concentration, temperature, shear forces and pH. Normally the unfolded structures will refold into their native conformation, but sometimes an unfolded structure will attach to another unfolded structure and start to form an aggregate. Proteins modified by partial proteolysis, glycation, oxidation and deamidation during storage or through a purification procedure have a tendency to form aggregates. The formation of aggregates can be problem for most protein researchers, but it is a problem that needs to be addressed in the purification and storage of therapeutic proteins. For example, the presence of aggregates in an injectable solution of humanised immunoglobulins may result in adverse reactions in the recipient patients.

Size exclusion chromatography, a separation technique based upon the molecular mass of proteins, has been used successfully to monitor and remove low levels of contaminating proteins and aggregates (see Figure 7.6). A chromatographic run using a SEC resin will have the benefit of separating the target protein from other proteins with a different size and shape as well as from any dimers and oligomers of the target protein. The disadvantage of using SEC for aggregate detection is that it may hide any insoluble aggregates in the sample, which will tend to lodge within the pores of the SEC resin as the sample progresses down the column. Soluble aggregates with a propensity to bind to or interact with the SEC resin will also not emerge from the column, giving the sample an incorrect clear bill of health.

To help establish that therapeutic proteins do not contain aggregates, additional methods can be used to demonstrate the homogeneity of a

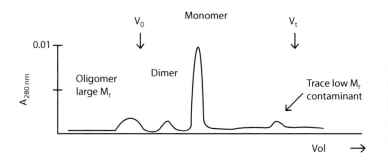

Figure 7.6 Size exclusion chromatography of a purified protein solution demonstrating the presence of the required monomer and contaminating oligomeric, dimeric and low molecular weight material.

protein sample. Electrophoresis in denaturing (see Section 8.3.4) and non-denaturing conditions (see Section 8.3.5) as well as capillary electrophoresis (see Section 8.6), reversed-phase chromatography (see Section 8.7), dynamic light scattering detectors (see Section 7.6) analytical ultracentrifugation and mass spectrometry can be useful additional methods to help determine the purity of a therapeutic protein sample. The methods listed above separate proteins based upon different principles (orthogonal analysis), and more than one method is required to establish that the sample is free from extraneous material (FDA Biosimilarity Guidance 2015).

7.5.3   Desalting (group separation)

At different stages in a purification protocol, a change of sample buffer may be required prior to the sample's application to another resin or prior to electrophoresis. The exchange of buffer ions can be achieved by dialysis (see Protocol 4.9), but the process is time-consuming. An alternative to dialysis is performing SEC using resins with a small pore size, which totally exclude the proteins in the applied sample from the porous space within the resin beads (see Protocol 7.1). The smaller ($M_r < 1500$) buffer or metal ions are totally included in the porous space within the beads. Sephadex G-25, or G-50 (GE Healthcare, UK) and Biogels P-6 or P-10 (Bio-Rad) resins can be used for desalting (or pre-packed columns of G-50 (PD-10) can be purchased (GE Healthcare, UK)). The pre-swollen resin (see Section 7.4) can be packed into a syringe with glass wool at the base (see Figure 3.7) (to prevent the resin leaving the column) and equilibrated with the buffer into which the protein sample will be exchanged. The sample in the original buffer that is no longer required is applied to the resin (sample volume:SEC resin volume ratio should be no less than 1:5) and fractions are collected. The protein will elute early, because it is excluded from the resin but it will now be in the new buffer; the buffer ions that are not required will elute later. Desalting requires significantly less time than dialysis and is favoured in the biotech industry for buffer exchange. Dilution of the sample with SEC porous beads will take place in both dialysis and desalting.

7.5.4   Refolding of denatured proteins

Prokaryotic protein expression systems will not have the necessary chaperones to correctly fold many eukaryotic proteins into their correct tertiary structure (see Chapter 2 for the protein structure and Section 6.12 for recombinant protein purification). Proteins that have been expressed in *E. coli*, for example, may form cytoplasmic aggregates called inclusion bodies. Extracting the expressed recombinant proteins from the inclusion bodies will require the use of chaotropic salts (e.g., urea) and detergents (e.g., SDS). After extraction, the solubilising agents will have to be removed to allow the proteins to fold into their correct conformation. The reduced diffusion in SEC has been used to promote the correct refolding of proteins by suppressing nonspecific protein-to-protein interactions. In addition, during SEC the high molecular weight aggregates and the buffers used for solubilising the inclusion bodies are removed in a single experiment.

7.6   DYNAMIC LIGHT SCATTERING

In recent years dynamic light scattering (DLS), also known as quasi-elastic light scattering (QELS), has been used to assess the size of chemical and biological polymers in solution. The technique is based upon the variations in light intensity as particles move in solution due to Brownian motion in a short time scale (0.1 μsec to 0.1 sec). Larger polymers move more slowly in solution due to frictional forces; therefore, variations in the light scattering over time will be related to a protein's radius. The DLS detectors provide a measure of the protein's radius or hydrodynamic diameter, but not the protein's relative molecular mass (M_r). To convert the hydrodynamic radius into a molecular weight estimation requires the Mark–Houwink equation and consideration of the viscosity of the buffer used in the experiment at the different temperatures at which measurements are made (Masuelli, 2014).

Dynamic light scattering instruments can be used to monitor the outflow from a SEC column, providing the means to obtain direct measurements of the protein sample's relative molecular mass (M_r) and any contaminants. Dynamic light scattering coupled with ultra-high pressure liquid chromatography (UHPLC) SEC (see Section 8.8) provides a rapid method of detecting contaminants in a protein sample, which can be useful in the biotechnology industry (see Section 7.5.2).

7.7   SUMMARY

Of all the techniques covered in this book, size exclusion chromatography most closely matches the definition of chromatography (i.e., a partition (or distribution) between two immiscible phases (see Section 3.2). The easy-to-calculate distribution K_{av} approximates closely the distribution coefficient K_D. Understanding the separation of molecules in size exclusion chromatography provides a path to understanding other forms of chromatography where the distribution between the two immiscible phases (the mobile and stationary phase) is not as clear. As useful as SEC is in providing insight into the mechanism of chromatography, its use in protein purification is limited. The technique is limited by medium to low resolution of the sample components, the small sample volumes that can be ideally applied and the fact that it dilutes the sample during its path through the chromatography resin. For these reasons, it is usually used towards the end of the purification schedule to remove trace amounts of contaminating proteins and any aggregates that may have formed. The one exception is in the purification of membrane proteins (see Sections 4.4.10 and 6.10). The other area that SEC excels in is rapid buffer exchange, as an alternative to the effective but time-consuming dialysis technique.

EXERCISE 7.1 PRACTISE CALCULATIONS FOR M_r ESTIMATION USING SIZE EXCLUSION CHROMATOGRAPHY (SEC)

A gel filtration column ($V_0 = 85$ ml and $V_t = 250$ ml) has been calibrated with five standard proteins of known molecular mass (M_r).

Standards	M_r	$Log_{10} M_r$	V_e(ml)	K_{av}
Aprotinin	6,500		215	
Trypsinogen	24,000		187	
Bovine serum albumin	66,000		150	
Alcohol dehydrogenase	150,000		103	
Amylase	200,000		94	

Calculate the K_{av} for the standard proteins and plot a calibration graph for the column ($Log_{10} M_r$ v K_{av}).

Using the same column the V_e for egg albumin was 135 ml.

Determine the K_{av} for egg albumin and using the calibration graph estimate the M_r of egg albumin.

- See Appendix 6 for the solution to these problems.

EXERCISE 7.2 THE DIFFERENCE BETWEEN ESTIMATING THE M_r OF A PROTEIN USING SEC AND SDS-PAGE (SEE CHAPTER 8 AND EXERCISE 8.1)

When a sample of haemoglobin and myoglobin are applied to a 10% SDS-PAGE gel both proteins produced a single band with a estimated M_r of 16,000.

When the samples were subjected to SEC, haemoglobin had an M_r of 64,000 and myoglobin an M_r of 16,000.

Please explain the difference between the result obtained by SDS-PAGE and SEC

- See Appendix 6 for the solution to these problems.

PROTOCOL FOR CHAPTER 7

Protocol 7.1 Desalting: The exchange of buffer ions in a protein sample using size exclusion chromatography

Size exclusion chromatography (SEC) is a rapid alternative to dialysis (see Protocol 4.9) in the removal of a high concentration of ions from a protein sample, e.g., to reduce or remove the high NaCl concentration after elution from an ion exchange experiment. The same procedure of desalting could be employed to exchange the buffer ions in a protein solution into different buffer ions for an assay, e.g., to exchange a phosphate buffer for a Tris/HCl buffer to avoid problems in the assay of a calcium dependent enzyme.

The technique is straightforward and can be undertaken using inexpensive materials. The low M_r exclusion limit of the size exclusion resins (e.g., G25 >1500) excludes proteins from the space within the resin beads. The ions in the protein sample are small enough to percolate into the space within the beads. The result is the protein elutes from the column first away from the buffer and salt ions it had previously been dissolved in. If the volume of SEC resin to the volume of sample is maintained in a ratio of 5:1, the result will be a complete exchange of the buffer ions in the protein sample. Normal SEC will also exchange the buffer ions in a sample and provide medium to low resolution of the components in a sample over a longer time period.

Requirements (see Section 3.6.1 and Figure 3.7) to exchange the 50 mM phosphate buffer pH 7.4 in a protein sample for 50 mM Tris/HCl ions:

- Pre-swollen G25 or G50 Sephadex (GE Healthcare, Ltd) or Biogel-P6 (Bio-Rad, UK)
- 5.0 ml syringe
- A small ball of glass wool
- Rubber tubing to fit to the end of the syringe and a clip to arrest the flow
- Microfuge tubes in a rack

The G25 Sephadex can be swollen for use by incubation in 50 mM Tris/HCl pH 7.5 buffer overnight at 4°C.

- Compress the ball of glass wool into the syringe to provide support for the G25 Sephadex.
- Load 5.0 ml of Sephadex G25 into the syringe until all the resin has been packed. The buffer running through can be allowed to go to waste.

- Wash the column with 10.0 ml of 50 mM Tris/HCl pH 7.5 (2 column volumes).
- Arrange the microfuge tubes in a rack.
- Allow the liquid in the G25 column to reach the surface of the G-25 resin, then arrest the flow.
- Carefully layer the 1.0 ml of sample (in 50 mM phosphate buffer pH 7.4) onto the surface of the resin.
- Allow the sample to flow onto the G25 Sephadex until the liquid reaches the top of the resin, then arrest the flow. As the sample flows into the column, start to collect the liquid emerging from the syringe in 0.5–1.0 ml fractions.
- Carefully add 5.0 ml of 50 mM Tris/HCl pH 7.5 to the top of the column and run this onto the column.
- Collect fractions throughout the run.

Measuring the $A_{280 \text{ nm}}$ (see Protocol 4.1) or using a protein assay (see Protocols 4.2–4.4) will confirm that the protein elutes in the early fractions.

The BCA or Coomassie Blue dye binding protein assay can be truncated to provide a qualitative assay by adding 50 µl of the fractions to the wells of a 96 well plate and also adding 50 µl of the standard working reagent for either protein assay.

A change of colour will quickly reveal the fractions containing protein.

A phosphate assay (e.g., the molybdate assay) will confirm that the target protein is free from phosphate buffer ions.

The protein fractions can be pooled and subjected to a quantitative protein assay.

It should be remembered that exchanging of ions using SEC or dialysis will increase the final volume that the target protein is dissolved in.

RECOMMENDED READING

Research papers

Batas, B. and Chaudhuri, J.B. (1995) Protein refolding at high concentration using size-exclusion chromatography. *Biotechnol Bioeng* 50:16-23.

De Bernardez Clark, E. (2001) Protein refolding for industrial processes. *Curr Opin Biotechnol* 12:202-207.

Goetz H., Kuschel, M., Wulff, T., Sauber, C., Miller, C., Fisher, S. and Woodward, C. (2004) Comparison of selective techniques for protein sizing, quantitation and molecular weight determination. *J Biochem Biophys Methods* 60:281-293.

Lathe, G.H. and Ruthven, C.R.J. (1956) The Separation of Substance and Estimation of their Relative Molecular Sizes by the use of Columns of Starch in Water. *Biochem J* 2:665-674.

Li, M., Su, Z.G. and Janson, J.C. (2004) In vitro protein refolding by chromatographic procedures. *Protein expr purif* 33:1-10.

Masuelli, M.S. (2014) Mark-Houwink parameters for aqueous-soluble polymers and biopolymers at various temperatures. *J Polymer Biopolymer Phys Chem* 2:37-43.

Porath, J. and Flodin, P. (1959) Gel filtration: a method for desalting and group separation. *Nature* 183:1657-1659.

Wang S., Chang, C. and Liu, H. (2006) Step change of mobile phase flow rates to enhance protein folding in size exclusion chromatography. *Biochem Eng J* 29:2-11.

Wen, J., Arakawa, T. and Philo, J.S. (1996) Size-Exclusion Chromatography with On-Line Light-Scattering, Absorbance, and Refractive Index Detectors for Studying Proteins and Their Interactions. *Anal Biochem* 240:155-166.

Books

Cutler, P. (Ed.) (2004) *Protein Purification Protocols*. 2nd ed. Humana Press, New Jersey, USA.

Deutscher, M.P. (Ed.) (1990) "Guide to Protein Purification." *Methods in Enzymology*, 182. Academic Press, London, UK.

Roe, S. (Ed.) (2001) *Protein Purification: Methods*. 2nd ed. Oxford University Press, Oxford, UK.

Rosenberg, I.M. (2005) *Protein Analysis and Purification*. 2nd ed. Birkhauser, Boston, USA.

Sahin, E. and Roberts, C.J. (2012) "Size exclusion chromatography with multi angle light scattering for elucidating protein aggregation mechanisms." *Therapeutic Proteins*. Springer Verlag, New York, USA.

Striegel, A., Yau, W.W., Kirkland, J.J. and Bly, D.D. (2006) *Modern Size Exclusion Liquid Chromatography: Practice of Gel Permeation and Gel Filtration Chromatography*. 2nd ed. Wiley, New Jersey, USA.

Mori, S. and Barth, H.G. (2013) *Size Exclusion Chromatography*. Springer Verlag, New York, USA.

Pasch, H. and Trathnigg, B. (2013) "Multi-detector size exclusion chromatography." *Multidimensional HPLC of Polymers*. Springer Verlag, New York, USA.

Wu, C.S. (Ed.) (2004) *Handbook of Size Exclusion Chromatography and Related Techniques*. 2nd ed. Marcel Dekker, New York, USA.

Web page

FDA Biosimilarity Guidance (2015). http://www.fda.gov/downloads/drugs /guidancecomplianceregulatoryinformation/guidances/ucm291134.pdf.

Methods for Monitoring the Purity of Protein Solutions

8

8.1 INTRODUCTION

In the previous seven chapters, we looked at how proteins/peptides may be extracted and purified using chromatographic methods. In all of these processes, the purity of the extracted protein relative to the total extract needs to be assessed. An integral part of the protein purification process is analysing the results of each chromatography experiment and making informed decisions about the next step in the protocol. Quality control checks are necessary to both assess the efficacy of the technique used and to determine an appropriate stage to call a halt to the procedures.

8.2 QUALITY CONTROL: INFORMATION FOR A PROTEIN PURIFICATION BALANCE SHEET

A protein purification balance sheet provides the data necessary to measure both the value of the chromatography run that has been performed and the overall effectiveness of the purification schedule. It records information on the volume of the pooled active fractions, the protein concentration and the activity relative to the amount of protein present (specific activity). It also provides data on the yield (% recovery [i.e., how much remains after a chromatographic technique compared to the amount present in the starting material]) and the degree (fold) of purification (a measure of the increase in specific activity after the chromatographic procedure).

The following calculations are required to complete a protein purification balance sheet. An example calculation can be found in Exercise 8.1.

The activity and total protein in the initial (crude) extraction (step 1) represents the maximal amount of activity that can be worked with during the purification schedule. The percent yield of the target protein in the crude extract is 100% and the fold purity is one. Therefore, the percent yield and the degree of purification in subsequent steps are relative to the activity and total protein determined in the initial extract. In an ideal world, during the purification the percent yield of the target protein will remain close to 100% and the degree of purification will increase rapidly. However, biologically active protein is lost at every step of the purification (see Section 3.5) and more rapidly during the later stages. It can be common to find an increase in the percent yield (i.e., >100%) in the purification step following the initial extraction. This may be due to conflicting enzyme activities or the presence of inhibitors in the initial extract that are removed during the first purification step. The net outcome is an underestimation of the total activity in the initial extract and not a cause for concern.

- Specific activity (SA) $= \dfrac{\text{units of enzyme activity ml}^{-1} \text{ of extract}}{\text{protein concentration (mg ml}^{-1})}$

  $= \text{units mg}^{-1}$ protein
- Total protein (TP) = protein concentration (mg ml^{-1}) × volume of extract or combined fraction (ml)

  $= \text{mg protein}$
- Total activity (TA) = units mg^{-1} protein × total protein (TP) or units ml^{-1} × total extract volume (ml)

  $= \text{units}$
- Degree of purification (Fold Purity) = SA step 2/SA step 1
- Yield (% recovery) = TA step 2/TA step 1 × 100

  Note:
- At every stage in the purification there is a loss of activity (see Figure 3.4).
- From Table 8.1 the ion exchange procedure typically produces a tenfold increase in specific activity with good yield (see Section 5.1).
- In Table 8.1 the highest increase in specific activity was recorded using affinity chromatography, which also produced the greatest loss of total activity. This possibly reflects the harsh elution condition that have to be employed to break the strong interaction between the protein and the affinity ligand or antibody (see Section 6.4).
- Size exclusion chromatography (see Table 8.1) produces a small increase in specific activity with little loss of yield, but it does dilute the sample. Another run on a small ion exchange column (e.g., Uno Q anion exchange polishing column, Bio-Rad, UK) could be used to quickly concentrate the sample (alternative procedures are discussed in Section 4.11).

Throughout the purification process the purity of the pooled target protein fraction should be monitored regularly. Denaturing polyacrylamide

Table 8.1 An example of a purification table for a hypothetical enzyme (the volume, protein concentration and enzyme activity were recorded after each chromatographic procedure).

Purification procedure	Vol (ml)	Protein concentration (mg ml⁻¹)	Total protein (mg)	Specific activity (units mg⁻¹)	Total activity	Fold purity	% Yield
Step 1. Crude homogenate after clarification	1500	12.0	18,000	1.1	20,000	1	100
Step 2. Ammonium sulphate precipitation 40–60% (sat)	550	11.0	6050	2.8	16,940	2.5	84.7
Step 3. Anion exchange chromatography	125	4.5	562	25.6	14,387	23.3	71.9
Step 4. Affinity chromatography	10	1.1	11.0	411.8	4530	374.4	22.6
Step 5. Size exclusion chromatography	15	0.35	5.25	826.7	4340	751.5	21.7

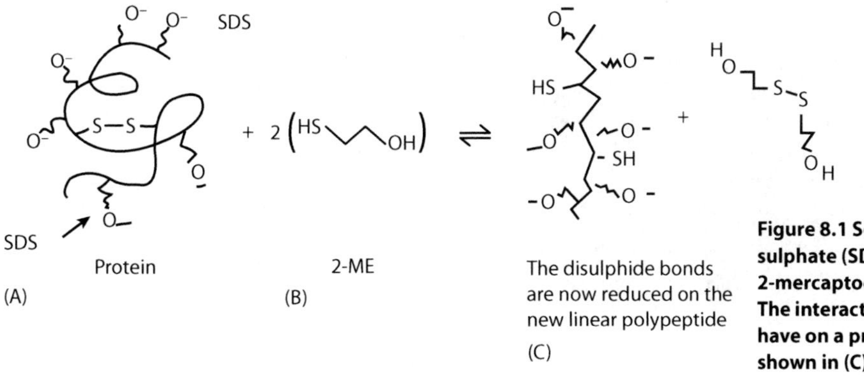

(A)

Protein

SDS

(B)

2-ME

(C)

The disulphide bonds are now reduced on the new linear polypeptide

Figure 8.1 Sodium dodecyl sulphate (SDS) (A) and 2-mercaptoethanol (2-ME) (B). The interaction these molecules have on a protein's structure is shown in (C).

gel electrophoresis (PAGE) is the most popular visually accessible technique used to monitor the purity of the pooled protein fractions. This technique denatures globular proteins into linear polypeptides using the detergent sodium dodecyl sulphate (SDS) and a reducing agent (e.g., 2-ME; 2-mercaptoethanol) (see Figure 8.1). The polypeptides are separated according to their relative molecular mass (M_r). A single band on an SDS-PAGE gel is a good indication of a homogeneous preparation of protein. However, because SDS-PAGE separates polypeptides on their M_r, a single band does not rule out the possibility that there are other polypeptides present in the sample with the same M_r. To verify the homogeneity of the protein preparation, alternative methods can be used in combination with denaturing SDS-PAGE. These supplementary techniques must exploit a physical parameter other than the molecular mass of polypeptides to increase the stringency of the analysis. For example, PAGE in the absence of a detergent (non-denaturing PAGE) will separate proteins according to both their hydrodynamic volume (related to M_r) and surface charge at a high pH. A homogeneous band on both denaturing and non-denaturing PAGE is a better indication of the purity of the protein fraction. Other techniques that exploit different properties of proteins include: isoelectric focusing (IEF), capillary electrophoresis (CE), analytical SEC or reversed-phase chromatography (RPC). Mass spectrometry could be utilised in combination with several of these techniques to help determine the purity of the fraction.

Another problem with SDS-PAGE is that the presence of low amounts of contaminating polypeptides with different M_r's may not be obvious with low sample loadings. To overcome this problem, it is possible to load a denaturing polyacrylamide gel with increasing amounts of the "homogeneous" protein. At the higher loadings, the presence of low levels of contaminating proteins should be visible. The alternative is to switch to a more sensitive protein stain, such as a silver stain or imidazole (see Protocols 8.5–8.7).

8.3   THE THEORY OF ELECTROPHORESIS

Charged molecules will move under the influence of an electrical field to an electrode of opposite charge. Anions (negatively charged molecules) will move to the anode (positively charged electrode), whereas cations (positively charged molecules) will move to the cathode (negatively charged electrode). In electrolysis the charged molecules move under the influence of an electrical field and may contact the electrode. Biological molecules would denature if they were allowed to contact an electrode. So, when biological molecules are subjected to movement in an electrical field, the experiment is terminated before the sample contacts the electrode. This process is termed "electrophoresis" and can be viewed as incomplete electrolysis.

In an electrical field, a charged molecule is subjected to both a propelling force determined by the field strength and charge on the molecule, and a retarding force determined by the size and shape of the molecule and the viscosity of the medium.

If two electrodes with a potential difference (v) of 100 volts are placed in a solution 0.1 m (10 cm) apart (l), the field strength

$$(E) = v/l = 100/0.1 = 1000 \text{ v m}^{-1}$$

If the net charge on a molecule is q coulombs, the propelling force on the molecule

$$(F) = E.q. = v/l.q \text{ newtons} \tag{8.1}$$

In solution, the retarding force on a molecule is comprised of friction and drag influenced by the size and shape of the molecule and the viscosity of the medium.

$$\text{The retarding force } (F) = 6\pi r \eta v \tag{8.2}$$

where F = drag force, r = radius of a spherical molecule, η = viscosity of the medium, v = velocity of the molecule.

The overall rate of migration, taking into account both the propelling force contributed by the field strength and charge on the molecule (Equation 8.1) and retarding force contributed by the size of the molecule and the viscosity of the medium (Equation 8.2), is given by:

$$E.q = 6\pi r \eta v$$
$$v = \frac{E.q.}{6\pi r \eta}$$

The movement of a charged molecule under the influence of an electrical field is proportional to the field strength and the charge on the molecule, but inversely proportional to the size/shape of the molecule and the viscosity of the medium.

To increase the net rate of movement of a charged molecule in an electrical field, it is possible to either reduce the viscosity of the medium or increase the field strength. In practise, increasing the field strength is the only sensible option; the drawback is that high field strengths generate heat, which can be damaging to a protein's structure. Some electrophoresis devices can be fitted with cooling setups to disperse the heat generated when the voltage is switched on. This is particularly important in non-denaturing PAGE, when biological activity is being measured *in situ* (see Section 8.3.5).

Proteins are derived from different genes, and thus have a different content of amino acids. This means they have different masses, fold into different three-dimensional shapes and are covered in different surface charges. The charge on a protein's surface is pH-dependent (see Section 1.5 in Chapter 1).

At a certain point on the pH scale, the overall charge on a protein's surface is zero. This is termed the isoelectric point (pI). When a protein is dissolved in a buffer at its pI, the protein will not move under the influence of an electrical field. At pH values above its pI, a protein will behave as an anion and at pH values below its pI, a protein will behave as a cation. (This is analogous to the requirements for a protein to bind to an oppositely charged ion exchange chromatography resin; see Section 5.5 in Chapter 5.)

8.3.1   Polyacrylamide gel electrophoresis (PAGE) of proteins

Electrophoresis using polyacrylamide is a popular method of analysing protein mixtures because the technique is both reproducible and flexible. The polyacrylamide gels are formed by the polymerisation of acrylamide monomers in the presence of the N,N′-methylene bis-polyacrylamide, which acts as the cross-linking reagent. The reaction is **free radical** catalysis, thus following initiation there is a period of polymer elongation and then termination.

Two catalysts are required to initiate the polymerisation of polyacrylamide: N,N,N′,N′-tetramethylenediamine (TEMED) and ammonium persulphate. The TEMED catalyses the decomposition of the persulphate ion to produce a free radical (indicated by the symbol * in the diagrams below).

$$S_2O_8^{2-} + e^- \rightarrow SO_4^{2-} + SO_4^{-*}$$

The reactive free radical (SO_4^{-*}) interacts with the acrylamide monomer, generating an acrylamide free radical that reacts with another acrylamide monomer, sequentially adding monomers to the free radical end to form a polymer. Occasionally the bis-polyacrylamide is added into the growing polyacrylamide chain, linking adjacent polyacrylamide chains together. Eventually, when all the monomers have been used up, two free radicals interact to terminate the polymerisation. The result is a solid polyacrylamide gel that is comprised of a porous network of cross-linked polyacrylamide polymers (see Figure 8.2).

This continues with monomer additions to build a large linear polymer. Occasionally, at random, the bis-polyacrylamide is added to cross-link adjacent chains.

The cross-linked chains can add more monomers or more cross-linkers to eventually produce the tangled mesh of polyacrylamide's porous network.

Figure 8.2 Diagram to show how the polyacrylamide network is built (FR is the free radical, acryl is the polyacrylamide monomer and ACRYL-ACRYL is the bis polyacrylamide cross-linking agent).

$$FR^* + Acryl \longrightarrow FRAcryl^*$$

$$FRAcryl^* + Acryl \longrightarrow FRAcrylAcryl^* \ etc$$

$$FRacrylacrylacryl^* \ + \ ACRYL \ \rightarrow \ FRacrylacrylacrylACRYL^*$$
$$| \qquad\qquad\qquad\qquad\qquad |$$
$$FRacrylacrylacryl^* \ + \ ACRYL \ \rightarrow \ FRacrylacrylacrylACRYL^*$$

Gels with different percentages of polyacrylamide can be cast to alter the fractionating properties of the gel. A polyacrylamide gel of 18% can be used to detect peptides as small as M_r 1000 (approximately 10 amino acids), a 5% polyacrylamide gel will fractionate proteins in the mass range 60,000 to 350,000 and a 10% polyacrylamide gel will fractionate proteins in the mass range 10,000 to 200,000.

It should be remembered that proteins with a mass larger than the upper limit of the polyacrylamide's fractionation range will not gain entry into the gel at the point of application. A gel with a small pore size will prevent the entry of large polypeptides/proteins into the **resolving** gel. This is called **molecular sieving** and is a drawback of SDS-PAGE that should be remembered when polyacrylamide gel results are analysed. You will not be viewing all the polypeptides in the sample, only the ones in the gel's fractionation range.

8.3.2   The stacking gel

A gel with a low percentage polyacrylamide (<5%), referred to as the **"stacking" gel**, is routinely cast on top of the main gel (resolving gel), which has a higher percentage polyacrylamide designed to fractionate the polypeptides in the sample. The purpose of the wide-pored stacking gel is not to fractionate the polypeptides in the samples but to concentrate them, so that all the polypeptides (irrespective of the volume applied) enter the resolving gel as a narrow band. This is achieved by using discontinuous buffers (see Figure 8.3). A popular discontinuous buffer system uses

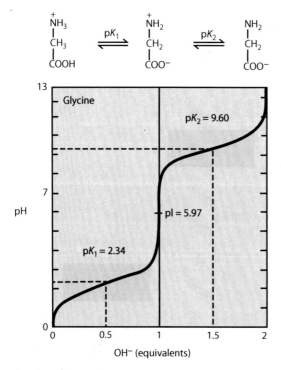

Titration of an amino acid. Shown here is the titration curve of 0.1 m glycine at 25°C. The ionic species predominating at key points in the titration are shown above the graph. The shaded boxes, centred at about $pK_1 = 2.34$ and $pK_2 = 9.60$, indicate the regions of the greatest buffering power.

Figure 8.3 The ionization of glycine.

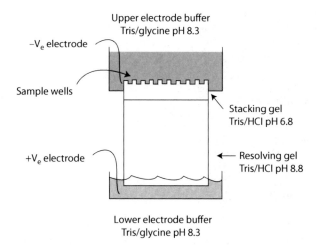

Upper electrode buffer
Tris/glycine pH 8.3

−V$_e$ electrode

Sample wells

+V$_e$ electrode

Stacking gel
Tris/HCl pH 6.8

Resolving gel
Tris/HCl pH 8.8

Lower electrode buffer
Tris/glycine pH 8.3

Figure 8.4 A diagram of a typical discontinuous buffer system used in PAGE.

Tris/HCl pH 8.8 as the resolving gel buffer, Tris/HCl pH 6.8 as the stacking gel buffer and Tris/glycine pH 8.3 as the electrode buffer (Leammli, 1970).

At the start of the experiment the glycinate ions (pH 8.3) in the upper buffer chamber and the chloride ions in the stacking gel (pH 6.8) are fully charged. When the experiment is initiated and the voltage has been applied, the glycinate ions from the buffer enter the stacking gel (pH 6.8) and the change in pH results in the loss of most of its charge (see Figure 8.4). The glycinate ions lose most of their negative charge and become less electrophorectically mobile than the negatively charged protein/polypeptide complexes and the chloride ion. The protein/polypeptide complexes are sandwiched between the fast-moving chloride ion and the slower-moving glycinate ion. The negatively charged protein molecules race towards the fast-moving chloride ion front but are unable to move past it. During the course of travelling through the stacking gel, the protein ions furthest from the chloride ion front are constantly trying to catch up to it. The result is that the protein ions in the sample focus into a narrow band as they progress through the stacking gel. When the resolving gel (pH 8.8) is reached, the glycinate ions return to being fully charged and start to move with the chloride ion with the dye front. The protein ions in the sample enter the smaller pores of the resolving gel and are fractionated during the course of the experiment. The progress of the polypeptides in the resolving gel depends upon the size of the polypeptide in an SDS-PAGE experiment (or on the size and charge of the proteins present in the sample in non-denaturing PAGE).

8.3.3 Denaturing polyacrylamide gel electrophoresis of proteins

The detergent (SDS) (see Figure 8.1) initially disrupts the hydrophobic content of a protein's structure. As the tertiary structure of the protein starts to unwind, the other weak forces (hydrogen bonds, salt bridges and van der Waal interactions; see Chapter 2) that hold a protein's structure together become diminished. The protein loses its globular/fibrous shape and starts to become a linear rod-like shape. The variable charge on a protein's surface (see Section 2.7.1) becomes swamped with the negative charge on the SDS detergent molecule, which binds every two amino acids. The net result is that a protein molecule with a tertiary structure that had a surface charge comprised of both positive and negative charges is now altered into a linear polypeptide with an overall negative charge (see Figure 8.5). Prior to the addition of the detergent SDS, the proteins in a sample have a wide variety of mass-to-charge ratios. After the addition of the detergent molecules, the proteins are converted into polypeptide chains, all with the same mass-to-charge ratio. The only difference among them will be the length of their polypeptide chains.

The detergent SDS will unravel the weak forces that hold a protein's structure together, but it will not break the covalent disulphide (S-S) bonds present in the structure of some proteins. In general, only proteins that are to be exported from the cell or processed in the endomembrane system for export have disulphide bridges. These provide the exported proteins with additional structural strength so they can endure the more onerous physicality of the extracellular environment. These exported proteins will have been synthesised into the lumen of the endoplasmic reticulum (ER), post-translationally processed through the Golgi bodies and possibly stored in vesicles below the plasma membrane, awaiting the signal for them to be exported from the cell.

In any cell/tissue extract there will be some proteins with disulphide bonds. To break the disulphide bonds and completely linearise all the proteins in a sample, a reducing agent (e.g., 2-ME:2-mercaptoethanol or DTT: dithiothreitol) is included in the SDS sample preparation buffer.

The sample is mixed with an equal volume of (2×) sample buffer (see Protocol 8.1) and heated for 5 min to completely linearise all the protein molecules into polypeptide chains prior to their application onto the gel. When the samples have been applied to the stacking gel, the SDS/polypeptide complexes become concentrated but migrate unhindered through the wide pores of the stacking gel (see Section 8.3.2 above). When the SDS/polypeptide complexes enter the resolving gel, small polypeptide chains migrate through the porous polyacrylamide network with relative ease. The movement of larger polypeptides through the gel is restricted due to their size, so they migrate more slowly. At the end of the experiment,

Before SDS (a globular structure with positive and negative charge)

Charged functional groups

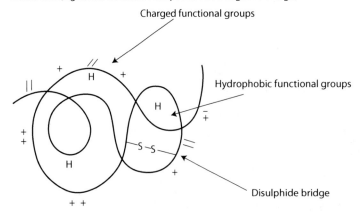

Hydrophobic functional groups

Disulphide bridge

After treatment with SDS, 2-ME and heat
(a linear pelypeptide with an overall negative charge)

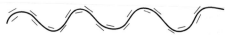

Figure 8.5 The structure of proteins before and after the addition of SDS and 2-ME.

when the bromophenol blue (the fastest running visible molecule) has come to within 0.5 cm of the end of the gel, the experiment can be stopped. The gel is removed from the electrophoresis tank and stained (see Section 8.3.5 below and Protocols 8.5–8.7) to visualise the samples applied.

8.3.3.1 Analysing the results of SDS-PAGE

The distance a polypeptide migrates in SDS-PAGE is inversely proportional to $\log_{10}$ of the polypeptide's relative molecular mass (M_r). It is common practise to load a series of standard proteins whose M_r has been characterised on a polyacrylamide gel at the same time as the samples. The relative migration distances of these standard polypeptides can be measured and plotted against the $\log_{10}$ of their molecular masses. The calibration graph can then be used to estimate the molecular masses of polypeptides in the samples (see Exercise 8.2 and Figure 8.6).

8.3.4 Non-denaturing (native) polyacrylamide gel electrophoresis

The electrophoresis of proteins in the absence of a detergent is described as non-denaturing PAGE or native PAGE (see Protocol 8.2). The proteins are applied to the gel and subjected to electrophoresis in their native conformations. The progress of a protein towards an electrode of opposite charge will depend upon two factors: (a) the overall surface charge on the protein, which is pH-dependent (the exact surface charge at any pH is determined by the amino acid composition of the protein and any post-translational modifications [e.g., phosphorylation]) and (b) the protein's hydrodynamic volume, with small compact structures migrating quicker than large disperse structures. Changes to the conformation of the protein can also influence the rate of migration (e.g., the formation of aggregates and post-translational modifications such as glycosylation). For example, if two proteins with an M_r of 30,000, protein X (containing four aspartate and glutamate amino acids) and protein Y (containing sixteen aspartate and glutamate amino acids), were subjected to non-denaturing PAGE at a pH above pH 7.0, protein Y would migrate further in the gel. Their masses are the same but the relative charge on protein Y is four times larger than protein X. Therefore, in non-denaturing PAGE, protein Y will migrate further in the gel because protein Y is more electronegative. An example of the use of non-denaturing PAGE is shown in Figure 8.7. Storage globulins (*Vicia faba*) were isolated from sown seeds at different days after the onset of germination. The isolated globulins have similar molecular masses, but they show increased electronegativity due to the loss of amide nitrogen (i.e., conversion of asparagine and glutamine to aspartate

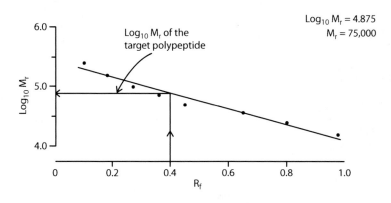

Figure 8.6 An SDS-PAGE calibration plot obtained from standard proteins.

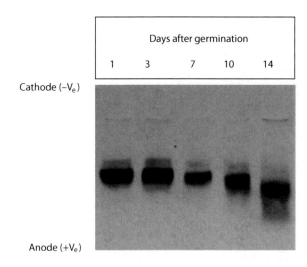

Cathode (–V$_e$)

Anode (+V$_e$)

Days after germination

1   3   7   10   14

Figure 8.7 Storage proteins isolated from *Vicia faba* seeds at different stages of germination subjected to non-denaturing (native) PAGE in a 7.5% gel.

and glutamate). The storage proteins have become more electronegative during the process of germination.

8.3.4.1 The different uses of non-denaturing PAGE

If, after purifying a protein, a homogenous band is visualised using SDS-PAGE (separation on size) and the same preparation shows a homogenous band after non-denaturing PAGE (separation on hydrodynamic volume and charge), this can be taken as a good indication of the purity of the fraction.

The electrophoretic progress of a protein in non-denaturing PAGE is determined in part by the protein's conformation. Changes in the conformation due to the formation of aggregates (dimers or oligomers) or the binding of ligands to generate more compact (or disperse) structures can be visualised on non-denaturing PAGE.

In non-denaturing PAGE, if the apparatus is cooled throughout the electrophoretic run, the proteins will retain their native conformation and their biological activity. An enzyme of interest can be identified *in situ* by incubating the gel in a chromogenic substrate solution or by including the chromogenic substrate in 1% (w/v) agarose and overlaying the agarose/substrate mixture on top of the polyacrylamide gel. Bands will appear in areas of the gel corresponding to where the enzyme has migrated. This can be a useful technique to identify isoenzymes, which may differ by only a few amino acid substitutions.

8.3.5   Visualising the polypeptides/Proteins in polyacrylamide gels

The most commonly used protein stain, after SDS-PAGE, is Coomassie blue dye binding (sensitivity approximately 100 ng per protein band; see Protocol 8.1) in a methanol/acetic acid mixture (used to precipitate the proteins within the gel, preventing them from diffusing away before analysis). The use of methanol and acetic acid mixtures can be avoided by purchasing proprietary aqueous Coomassie protein gel stains (e.g., "Safe stain" Coomassie; Bio-Rad, Expedeon, Sigma and Thermo Fisher, UK). Compared to solvent-based stains, water-based stains allow the protein bands develop more quickly, increase the level of protein detection and are less hazardous to dispose of.

Silver staining (see Protocol 8.5) increases the level of detection compared to Coomassie based stains approximately 100-fold, detecting down to 1.0 ng of protein in a band. Silver staining can be used instead of, or after, Coomassie blue staining to increase the levels of detection. This is a popular stain in the field of proteomics after 2D-PAGE. Fluorescent stains such as Sypro® red (Invitrogen; see Protocol 8.6) give a comparable level of sensitivity to silver. A rapid and sensitive stain for polypeptides after SDS-PAGE involves using zinc ions and imidazole (see Protocol 8.7).

The post-experimental staining of gels can be circumvented by including 0.5% (v/v) trichloroethanol (TCE) in the polyacrylamide mixture (see Protocol 8.8) prior to polymerisation (Ladner et al., 2004). After electrophoresis the polypeptides can be visualised by exposure to ultraviolet light for 5 minutes, which catalyses a reaction between tryptophan and TCE to produce a fluorescent image that can be captured using a light-sensitive camera in gel documentation systems. Following the image capture, the gel can then be used for other analytical techniques, such as Western blotting (see Section 8.4 below and Protocol 8.3).

8.4   PREPARATIVE GEL ELECTROPHORESIS AND METHODS TO ISOLATE PROTEINS FROM POLYACRYLAMIDE GELS

Electrophoresis is a highly resolving technique, routinely used to monitor the purity of pooled protein fractions produced by chromatographic separations (see Section 8.3 above). Analytical electrophoresis can be viewed as incomplete electrolysis because the experiment is stopped before the protein/polypeptide sample reaches the electrode. The samples within the gel are visualised by post-electrophoresis staining. If a polyacrylamide gel electrophoresis experiment is allowed to proceed (after the bromophenol blue tracking dye has run off the end of the gel), the proteins within the applied sample will continue to travel towards the anode. They will emerge from the bottom of an analytical gel, enter the anodic buffer chamber and eventually be denatured when they physically contact the anode electrode. Preparative gel electrophoresis takes advantage of the high resolving power of polyacrylamide gels by coupling it with the detection and fraction collection of chromatographic systems.

Preparative electrophoresis is analogous to a chromatographic separation but not directly comparable. In chromatography, the separation of molecules is based upon a partition coefficient (K_D) between two immiscible phases; in electrophoresis the separation through the complex network of cross-linked polyacrylamide polymers is based upon relative mobility. Maizel (1964) first described a preparative polyacrylamide gel electrophoresis (PAGE) system for the separation of proteins. The proteins applied to the top of a polyacrylamide gel were eluted from the bottom of the gel and collected in a fraction collector. There are a number of proprietary apparatuses available for the purification of proteins using either non-denaturing or denaturing polyacrylamide gel electrophoresis. In preparative electrophoresis systems, the protein sample is applied to a column of polyacrylamide and run through the gel using conventional buffer systems (see Protocols 8.1 and 8.2). The end of the polyacrylamide column rests upon a sintered glass disc (see Figure 8.8), through which a buffer flows tangentially to the bottom of the acrylamide column, gathering protein/polypeptides as they emerge from the bottom of the

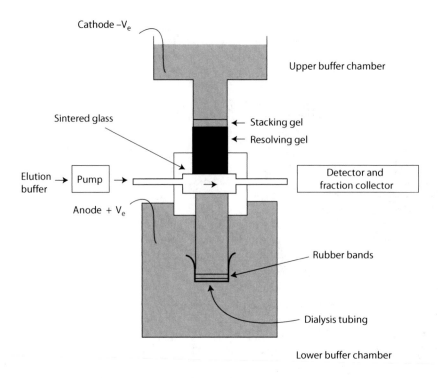

Cathode $-V_e$

Upper buffer chamber

Sintered glass

Stacking gel ←
Resolving gel ←

Elution → | Pump | →
buffer

Detector and
fraction collector

Anode $+ V_e$

Rubber bands

Dialysis tubing

Lower buffer chamber

Figure 8.8 A typical preparative polyacrylamide gel electrophoresis setup.

polyacrylamide gel and transferring them to a fraction collector. Proteins
are prevented from contacting an electrode by the use of dialysis tubing,
which also maintains the electrical integrity of the system.

A preparative gel apparatus rarely matches the excellent resolution of bands
that appear on analytical polyacrylamide gels. This is because as the bands
emerge from the bottom of the polyacrylamide column, mixing takes place
in the eluting buffer; reducing both the amount of sample applied and the
dead volume between the preparative PAGE apparatus and the fraction collector can help reduce sample mixing. For these reasons, it is not an ideal
technique to use in the early stages of a purification protocol, when the target
protein is usually a small percentage of the total protein. However, it can be
used successfully in the later stages of a purification protocol to remove the
trace protein/polypeptide contaminants that are usually present. If the temperature is controlled during a non-denaturing preparative PAGE experiment (separation based upon mass and charge), the sample will emerge from
the experiment in an active conformation. If the purity of the sample is still
not acceptable, the active fractions can be concentrated (see Section 4.11),
incubated with SDS and 2-ME and rerun on the same polyacrylamide column (the electrode buffers would require changing for denaturing PAGE),
isolating the sample this time based solely on relative molecular mass.

If the target protein can be identified on an analytical gel using an antibody to the target protein (see Protocol 8.5; Western blotting), detecting
the protein's activity *in situ* (see Section 8.3.4; non-denaturing PAGE), or
using the M_r of the target protein (see Section 8.3.3; denaturing PAGE), the
band containing the target protein can be excised from the gel. Preparative
well-forming combs coupled with wider gel forming spacers (1.0 mm and
1.5 mm) will enable larger amounts of the target protein to be applied to

the gel. Remember that there is an upper limit to the amount of protein that can be applied to any polyacrylamide gel that depends on the number and relative amounts of protein/polypeptides in the sample. As the protein concentrates within the gel during the electrophoresis run, localised heat spots can be generated at high protein loadings, resulting in band distortion.

8.4.1 Electroelution of proteins from polyacrylamide gels

A proprietary polyacrylamide gel electroeluting apparatus can be used that moves the sample from an excised polyacrylamide gel by electrophoresis into a collection chamber. The sample is prevented from contacting the anode by dialysis membrane. Alternatively, gel slices can be placed into a dialysis bag in buffer and then draped over a horizontal electrophoresis apparatus. Minimum buffer can be used in the dialysis bag to contact the two electrodes. The protein within the gel will migrate into the buffer, where it can be collected. While the electrical field is in place, the proteins will continue to move towards the anode. Over time, this can result in proteins contacting the dialysis membrane. To overcome this, at the end of the electroelution the polarity of the current should be reversed for 2 minutes to propel the proteins from the dialysis membrane back into the buffer. Stained and unstained proteins can be electroeluted effectively, and the recovery of protein is usually higher when SDS is included in the electrode buffers. Any detergent molecules in the sample (e.g., SDS) can be removed by dialysis (see Protocol 4.9) or SEC (see Sections 7.5.3–7.5.4 and Protocol 7.1).

8.4.2 Gel homogenisation

The polyacrylamide gel slices containing a target protein can be fragmented to increase the diffusible gel surface area prior to, for example, electroelution (see Section 8.4.1, above). The polyacrylamide gel slices can be fragmented by finely chopping with a scalpel or by centrifugation through copper wire. The gel fragments are then put into a suitable buffer to allow diffusion of the target protein to take place. The target protein can be recovered from the gel fragments by centrifugation or by centrifugation through **silanised** glass wool (see Protocol 8.9). To improve the recovery of the target protein, fresh buffer can be added to the gel fragments and the process repeated. Inclusion of 0.05–0.1% (w/v) SDS in the diffusion buffer will improve recoveries. If required, the pooled fractions can be concentrated and the SDS removed using precipitation (see Protocol 4.10), dialysis (see Protocol 4.9) or SEC (see Sections 7.5.3–7.5.4 and Protocol 7.1).

8.4.3 Gel solubilisation

Polyacrylamide gel slices can be solubilised in 30% (v/v) hydrogen peroxide at 50°C overnight. This treatment will be damaging to proteins, which makes the resultant material suitable only for scintillation counting of radioactively labelled proteins.

8.5 INTRODUCTION TO WESTERN BLOTTING

After either denaturing or non-denaturing PAGE, individual polypeptides/proteins can be identified using Western blotting. This involves the electrophorectic transfer of polypeptides separated by SDS-PAGE (or proteins by non-denaturing PAGE) onto a nitrocellulose membrane filter (see Figure 8.9). The transfer can be completed in a "wet" blotter, in which the gel membrane sandwich is immersed in continuous transfer buffer (CTB), or a "semi dry" blotter, which uses only sufficient buffer to complete the electrical circuit (see Protocol 8.3). Rapid Western blot transfer systems are available to purchase (e.g., Bio-Rad, UK) that can facilitate the transfer of the abundant proteins in a polyacrylamide in shorter time periods (5–15 min).

The Western blot produces a replica of the pattern of polypeptides/proteins that have run through the polyacrylamide gel onto the nitrocellulose membrane. This renders the separated polypeptides/proteins more accessible to probing with a specific antibody (either monoclonal or polyclonal). Before the probing with an antibody can begin, it is essential that the vacant protein binding sites on the nitrocellulose membrane are masked with another "neutral" protein (e.g., BSA or powdered milk protein). This masking of the nitrocellulose membrane prevents the primary antibody (also a protein) from binding non-specifically to the membrane. When the blocking has been completed, the Western blot can be probed with the primary (1°) antibody at an appropriate dilution in phosphate buffered saline containing a detergent (e.g., 0.1% [v/v] Tween 80). Several washing steps need to be included between each stage of the procedure to ensure that all the proteins from the previous stages have been removed and will not interfere with the subsequent stages. After probing the blot with the primary antibody, the polypeptide-antibody complex can be visualised using a secondary (2°) antibody raised against the IgG fraction of the primary antibody species (e.g., anti-mouse IgG (whole molecule)

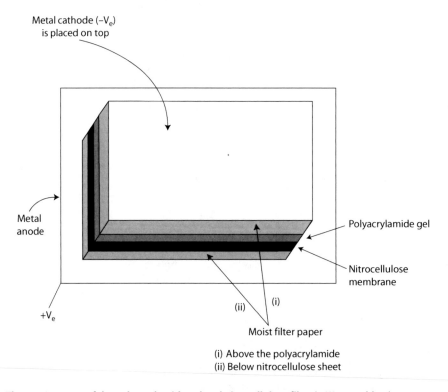

Metal cathode (−V$_e$)
is placed on top

Metal
anode

Polyacrylamide gel

Nitrocellulose
membrane

+V$_e$

(ii)   (i)

Moist filter paper

(i) Above the polyacrylamide
(ii) Below nitrocellulose sheet

Figure 8.9 The arrangement of the polyacrylamide gel and nitrocellulose filter in Western blotting.

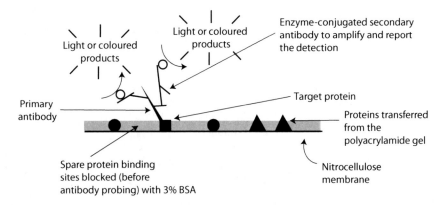

Figure 8.10 The use of primary antibodies in Western blotting to detect the protein of interest on nitrocellulose and the use of conjugated secondary antibodies to report and amplify the detection.

raised in rabbit) and conjugated to an enzyme (e.g., horseradish peroxidase [HRP] or alkaline phosphatase), a radioactive molecule (e.g., ^{125}I) or a fluorescent molecule (e.g., fluorescein isothiocyanate FITC). Many conjugated secondary antibodies are polyclonal antibodies, resulting in multiple binding of the conjugated secondary antibodies to the primary antibody, which in turn amplifies the detection (see Figure 8.10).

Enhanced chemiluminescence (ECL) is a popular method of visualising protein/antibody complexes on nitrocellulose after Western blots because it is cost-effective, safe, sensitive and easy to use. After probing the immunoblot with the primary antibody, the HRP-conjugated secondary antibody can be used with hydrogen peroxide, luminol and chemical enhancers to generate light (see Protocol 8.3). The area on the nitrocellulose producing the light can be detected almost immediately with a luminescent image analyser or after incubation on an X-ray film.

8.5.1   Recovery of proteins from nitrocellulose

After Western blotting, proteins can be visualised on the nitrocellulose by using reversible stains such as copper pthalocyanine (see Protocol 8.3). If the area on the blot occupied by the target protein can be identified (e.g., by M_r), it can be excised. Alternatively, a strip from the blot can be blocked and probed with an antibody raised to (or cross-reacted with) the target protein. After visualisation (see Protocol 8.3), the nitrocellulose membrane strip can be aligned with the membrane that has not been stained to subsequently excise the correct area corresponding to the target protein. The protein can be recovered from the nitrocellulose by using a buffer containing either detergents (e.g., 0.1–1.0% [w/v] SDS or 20% [v/v] acetonitrile or pyridine). After this treatment the proteins can be recovered from the solvents by precipitation using acetone (see Protocol 4.10) or from the detergents by dialysis (see Protocol 4.9) or using SEC (see Sections 7.5.3–7.5.4).

8.6   INTRODUCTION TO ISOELECTRIC FOCUSING

In isoelectric focusing (IEF), a pH gradient is generated in a polyacrylamide (4%) gel (agarose gels can be used for proteins with high molecular masses) by the inclusion of **ampholytes** in the monomer mixture prior to polymerisation. The pH gradient is established within the polymerised polyacrylamide by the application of an electrical field across the gel for a short period of time. A sample can then be applied and the electrical field switched back on. The proteins in the sample will move towards the oppositely charged electrode, gradually approaching their isoelectric point (pI). As they near their isoelectric point, the rate of migration will slow down as the proteins lose surface charge. When the proteins reach their pI, they will have no charge and will remain immobile within the gel (see Figure 8.11). When the experiment has finished, the gel is washed with 10% (w/v) trichloroacetic acid to fix the proteins in the gel and wash away the ampholytes. The gel can then be stained with Coomassie blue (see Protocol 8.1) to visualise the samples.

In IEF, some proteins will move towards their pI and retain their conformation and others will denature. The former can be visualised *in situ* using chromogenic substrates (see Section 8.3.4.1 above). Standard proteins with different pI's can be purchased and loaded onto the same gel as the sample. The progress of the experiment can be monitored by the movement of the coloured standards, and a calibration graph can be prepared by measuring the distance moved by the coloured standards from an electrode and plotting this migration distance against the pH. The migration distance of the unknown proteins present in the sample can then be measured and their pI can then be determined.

Ampholytes can be purchased to generate gradients with different pH ranges. This allows better resolution of the target protein from other proteins present around the pI of the protein of interest. Alternatively, IEF gel strips can be purchased with immobilised ampholytes present within the gel. These strips are rehydrated in the presence of the sample, which becomes absorbed into the entire length of the gel. When the electrical field is applied, the proteins will migrate towards their pI no matter where the sample is placed (see Figure 8.11).

Isoelectric focusing is a highly resolving technique that can separate proteins with as little as 0.01 pH difference in pI values. This makes it ideal for

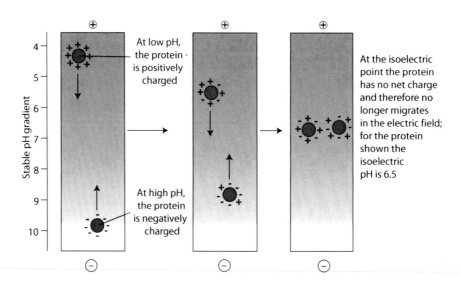

Figure 8.11 Isoelectric focusing of proteins.

visualising any contaminating proteins that might be present in a sample that has been purified to apparent homogeneity. In addition, IEF is able to identify **isoenzymes** (different forms of the enzyme that may differ by a single amino acid) or show micro-heterogeneity (a protein may exist as a phosphorylated and non-phosphorylated form). Isoenzymes and proteins with micro-heterogeneity would migrate to the same point on an SDS-PAGE gel because the mass differences would be small, but the change in charge would be sufficient to show different bands or a smear on an IEF gel.

Isoelectric focusing can be combined with SDS-PAGE in a technique known as two-dimensional polyacrylamide gel electrophoresis (2D-PAGE). The sample is subjected to IEF in the first dimension, separating proteins according to their charge. The IEF strip is then layered onto a precast well in a SDS-PAGE gel. The proteins in the IEF strip emerge and move towards the anode through the SDS polyacrylamide gel. Their migration is now related to their size, producing a highly resolving gel of the components in a sample. This would be a very good method of establishing that a purified sample is homogeneous. The polypeptide spots can be excised from the gel and treated with trypsin to generate peptides from the polypeptide. The fragments of peptide can be concentrated and presented to a mass spectrometer to establish the isotopic masses of the peptides present in the sample. Selected peptide fragments can be subjected to additional energy within the mass spectrometer and the fragmentation pattern analysed to provide the sequence of the selected peptide. A bioinformatics search with mass analysis software (e.g., MASCOT; http://www.matrixscience.com/) will provide proposed identities for the parent protein. The presence of a single spot in the gel after a 2D-PAGE experiment would be good confirmation of the homogeneity of the purified sample. The identification of the single component (hopefully your target protein) in the sample after 2D-PAGE and mass spectrometry again would be confirmation of a homogeneous sample. The identity of the target protein could be confirmed by Western blotting after 2D-PAGE and probing with a specific monoclonal antibody to the target protein.

8.6.1   Preparative isoelectricfocusing (IEF)

Isoelectric focusing separates proteins according to their charge (see Section 8.5). Preparative IEF apparatus (Rotofor or mini Rotofor; Bio-Rad) can be used to concentrate and fractionate proteins by liquid-phase IEF. The sample proteins (μg-g amounts) are focused into chambers and collected under vacuum into fractions spanning the pH scale used in the experiment. The proteins will be in their native conformation and may start to precipitate at their pI, but the inclusion of non-ionic detergents (e.g., Nonindet, Tween or Triton) can improve any solubility problems. By initially using a wide pH range (3–10) followed by a narrow pH range (1.0 pH scale spanning the pI of the target protein), highly purified fractions can be obtained that can then be subjected to additional chromatographic or electrophoretic techniques.

8.7   INTRODUCTION TO CAPILLARY ELECTROPHORESIS (CE)

Electrophoresis in a narrow bore glass capillary (typically 50–100 cm with a 50 μm internal diameter) using high voltages (10–50 kV) is termed "capillary electrophoresis." The ends of the capillary are submerged into two separate buffer chambers containing either the anode or cathode connections (see Figure 8.12). Depending on the instrument, the sample can be injected into one end of the capillary by syphoning, high-pressure or high voltage. The capillary is then removed from the sample and replaced in the buffer chamber before the application of a high voltage to commence the separation.

The surface of the glass walls of the capillary contain silanol (Si-OH) groups that become ionised above pH 2.0, coating the internal walls of the capillary in a negative charge. This negatively charged surface becomes attractive to positively charged hydrated ions (e.g., hydronium ions (H_3O^+); see Section 1.4), which move towards the cathode when an electrical field is applied. In capillary zone electrophoresis, this electroendosmotic flow of positively charged hydronium ions is greater than the electrophoretic velocity of the charged components in the sample, propelling all of the components towards the cathode irrespective of their charge. In a complex mixture the cations will migrate the quickest, followed by neutrally charged species and finally the anionic components. In contrast to chromatography there are no spherical beads for the sample to move around during progress through the capillary so all the components migrate in a narrow band, giving excellent resolution of complex mixtures in short time frames.

Capillary zone electrophoresis of free solutions is the most widely practised technique, particularly of molecules with relatively small M_r. However, the charged internal surface of the capillary does not make the technique generally applicable to proteins. When a protein solution is loaded onto a capillary, the proteins that have charge at all pH values can adsorb to the charged internal surface of the capillary and leak from the surface when the high voltage is applied. This leads to band broadening or the total loss of the sample. Chemically modified capillaries can be used, in which the silanol groups are capped with a neutrally charged molecule that prevents the protein from binding to the capillary's internal surface. The capped silanol residues will eliminate the electroendosmotic flow, and the charged species will migrate towards the oppositely charged electrode. The detector (UV/visible, fluorescence and mass spectrometry) is usually placed at one end of the capillary (see Figure 8.12) and will only detect the charged species flowing towards that electrode. By controlling the pH of the buffer, proteins can be made to migrate to the chosen electrode. In general, there is poor resolution of a complex protein sample in capped capillaries.

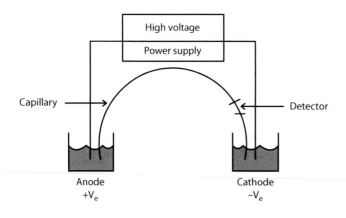

Figure 8.12 A typical capillary electrophoresis setup.

Capillaries can be filled with a gel (either agarose or polyacrylamide) and separations undertaken that are similar to SDS-PAGE or IEF. A single peak on a polyacrylamide-filled capillary in the presence of SDS and a single peak on a free solution capillary run would be another good indication of the purity of a protein sample.

The advantages of CE include fast separation times, low sample volumes (nanolitre), high sensitivity (femtomol detection) and excellent resolution. The disadvantage is that the equipment can be expensive.

8.8   INTRODUCTION TO REVERSED-PHASE HIGH-PRESSURE LIQUID CHROMATOGRAPHY OF PROTEINS

Reversed-phase high-pressure liquid chromatography (RP-HPLC) can be a useful technique in the isolation and analysis of peptides and proteins. Aliphatic groups (e.g., C_8, C_{12} or C_{18}) bonded to a silica resin form the stationary phase in the column. There are many resins specifically manufactured for use with proteins and peptides (see Appendix 8; the list of chromatography suppliers). At the start of the chromatographic run, the mobile phase is a polar solvent. When a protein sample is applied to the reversed-phase resin, the hydrophobic regions in the protein's structure interact with the hydrophobic stationary phase (see Section 2.7.2). The proteins or peptides will remain bound to the stationary phase while the polarity of the initial mobile phase is high (i.e., low solvent concentration). To elute the bound proteins, the concentration of solvent in the mobile phase is gradually increased. The proteins with the highest hydrophobic content will elute later in the elution profile.

To increase the amount of the bonded phase and reduce the height equivalent to a theoretical plate (HETP; see Section 3.3.2) in a reversed-phase (RP) column, the particle diameter (normally 5 μm) can be reduced to 2 μm. Elevated pressures (20,000 psi) are required to move the mobile phase through the small diameter resins designated ultra-pressure systems (UHPLC). The high-pressure pumps can be software-controlled to produce a linear solvent gradient (see Section 3.7). A detector capable of monitoring in the ultraviolet (UV) region is also required, as proteins absorb UV light at 280 nm (due to the presence of the amino acids tyrosine and tryptophan) and at 210 nm (due to the presence of the peptide bond). A fluorescence detector can be used (excitation wavelength 280 nm and emission wavelength of 320 nm for tyrosine or 340 nm for tryptophan), which will increase the sensitivity of the detection. In addition a mass spectrometer detection system can be coupled to RP-HPLC or RP-UHPLC to monitor the output of the experiment.

The solvents used in RP-HPLC (e.g., methanol and acetonitrile) are volatile and can be easily removed from the sample at the end of the chromatographic run by using a centrifugal evaporator. However, the tertiary structure of a protein will be altered due to the solvents in the mobile phase and the interaction with the stationary phase, which has a high ligand density resulting in multiple interactions between the protein and the stationary phase. This will almost certainly mean that the proteins, when they are eluted from the stationary phase, will not fold back into their native conformation, resulting in loss of biological activity. The loss of biological activity may be minimised by reducing the run times and by switching to a less damaging solvent. The loss of biological activity may be a problem if RP-HPLC is being used to purify a target protein, but it is not a problem when the technique is used to monitor the purity of protein fractions, or when a protein is being prepared for the production of antibodies.

8.9   SUMMARY

After each stage in the purification process, a visual as well as a quantitative assessment of the purification process is essential to assess the efficacy of each purification step. If the target protein is an enzyme, a measure of the volume, activity and protein concentration will provide the numbers to assess the fold purification and percentage recovery. These numbers allow the operator to judge the value of each procedure with reference to the goals determined at the start of the purification process. Routine visible assessment of the purification can be undertaken with SDS-PAGE, which is quick and reliable. An increase in the intensity of a band at the molecular weight of the target protein is reassuring. When SDS-PAGE is combined with Western blotting, the increase in a band at the correct molecular weight that also interacts with a monoclonal antibody against the target protein provides additional visual evidence of experimental progress. However, a single band on an SDS-PAGE gel is only evidence that in the sample there are polypeptides of a similar molecular mass in the sample to the target protein, and Western blotting will confirm that some but maybe not all of them are the target protein. Additional techniques (e.g., size exclusion chromatography, isoelectric focusing, capillary electrophoresis or reversed-phase chromatography) that exploit other characteristics of proteins can be used to support the contention that the final sample is indeed homogeneous.

EXERCISE 8.1 WORKING OUT THE CALCULATIONS NECESSARY TO COMPLETE A PROTEIN PURIFICATION TABLE

A liver extract in 0.1 M Tris/HCl pH 8.0 was assayed for the activity of a proteolytic enzyme. The total volume of the extract was 125 ml and the protein concentration was 5.2 mg ml^{-1}.

The substrate Benzoyl-arginine-p-nitroanalide (BAPNA) can be cleaved by proteolytic enzymes with a preference for arginine/lysine releasing a vivid yellow-coloured p-nitroanalide with a molar absorptivity coefficient of 16,000 at 410 nm.

A 100 μl of the liver extract was assayed in a reaction volume of 1.0 ml at 37°C with BAPNA to give an absorbance of 0.25 over a 10 min reaction period.

Calculate

(a) The rate of reaction in ΔA_{410nm} min^{-1}
(b) The rate of reaction in international enzyme units (μmol of product formed min^{-1})
(c) The number of units ml^{-1} of enzyme extract
(d) The specific activity (SA) = units mg^{-1} of protein
(e) The total number of units (TA) = total units in the extract volume

The pH of the liver extract was adjusted to pH 8.5 and the extract was centrifuged at 13,000 × g for 30 min to clarify the extract. The supernatant from the centrifugation step (122 ml) was diluted to a final volume of 500 ml in 25 mM Tris/HCl pH8.5.

Step 1: Work out the rate of reaction which is a change in absorbance min^{-1} = ΔA_{410nm} min^{-1}.

Insert the answer

Step 2: There is a linear relationship between absorbance and concentration given by the **Beer-Lambert law**.

$$A = L * \varepsilon * C$$

where L = the path length of the cuvette (the standard length is 1.0 cm unless you are using a flow cell in an on line spectrophotometer).

ε = the molar absorptivity coefficient in L mol^{-1} cm^{-1} (This can be found from books and represents the theoretical absorbance of a molar solution. It is only true for a specific wavelength number)

C = concentration in mol L^{-1}.

Step 3: Return to the example:

$$0.025 = 1 * 16,000 * C$$

Therefore, C= 0.025/16,000

Insert your answer

The answer is C= 0.0000016 M min^{-1}.

Step 4: Change this to the appropriate unit used in biology.

Insert the answer

Step 5: Molar solutions are mol L^{-1} (or in a 1000 ml); we did not use a reaction volume of a 1000 ml but of 1 ml.

Therefore, we need to adjust for the volume which will give us the amount of product formed in the reaction cuvette over the 10 min time period from 100 µl of extract.

Adjust the units:

Insert the answer

We now have an amount of product formed per min by the enzyme catalysed reaction (*remember that a **mol** is the molecular weight in g of that chemical*).

Step 6: Convert to International Units of enzyme activity (I.U. = 1.0 µmol of product formed min^{-1}). This a physical weight of product formed or substrate consumed by 100 µl of extract.

Insert the answer

Step 7: Convert the units from 0.1 ml to 1.0 ml of extract.

Insert the answer

Step 8: Specific activity = units of enzyme mg^{-1} of protein (how much of the protein contains the enzyme of interest)

$$= \frac{\text{units of enzyme } \cancel{ml^{-1}} = \text{of extract}}{\text{protein in mg } \cancel{ml^{-1}} = \text{of extract}}$$

$$= \text{units of enzyme } mg^{-1} \text{ of protein}$$

Insert the answer

Step 9: Total protein in the 125 ml of extract:

Protein mg ml^{-1} * vol of extract

Insert the answer

Step 10: Total activity in the extract is units mg^{-1} * total protein.

Insert the answer

The other two columns in most purification tables are (a) % yield and (b) fold purity.

Step 11: % yield is the amount of activity left after a purification run compared to the total activity in the initial fraction. It is a % and will generally **decrease** as the purification proceeds.

Step 12: Fold purity is the increase in purity compared to the initial extract which is always 1. Therefore, fold purity will **increase** as the target enzyme in the extract becomes enriched through the purification.

Specific activity in the current purification fraction divided by specific activity in the initial extract.

EXERCISE 8.2 THE MOLECULAR WEIGHT CALCULATIONS ASSOCIATED WITH SDS-PAGE

The relative mobility (R_f also known as the retention factor) is the mobility of the standards/samples relative to the mobility of the dye front.

Relative mobility (R_f) is a value between 0 and 1.0 (i.e., if the sample remains at the origin it will have a R_f value of 0 and if it runs with the dye front it will have a value of 1.0). There can be no resolution of the polypeptides in the sample if they have an R_f of zero or one.

$$R_f = \frac{\text{the distance moved by the sample}}{\text{the distance moved by the dye font}}$$

The distances should be measured from the point of sample application (origin) to the mid-point of either the dye front or the relative molecular mass of the standard proteins bands in the gel.

For example: A 10% polyacrylamide gel has been run with standard proteins in lane A and a salmon muscle sample in lane B.

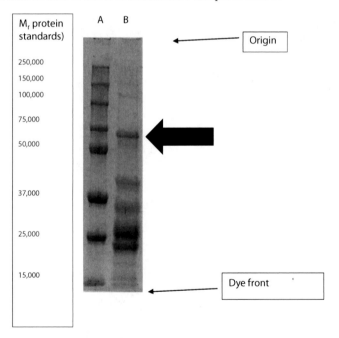

Analysis of the SDS-PAGE experiment to determine the approximate molecular mass of a polypeptide in the sample (the answers to Exercise 8.2 can be found in Appendix 6).

A. Calculate the R_f values for the standard proteins and plot the calibration graph for the experiment (this should be a plot of Log_{10} M_r of the standard proteins versus their R_f value).

B. Using the calibration graph determine the relative molecular mass (M_r) of the protein in sample B highlighted by the big black arrow.

PROTOCOLS FOR CHAPTER 8

Protocol 8.1 The procedure and solutions for denaturing PAGE

Note: (a) Prepare buffers fresh or from frozen stocks and use the highest reagent grade available. (b) Check the data sheets provided by the reagent's manufacturers and take appropriate health and safety precautions.

Running Buffer for SDS-PAGE: pH 8.3 (10× stock)

Tris base 30.3 g, glycine 144 g, SDS 10.0 g. Dissolve into 1000.0 ml with dH_2O. There is no need to adjust the pH of this buffer as it normally dissolves to exactly pH 8.3.

Reagents

(A) Resolving Buffer	1.5 M Tris/HCl pH 8.9
(B) Stacking Buffer	0.5 M Tris/HCl pH 6.7
(C) Acrylamide Solution*	30% (w/v) (29.2% acrylamide, 0.8% bis-acrylamide)

*The acrylamide monomer solution is very toxic and should be handled with due care (refer to your local health and safety documentation). Pre-prepared stock solutions of different acrylamide mixtures are available and should be used in preference to the acrylamide powder.

The detergent sodium dodecyl sulphate (SDS) is only required in the running buffer and sample buffer; it does not need to be included in the gel mixtures. These gel mixtures can be used for both denaturing (SDS) and non-denaturing PAGE.

Proprietary pre-caste acrylamide gels are available in a number of formats.

Resolving gel mixture	7.5% (ml)	10.0% (ml)	12.0% (ml)
(A)	5.0	5.0	5.0
(C)	5.0	6.7	8.0
H_2O	9.9	8.2	6.9
+10% (w/v) Ammonium persulphate	0.06	0.06	0.06
TEMED	0.04	0.04	0.04
Total	20.0	20.0	20.0

Stacking gel mixture	(ml)
(B)	5.0
(C)	2.5
H_2O	12.4
+10% (w/v) Ammonium persulphate	0.06
TEMED	0.04
Total	20.0

Preparing the gel:

- Pour resolving gel to approximately 1.0 cm below the distance that the well-forming comb extends into the gel setup. Overlay the resolving gel acrylamide and buffer mixture with isopropanol (or isobutanol) and allow to the gel mixture to polymerise. This could take between 30–60 minutes, depending on the ambient temperature of the laboratory.
- Remove the solvent and wash with distilled water. Remove the water using filter paper or tissue paper (without touching the resolving gel).
- Insert the Teflon well-forming comb, add the catalysts to the stacking gel mixture and pour onto the resolving gel until the stacking gel mixture reaches the top of the glass plates. Overlay with a minimal volume of isopropanol (approximately 50–100 µl) and allow to polymerise.
- When the polymerisation has completed, gently remove the well-forming comb. Wash the sample wells with distilled water to remove any acrylamide that has not polymerised. Then add a small volume of running buffer until the liquid reaches just below the top of the wells.

Denaturing PAGE sample buffer (2× stock):

5.0 ml (B) + 1.0 ml 20% (w/v) SDS + 1.0 ml 2-ME + 2.0 ml of glycerol + 10.95 ml H_2O + 0.05 ml of a saturated solution of bromophenol blue (add a small amount of bromophenol blue dye to a 1.5 ml microfuge tube and make up to 1.0 ml with distilled water. Vortex mix and allow the dye powder to settle. Pipette the liquid from above the remaining solid).

Prepared stocks of 2× denaturing (Laemmli sample buffer) are available from suppliers.

Sample preparation for denaturing PAGE:

> Add the denaturing sample buffer to an equal volume of sample in a 1.5 ml microfuge tube. Heat the mixture at 95°C for 5.0 minutes in a heating block (with the microfuge lid anchor in place) to denature the proteins in the sample. The resultant polypeptides will be coated with SDS and have a linear conformation before application to the gel. After boiling in sample buffer, the sample can be stored at room temperature until required.

Running the electrophoresis experiment for denaturing PAGE:

- A small volume (2 μl) of pre-stained protein standards is normally applied into the edge wells of the gel to calibrate the experiment and provide the means to calculate the relative molecular mass of a polypeptide in the samples (see Exercise 8.1).
- Apply the samples and run the gel at 40 ma per gel (this may need adjusting to avoid going over 200 volts and overheating).
- Stop the experiment when the bromophenol blue reaches approximately 0.5 cm from the end of the gel.
- Remove the gel from the gel cassette, place in a tray and cover with distilled water for 5.0 min.
- Place the gel in stain for the required period.
- Remove from the stain and place in destain until the background is clear enough to visualise and record the samples and/or standards.

Staining the gel:

> There are many different staining methods to visualise proteins and polypeptides in polyacrylamide gels. A simple stain using Coomassie blue dye is outlined below but other proprietary Coomassie blue stains for gels without solvents (described as "safe stains") are available to buy. These "safe stains" have several advantages: they are sensitive, relatively quick and destained in distilled water.
>
> Other more sensitive stains (e.g., fluorescent stains) are available and many are also compatible with mass spectrometry (see Protocols 8.3 and 8.4).

Stain

> 1.25 g Coomassie blue R (PAGE BLUE 83) dissolved in 225 ml methanol and 225 ml distilled water. Stir for a couple of hours and filter through Whatman No. 1 filter paper. Add 50 ml of acetic acid and store in a dark bottle at room temperature.
>
> When a gel requires staining, place the gel into a suitable tray and cover the gel with the Coomassie stain. Leave the gel on a rotating platform for 60 min before removing the stain. Wash the gel in distilled water and then place the gel in destain (see below). Several changes of destain may be required to clear the background in the gel to a suitable level for photography.
>
> Small balls of tissue paper can be added to the destain to expedite the removal of excess stain from the gel. The cellulose binds Coomassie blue irreversibly, thus acting to prevent the dye in the gel and destain reaching an equilibrium.
>
> Destain: 25% (v/v) methanol (or ethanol) + 10% (v/v) acetic acid

Protocol 8.2 The procedures and solutions to run non-denaturing PAGE

Note: (a) Prepare buffers fresh or from frozen stocks and use the highest reagent grade available. (b) Check the data sheets provided by the reagent's manufacturers and take appropriate health and safety precautions.

Running Buffer for non-denaturing PAGE: pH 8.3 (10× stock)

Tris base 30.3 g, glycine 144 g. Dissolve into 1000.0 ml with ddH$_2$O. There is no need to adjust the pH of this buffer as it normally dissolves to exactly pH 8.3.

Reagents

(A) Resolving Buffer	1.5 M Tris/HCl pH 8.9
(B) Stacking Buffer	0.5 M Tris/HCl pH 6.7
(C) Acrylamide Solution*	30% (w/v) (29.2% acrylamide, 0.8% bis-acrylamide)

*The acrylamide monomer solution is very toxic and should be handled with due care (refer to your local health and safety documentation). Pre-prepared stock solutions of different acrylamide mixtures are available and should be used in preference to the acrylamide powder.

Proprietary pre-caste acrylamide gels are available in a number of formats.

Resolving gel mixture	7.5% (ml)	10.0% (ml)	12.0% (ml)
(A)	5.0	5.0	5.0
(C)	5.0	6.7	8.0
H$_2$O	7.9	6.2	4.9
Glycerol	2.0	2.0	2.0
+10% (w/v) Ammonium persulphate	0.06	0.06	0.06
TEMED	0.04	0.04	0.04
Total	20.0	20.0	20.0

Stacking gel mixture	(ml)
(B)	5.0
(C)	2.5
H_2O	12.4
+10% (w/v) Ammonium persulphate	0.06
TEMED	0.04
Total	20.0

Preparing the gel:

- Pour resolving gel to approximately 1.0 cm below the distance that the well-forming comb extends into the glass gel casting setup. In this gel mixture the presence of glycerol makes the resolving gel solution denser than the stacking gel mixture. The stacking gel solution can be initiated to polymerise and poured with care directly onto the resolving gel mixture to the top of the gel plates.
- Insert the Teflon well-forming comb and overlay with a minimal volume of isopropanol (approximately 50–100 µl) and allow the gels to polymerise. The resolving gel and the stacking gel will polymerise together, saving time.
- After 30–60 min remove the Teflon comb and wash the wells with distilled water to remove the solvent and any acrylamide solution that has not polymerised.
- Add a small volume of running buffer until the liquid reaches just below the top of the wells.

Non-denaturing PAGE sample buffer (2× stock):

5.0 ml (B) + 2.0 ml of glycerol + 12.95 ml H_2O + 0.05 ml of a saturated solution of bromophenol blue (see Protocol 8.1).

Sample preparation for non-denaturing PAGE:

Add the non-denaturing sample buffer to an equal volume of sample in a 1.5 ml microfuge tube. Vortex mix and store the samples on ice until they are applied to the gel.

Running the electrophoresis experiment for non-denaturing PAGE:

- There is no requirement to apply prestained standards to non-denaturing PAGE gels. The separation is based upon the charge and mass of the proteins applied.
- Apply the samples and run the gel at 40 ma per gel (this may need adjusting to avoid going over 200 volts and overheating).
- If the non-denaturing PAGE has been run to detect enzymes in the gel, then the electrophoresis apparatus should be cooled to 4°C throughout the run. This is easily achieved by ensuring the Tris/glycine pH 8.3 running buffer in the lower buffer chamber covers most of the non-denaturing gel in the lower buffer chamber.

- Place a stirring bar into the lower buffer reservoir and after loading the samples place the electrophoresis setup into a deep tray containing ice.
- Place the cooling setup onto a magnetic stirrer and commence stirring before connecting to the power supply.
- Stop the experiment when the bromophenol blue reaches approximately 0.5 cm from the end of the gel.
- Remove the gel from the gel cassette, place in a tray and cover with distilled water for 5.0 min.
- If the denaturing gel has been run to detect enzymes, the polyacrylamide gel should be incubated *in situ* with appropriate reagents to detect the required enzymes. Many different enzymes (isoenzymes) can be detected using this method (Gabriel, 1971).
- If the gel has been run to observe changes in protein mass or charge in the sample, then place the gel in stain for the required period (see Protocols 8.1 and 8.4–8.6).
- Remove from the stain and place in destain until the background is clear enough to visualise and record the samples and/or standards (see above Protocol 8.1).

Protocol 8.3 Western blotting using a semi-dry blotter

Materials

- 12 pieces of 3 MM filter paper cut slightly larger than the gel itself (i.e., 8 cm × 9 cm for mini gels)
- 1 piece of nitrocellulose membrane filter (6 cm × 9 cm for mini gels)
- Tris buffered saline (TBS): 0.5 M **Tris** pH 7.6 containing 9% (w/v) NaCl
- Continuous transfer buffer (CTB): dissolve 5.81 g Tris, 2.89 g glycine, 0.315 g SDS in 800 ml distilled H_2O and add 200 ml methanol
- 0.05 % (w/v) copper pthalocyanine
- 3% (w/v) bovine serum albumin (BSA) in TBS (BSA/TBS)
- 0.05% (v/v) Tween 20 in TBS (TBS/Tween)
- Primary and secondary antibodies at appropriate dilutions in BSA/TBS

Procedure for Use with a Semi-Dry Blotter

- After the completion of PAGE (see Protocols 8.1 and 8.2), remove the polyacrylamide gel from the cassette and soak briefly in CTB.
- Moisten the top and bottom (cathode and anode) surfaces of the blotter with CTB.
- Soak 6 pieces of blotting paper in CTB, remove any excess, and then place on the anode plate of the blotting apparatus. Remove any air bubbles by rolling the filter papers with a glass rod. After soaking the nitrocellulose in CTB, place the nitrocellulose membrane on top of the filter papers.
- Transfer the polyacrylamide gel from CTB onto the surface of the nitrocellulose membrane filter.
- Soak another 6 pieces of 3MM paper in CTB and place on top of the gel. Remove any air bubbles with a glass rod.
- Position the cathodic plate of the blotting apparatus on to the filter paper/gel sandwich.
- Connect to the power supply and run the transfer at a current of 45 mA per gel for 50 min.
- If coloured standards have been included in the PAGE experiment, the transfer can be checked by gently lifting the gel over the standards. If the standards have not completely transferred, carefully reset the gel and the filter paper and resume the transfer.
- If coloured standards have not been included, the nitrocellulose can be reversibly stained with 0.05% (w/v) copper pthalocyanine. The image can be recorded before destaining in a solution of 12 mM NaOH until the dye has been cleared. The nitrocellulose membrane can be neutralised in several washes of TBS.
- To prevent the binding of primary antibody to the nitrocellulose membrane during probing, the unbound sites on the membrane are blocked by incubation for at least one hour at room temperature in either 3% (w/v) BSA or 3% (w/v) milk powder in TBS (the blots can be left at this stage for days at 4°C if a bactericide such as 0.05% (w/v) sodium azide is included).
- Wash the blot in several changes of TBS/Tween (minimum of 6 × 10 min washes) before incubation, with an appropriate dilution of primary antibody for at least 2 hours at room temperature,

but preferably overnight at 4°C (the blots can be left at this stage for days at 4°C if a bactericide such as 0.05% (w/v) sodium azide is included).

- Wash the blot in several changes of TBS/Tween (minimum of 6 × 10 min washes) to remove unbound primary antibody.

- Incubate with alkaline phosphatase-**conjugated** secondary antibody at an appropriate dilution in 3% (w/v) BSA in TBS (usually 1/1000 to 1/2000). This incubation should be conducted for at least 2 hours at room temperature, but preferably overnight at 4°C (the blots can be left at this stage for days at 4°C if a bactericide such as 0.05% (w/v) sodium azide is included).

- Wash as above to remove unbound secondary antibody and rinse the blot in substrate buffer for 2 min (0.2 M Tris pH 9.5). Then develop to reveal antibody-antigen binding in the following substrate mixture:

- 33 μl BCIP (5-bromo-4-chloro-3-indolyl phosphate; 50 mg ml^{-1} in DMF [dimethyl formamide]) and 44 μl NBT (nitroblue tetrazolium; 75 mg ml^{-1} in 70% [v/v] DMF) in 20 ml 0.2 M Tris pH 9.5.

- The colour development normally takes up to 30 min but may take up to several hours. Rinse the developed blots in distilled water and dry on filter paper.

- As an alternative, the secondary antibody mixture may be conjugated to horseradish peroxidase and reactivity revealed using a variety of substrates such as 4-chloronaphthol (2.0 ml at 5 mg ml^{-1} in ethanol plus 10 ml TBS and 10 μl 30% (v/v) H$_2$O$_2$, freshly mixed).

- For greater sensitivity, antibody reactivity can be detected using enhanced chemiluminescence (ECL). In this case, the washed and probed blot is placed on a clean glass plate and excess buffer removed with filter paper.

- A 1:1 mixture of ECL reagents (GE Healthcare; Bio-Rad; Perbio, Pierce Ltd) A + B (usually ~2 ml total volume for a mini gel blot) is spread evenly on the surface of the blot and left for 1 min at room temperature. Excess reagent is removed with filter paper and the blot covered with a sheet of cling film. The blot is then exposed in the dark room for at least 10 seconds onto Hyper film ECL and the image revealed using X-ray developer. Alternatively, the image can be recorded using a gel documentation system with the appropriate software.

- The reagents for ECL are given in Protocol 8.4.

Protocol 8.4 The preparation of enhanced chemiluminescent (ECL) reagent for developing Western blots probed with horseradish peroxidase conjugated secondary antibodies

Make a 250 mM Luminol and 90 mM p-Coumaric acid solution in DMSO and store these two solutions in separate dark bottles in the freezer.

When required, use two dark plastic bottles and label one *A* and the other *B*. Both of these ECL working solutions have a shelf life of 1–3 months if stored in a fridge.

Note: Never cross-contaminate solution A with solution B.

Bottle A

1.0 ml of the luminol solution

0.44 ml of the p-Coumaric acid

10.0 ml of 1.0 M Tris/HCl pH 8.5 and make the volume up to 100 ml with distilled water.

Bottle B

64 ml of 30% (v/v) H_2O_2

10 ml of 1.0 M Tris/HCl pH 8.5 and make the volume up to 100 ml with distilled water.

When required, mix 1.0 ml of reagent *A* with 1.0ml of reagent *B* in a 2.0 ml microfuge tube. Then pipette the mixture onto the surface of the nitrocellulose membrane (after the transfer and probing with appropriate antibodies; see Protocol 8.3). Spread the mixture evenly over the surface of the membrane and then place the nitrocellulose membrane in the imaging system to record the image. Many systems allow the operator to take an image without activating the luminescence. This will record the position of the coloured molecular weight markers. This image can then be overlaid onto the subsequent luminescent image to confirm the molecular weight of the target protein.

Protocol 8.5 Silver stain (adapted from GE Healthcare protocol) compatible with mass spectrometry

After electrophoresis (see Protocols 8.1 and 8.2), the polyacrylamide gel can be placed sequentially in the following solutions.

Fixation:

Place the gel in a solution of 40% (v/v) ethanol and 10% (v/v) acetic acid for 30 min.

Sensitizing:

Place the gel in a solution of 7% (w/v) sodium acetate, 5% (w/v) sodium thiosulphate, 30% (v/v) ethanol and 0.5% (v/v) glutaraldehyde (25% w/v) for 30 min.

Note: If the silver stained polypeptides in the gel are required for mass spectrometry, then omit the glutaraldehyde addition.

Wash:

Place the gel in ultra pure water (3 × 5 min per wash).

Silver staining:

Place the gel in a solution of 10% (v/v) silver nitrate (2.5% w/v), 0.04 % formaldehyde (37% w/v) for 20 min.

Wash:

Place the gel in ultra pure water (2 × 1 min per wash).

Developing:

Place the gel in a solution of 2.5 % (w/v) sodium carbonate. Add 40 μl of formaldehyde if the polypeptides in the gel are required for mass spectrometry and 20 μl of formaldehyde if they are not required for mass spectrometry. The developing should take between 2–5 min.

Stopping:

Place the gel in a solution of 1.5% (w/v) EDTA for 10 min.

Wash:

Place the gel in ultra pure water (3 × 5 min per wash).

Storage:

Place the gel in a solution of 4.6% (v/v) glycerol (87% w/w) and 30% (v/v) ethanol (2 × 30 min).

Protocol 8.6 Fluorescent staining for polypeptides in polyacrylamide gels

The fluorescent stains Sypro Red and Sypro Orange (Molecular Probes, USA; available through Thermo Fisher) are available to facilitate the detection of polypeptides after SDS-PAGE. This stain is sensitive and easy to use but requires overnight incubation to maximise sensitivity.

Method

- Use 0.05% (w/v) SDS in the electrophoresis running buffer instead of the usual 0.1% (w/v) SDS (see Protocol 8.1).
- During staining, the dye front gathers intense fluorescence. To avoid this, run the dye front from the bottom of the gel or remove the dye front with a scalpel.
- Typically for a mini gel mix 10 μl of the Sypro stain in 50 ml of 7.5% (v/v) acetic acid. For low percentage gels and to detect polypeptides with low M_r, use 10% (v/v) acetic acid.
- Wash and rinse the staining tray, then place the gel in the tray with the staining solution (a plastic bag with a seal can also be used).
- Cover the tray in aluminium foil or place the tray in a dark area.
- Abundant polypeptides will appear within 60 minutes but overnight staining may be required to detect the low-abundance polypeptides in the gel.
- The stain may be recovered and used again (up to 4 times). This may compromise the sensitivity of the stain but the detection of abundant proteins will be acceptable.
- Before recording the image, rinse the gel in 7.5% (v/v) acetic acid for 10–30 min to reduce the background fluorescence.
- Record the image on a 300 nm UV Trans illuminator.
- The gel should be stored in the dark to retain the sensitivity of the image.

Protocol 8.7 SDS-Imidazole zinc stain for polypeptides in polyacrylamide gels

This stain is approximately ten times more sensitive than silver stain. It is rapid, reversible so the same gel can be used for Western blotting, and compatible with mass spectrometry. However, it works in the presence of the detergent SDS so a non-denaturing PAGE gel must be pre-soaked for 5–10 min in 0.1M Tris pH 8.5 containing 0.1% (w/v) SDS before commencing the zinc imidazole treatment. This may impede any subsequent *in situ* staining for enzymes in the non-denaturing PAGE gel.

Method

- Rinse the gel for 5 min in distilled and deionised water.
- Incubate the gel for 10 min in 0.2 M imidazole and agitate on a rotating platform.
- Transfer the gel to a solution of 0.3 M $ZnCl_2$ and start to observe the stain development against a dark background. Protein bands appear transparent against a white background gel stain. The image contrast is enhanced with gels that are 1.5 mm thick.
- When the image has developed, discard the zinc solution and rinse the gel briefly in distilled water.
- The gel should be photographed in epiwhite light against a dark background.
- To destain the gel for further analysis (e.g., Western blotting [see Protocol 8.3]), agitate the gel in 2% (w/v) citric acid with several changes of liquid.
- The gel can be also stained with Coomassie blue if required.

Protocol 8.8 The detection of polypeptides in SDS-PAGE gels without the use of additional staining reagents (Ladner et al., 2004)

A rapid and sensitive method of visualising polypeptide bands in gels is achieved by the addition of 0.1 ml trichloroethanol to 20 ml of acrylamide mixture prior to the addition of the catalysts ammonium persulphate and TEMED (see Protocol 8.1).

The trihalogen reagent in the presence of UV light (5 min on a UV trans illuminator) reacts with the tryptophan residues in the polypeptides in the acrylamide gel to produce a fluorescent product. Once the image has been recorded, the gel can be used for other analytical techniques, such as Western blotting (see Protocol 8.3).

Protocol 8.9 Homogenisation of polyacrylamide gels containing a target protein

Requirements

- Two 1.0 ml pipette tips cut in half
- Copper wire from an electrical cable (10 × 15 mm pieces) compressed in a small ball
- 1.5 ml microfuge tube
- A small amount of silanised glass wool

Place the compressed copper wire in the bottom half of the 1.0 ml pipette tip and put the tip into a 1.5 ml microfuge tube. The acrylamide gel slice is placed on top of the copper wire and centrifuged at 12,000 × g for 15 seconds. The homogenised gel can be incubated in a suitable buffer for a period of time (2–16 hr) with mixing to allow the polypeptides in the gel fragments to diffuse into the buffer. The target protein can be recovered from the fragmented gel by repeating the above procedure, substituting silanised glass wool for the copper wire in the cut 1.0 ml pipette tip. After centrifugation at 12,000 × g for 15 seconds, the supernatant will be free from acrylamide and can then be subjected to further analysis.

RECOMMENDED READING

Research papers

Cameselle, J.C., Cabezas, A., Canales, J., Costas, M.J., Faraldo, A., Fernandez, A., Pinto, R.M. and Ribeiro, J.M. (2000) The simulated purification of an enzyme as a "dry" practical within an introductory course of biochemistry. *Biochem Educ* 28:148-153.

Davis, B.J. (1964) Disc electrophoresis. *Ann NY Acad Sci* 121:321-349.

Fountoulakis, M, and Juranville, J.F. (2003) Enrichment of low abundance brain proteins by preparative electrophoresis. *Anal Biochem* 313:267-282.

Gabriel, O. (1971) Locating enzymes on gels. *Methods in Enzymology* 22:578-604.

Gee, C.E., Bate, I.M., Thaomas, T.M. and Ryaln, D.B. (2003) The purification of IgY from chicken egg yolk by preparative electrophoresis. *Protein expr purif* 30:151-155.

Kobayashi, M., Hiura, N. and Matsuda, K. (1985) Isolation of enzymes from polyacrylamide disk gels by a centrifugal homogenisation method. *Anal Biochem* 145:351-353.

Laemmli, U.K. (1970) Cleavage of structural proteins during the assembly of the head of bacteriophage T4. *Nature* 227:680-685.

Ladner, C.L., Yang, J., Turner, R.J. and Edwards, R.A. (2004) Visible fluorescent detection of proteins in polyacrylamide gels without staining. *Anal Biochem* 326:13-20.

Maizel Jnr, J.V. (1964) Preparative electrophoresis of proteins in polyacrylamide gels. *Ann N Y Acad Sci* 121:382-390.

Ornstein, L. (1964) Disc electrophoresis-I Background and theory. *Ann N Y Acad Sci* 121:321-349.

Petersen, J.R., Okorodudu, A.O., Mohammad, A. and Payne, D.A. (2003) Capillary electrophoresis and its application in the clinical laboratory. *Clin Chim Acta* 330:1-30.

Thomas, T.M. Shave, E.E., Bate, I.M., Franklin, S.C. and Rylatt, D.B. (2002) Preparative electrophoresis: A general method for the purification of polyclonal antibodies. *J Chromatogr A* 944:161-168.

Vegvari, A. (2005) Peptide and proteins separations by capillary electrophoresis and electrochromatography. *Comp Anal Chem* 46:149-252.

Books

Catsimpoolas, N. (2013) *Biological and Biomedical Applications of Isoelectric Focussing*. Springer Verlag, New York, USA.

Cutler, P. (Ed.) (2004) *Protein Purification Protocols*. 2nd ed. Humana Press, New Jersey, USA.

Dunn, M.J. (2014) *Gel Electrophoresis of Proteins*. Butterworth-Heinemann, Oxford, UK.

Hames, B.D. (1998) *Gel Electrophoresis of Proteins: A Practical Approach*. 2nd ed. Oxford University Press, Oxford, UK.

Kurien, B.T. and Scofield R.H. (Eds.) (2015) *Western Blotting: Methods and Protocols*. Humana Press, New Jersey, USA.

Lundes, E., Reubsaet, L. and Greibrokk, T. (2014) *Chromatography: Basic Principles, Sample Preparations and Related Methods*. Wiley-VCH, Weinheim, Germany.

Oliver, R.W.A. (1998) *HPLC of Macromolecules: A Practical Approach*. 3rd ed. Oxford University Press, Oxford, UK.

Rosenberg, I.M. (2005) *Protein Analysis and Purification*. 2nd ed. Birkhauser, Boston, USA.

Tran, N.T. and Taverna, M. (Eds.) (2016) *Capillary Electrophoresis of Proteins and Peptides*. Humana Press, New Jersey, USA.

Westermeier, R. (2005) *Electrophoresis in Practise*. 4th ed. Wiley-VCH, New York, USA.

Wilson, K. and Walker, J. (Eds.) (2017) *Principles and Techniques of Biochemistry and Molecular Biology*. 8th ed. Cambridge University Press, Cambridge, UK.

APPENDIX 1: The Laws of Thermodynamics and the Gibbs Free Energy Equation

- The first law of thermodynamics states that the total energy of a system is constant. (Energy cannot be created or destroyed.)
- The second law of thermodynamics states that entropy (S) (measure of the randomness of a system) tends to increase over time.

The change in free energy (ΔG) within a system (the system in this context could be the flask containing water and oil) can be described by the Gibbs free energy equation.

Gibbs free energy equation $\quad \Delta G = \Delta H - T\Delta S$

Where:

Temperature (T) in degrees Kelvin.

Enthalpy (H) is a summation of the kinetic and potential energies of the molecules contained within the system at constant pressure (ΔH can be thought of as a measure of the heat generated within the system, which results in a positive (ΔH) for endothermic reactions and a negative (ΔH) for exothermic reactions).

Entropy (S) is a measure of the randomness of the system. For example, when water is frozen the molecules are organised into a crystal structure. There is less entropy in the ice water molecules because they are restricted in their movements. When the temperature of the system increases, the frozen water moves into the liquid phase, and the water molecules have more freedom of movement. If the temperature increases to boiling point, the liquid water molecules move into the gas phase, again with more freedom of movement.
When the Gibbs free energy equation gives a positive free energy change ($+\Delta G$) the reaction is said to thermodynamically unfavourable. If the Gibbs free energy equation gives a negative free energy change ($-\Delta G$) the reaction is said to thermodynamically favourable. When a system is at equilibrium the Gibbs free energy equation is resolved to be zero ($\Delta G = 0$).

APPENDIX 2: Properties of Amino Acids

Name	Single letter code	Solubility (g/100g, 25°C)	Crystal density (g/ml)	pI at 25°C
Alanine (Ala)	A	16.65	1.401	6.107
Arginine (Arg)	R	15	1.1	10.76
Aspartic Acid (Asp)	D	0.778	1.66	2.98
Asparagine (Asn)	N	3.53	1.54	–
Cysteine (Cys)	C	very	–	5.02
Glutamic Acid (Glu)	E	0.864	1.460	3.08
Glutamine (Gln)	Q	2.5	–	–
Glycine (Gly)	G	24.99	1.607	6.064
Histidine (His)	H	4.19	–	7.64
Isoleucine (Ile)	I	4.117	–	6.038
Leucine (Leu)	L	2.426	1.191	6.036
Lysine (Lys)	K	very	–	9.47
Methionine (Met)	M	3.381	1.340	5.74
Phenylalanine (Phe)	F	2.965	–	5.91
Proline (Pro)	P	162.3	–	6.3
Serine (Ser)	S	5.023	1.537	5.68
Threonine (Thr)	T	very	–	–
Tryptophan (Trp)	W	1.136	–	5.88
Tyrosine (Tyr)	Y	0.0453	1.456	5.63
Valine (Val)	V	8.85	1.230	6.002

APPENDIX 3: The Common Units Used in Biology

- One **mole** of a compound is the molecular weight in grams.
- One mole of any compound contains the same number of molecules (Avagadro's number = 6.023×10^{23}).
- A **molar** solution is one mole of a compound dissolved in a litre of water.

	1.0	1.0×10^{-3}	1.0×10^{-6}	1.0×10^{-9}	1.0×10^{-12}
Concentration	molar M	millimolar mM	micromolar µM	nanomolar nM	picomolar pM
Amount	mole	millimole mmoles	micromole µmoles	nanomole nmoles	picomole pmoles
	gram g	milligram mg	microgram µg	nanogram ng	picogram pg
Volume	litre(dm^3) L	millilitre (cm^3) ml	microlitre µl	nanolitre nl	picolitre pl

APPENDIX 4: Chromatographic Runs

The process of purifying a protein can be broken down into a series of separate but interrelated stages (see Figure 3.5).

(A) Starting conditions: Prior to embarking on a chromatographic run, it is a good idea to spend some time getting to know the enzyme you are working with. This will provide valuable information about some of the protein's properties, such as the pH optimum for catalytic activity, pH optimum for storage and thermal stability. These properties will then provide a guide to the starting conditions of the chromatographic run. The proteolytic profile of the extract and the effect of activators and inhibitors on these properties can be evaluated in small scale experiments to help guide the starting conditions for a chromatographic run (see Protocol 3.1).

(B) Pre-equilibrate the resin: Chromatographic resins are usually stored at 4°C in a preservative (0.1% (w/v) thiomersal; 0.05% (w/v) sodium azide or 20% (v/v) ethanol). The preservative needs to be removed and the resin needs to be equilibrated in a buffer that encourages the protein of interest to bind to the resin (e.g., a low salt buffer for IEX or a high salt buffer for HIC). This can be conveniently achieved using a Buchner flask connected to a vacuum to which a funnel with a sintered glass mesh is attached.

(C) The chromatographic resin can be poured onto the glass mesh and the vacuum started. The preservative is quickly removed and the resin can then be washed in start buffer.

(D) Allow the vacuum to remove most of the buffer and then switch off the vacuum.

(E) Resuspend the resin in start buffer (2× the resin volume) and allow the resin to settle. Particles that do not settle ("fines") should be removed by aspiration. If the fines are not removed, they can lodge themselves into spaces in the resin. This will increase the back pressure and may block the flow of the mobile phase. Once the fines have been removed the resin can be degassed under vacuum before being packed into the column.

(F) Prior to the assembly of the column, it is recommended that the mesh at the ends of the column (or flow adaptors), which prevents the resin from leaving the column, is checked for holes in the fabric and cleaned by sonication in water (or, if visibly dirty, sonicate first in 5% (w/v) SDS in 0.1 M NaOH and then in water) for 5 minutes.

(G) Distilled water should be flowed through the assembled chromatographic column to check for leaks in the column seals and the connections between the column and the pump. Connections from the pump through the detector to the fraction collector should also be checked for leaks.

(H) Once the integrity of the column has been verified, a small volume of start buffer should be placed into the bottom of the column and run from the outlet to liberate trapped air beneath the mesh. Gentle tapping on the column should help. Additional start buffer can then be added to cover the end mesh.

(I) The column should be tilted at an angle and the degassed resin slurry introduced to the column by running the slurry down the sides of the column until the column is full.

(J) The column should be placed into a vertical position and the resin packed into the column at a flow rate marginally faster than the anticipated flow rate for the experimental run. (This will prevent a reduction in the column's volume when the sample is applied). Remember that the resin has been introduced to the column as a slurry (i.e., there is more liquid than resin) and this may require the introduction of more resin from the slurry to achieve the desired bed volume.

(K) When the required bed volume has been packed, the flow of liquid is stopped and the upper column connector can be attached. Take care at this stage to ensure that there is no air trapped within the system. Running the column in the reverse direction at a relatively low flow rate can be used to facilitate removal of the trapped air at the top of the column.

(L) The resin within the column can then be equilibrated with the starting buffer at the required experimental flow rate.

(M) The column should ideally be packed at the temperature at which the chromatographic run is to be conducted. Remember that buffers stored at 4°C will have more dissolved gas that will be released as the temperature rises. The choice of temperature will be guided by the thermal stability of the enzyme, the estimated run time and the presence of proteolytic enzymes, particularly in crude extracts. Most modern resins have quite rigid structures, which allow the columns to be run at relatively high flow rates (>5.0 ml min^{-1}). This significantly reduces chromatographic run times, and most experiments can be conducted at room temperature unless the target protein is particularly unstable.

(N) After at least two column volumes of the starting buffer has been run through the column, and if there are no leaks, the sample can be applied either through an inline three-way valve or using a sample loop (see Figure 1.2). If a large volume of sample is to be applied, stop the pump delivering the start buffer, transfer the start buffer tube to the sample and use the pump to apply the sample to the column (taking care to avoid air bubbles when transferring the tube between buffer and sample). When the sample has been applied, stop the pump and reconnect the system to the start buffer. As soon as the sample has been applied to the top of the column, fractions from the column outlet should be collected, and they should be collected throughout the chromatographic run.

(O) The sample will interact with the selected resin and as a result of the start conditions, some protein will bind to the resin, while other proteins will not interact and will percolate through the column as unbound material. The unbound material should be eluted from the column using the start buffer until the absorbance at 280 nm monitoring the emergence of the unbound material reaches a background level. The elution conditions can then be applied and the eluted protein should be collected in fractions.

(P) The resin within the column can then be washed according to the manufacturer's instructions and then re-equilibrated in the start conditions for another run.

(Q) If the column is not to be reused for a period of time, the column may be dismantled and the resin stored in preservative. Alternatively, the column should be washed with two column volumes of water followed by two column volumes of a preservative.

(R) The fractions collected should be assayed for the protein of interest (enzyme assay or antibody) and the peak fraction(s) identified and pooled.

(S) The volume, the protein concentration (see Protocols 4.1–4.5) and the activity of the pooled fractions should be measured. The information obtained can then be recorded on the purification balance sheet (see Table 8.1).

(T) In addition to measuring the % yield and fold purity at each stage, it may be expedient to determine the purity by other techniques. The most popular method is denaturing (in the presence of the detergent sodium dodecyl sulphate (SDS)) polyacrylamide gel electrophoresis (PAGE). A single polypeptide band on an SDS-PAGE gel stained with Coomassie blue dye is a usually taken to be good indication of a homogeneous preparation (see Section 8.3). But it should be remembered that SDS-PAGE separates polypeptides based on relative molecular mass (M_r). A single band on an SDS-PAGE gel does not necessarily mean a homogenous preparation, because contaminants of a similar M_r may have co-purified with the target protein of interest, or contaminants may be present at low levels not detectable with the stain. It is possible to load a gel with increasing amounts of the "homogeneous" protein to try and visualise the presence of these low levels of contaminants or to switch to a more sensitive stain (e.g., silver stain; see Protocol 8.5). An alternative approach is to run the "homogeneous" preparation on a different electrophoretic technique (e.g., non-denaturing PAGE [see Section 8.3.6 and Protocol 8.2], capillary electrophoresis [see Section 8.7], or isoelectric focusing [IEF] [see Section 8.6]) or analytical chromatographic techniques (e.g., size exclusion chromatography [SEC] [see Section 7.5.2] or reversed-phase high-pressure chromatography [RP-HPLC; see Chapter 8.8]). The combination of a single band on SDS-PAGE at different loadings and a single band on non-denaturing PAGE or IEF (or a single peak after SEC or RP-HPLC) is a good indication of the homogeneity of the preparation.

(U) Tryptic digestion followed by ESI-RP-HPLC, sequence analysis of a number of peptide fragments by MS/MS and database searching will confirm the identity of the final protein sample.

The stages outlined (A-U) apply to a column that requires packing with resin. Pre-packed columns bought from a manufacturer can enter this scheme from (K-U). These proprietary columns may be able to tolerate the odd air bubble, but to make sure that the purification run is trouble-free, it is a good idea to check that there are no air bubbles or leaks in the system before applying the sample.

APPENDIX 5: Determining the Concentration of a Compound in a Solution in PPM

This method of calculating the concentration of a compound dissolved in a liquid (water/buffer or solvent) is popular among analytical chemists when the concentration of a compound is low.

$$\text{Parts per million (ppm)} = \frac{\text{grams of the compound}}{\text{grams of the solution}} \times 1{,}000{,}000$$

For example: When 50 mg of alanine is dissolved in a litre of water what is the concentration in parts per million?

$$\text{Answer:} \quad \text{Parts per million} = \frac{0.05}{1000} \times 1{,}000{,}000$$
$$= 50 \text{ ppm}$$

Remember to add the weight of the solute to the weight of the final liquid, although it makes little difference in the final answer.

$$\text{Parts per million} = \frac{0.05}{1000 \text{ g} + 0.05 \text{ g}} \times 1{,}000{,}000$$
$$= 50 \text{ ppm}$$

APPENDIX 6: The Answers to the Exercises in the Various Chapters

Answers to Exercise 4.1
A bench centrifuge at 3000 rpm with a rotor that had a radius of 95 mm. What is the RCF?

$$RCF = 1.118 \times 95 \times (5000/1000)^2$$
$$RCF = 1.118 \times 95 \times (5)^2$$
$$RCF = 2655 \times g$$

Answers to Exercises 7.1 and 7.2

Exercise 7.1 M_r estimation using size exclusion chromatography (SEC)

A column containing a size exclusion resin ($V_0 = 85$ ml and $V_t = 250$ ml) has been calibrated with five standard proteins of known molecular mass (M_r).

Standards	M_r	$Log_{10} M_r$	V_e (ml)	K_{av}
Amylase	200,000	5.30	94	0.05
Alcohol dehydrogenase	150,000	5.18	103	0.11
Bovine serum albumin	66,000	4.82	142	0.35
Trypsinogen	24,000	4.38	187	0.62
Aprotinin	6,500	3.81	215	0.79

$$K_{av} = \frac{V_e - V_0}{V_t - V_0}$$

Calculate the K_{av} for the standard proteins and plot a calibration graph for the column ($Log_{10} M_r$ [standard proteins] v K_{av}).

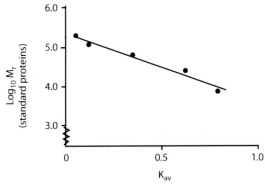

- Using the same column the V_e for egg albumin was determined to be 152 ml.
- Establish the K_{av} for egg albumin and using the calibration graph estimate the M_r of egg albumin.

Points to remember when drawing a size exclusion chromatography calibration plot

- Plot a line of "best fit" through the data.
- K_{av} is a value between 0.0 and 1.0.

- Do not attach the line to either axis. If the line is attached to the y-axis that indicates that the protein eluted in the total volume of the column (V_t). If the line is attached to the x-axis this gives a value of 1.0, which is the void volume (V_0) of the column indicating that the protein is large. An alternative SEC resin should be selected with a larger pore size (see Table 7.1).
- The egg albumin has an K_{av} of 0.41.
- Using the calibration plot this can be converted into a M_r for the protein of 44,668. Size exclusion chromatography is not that accurate so round the value to the nearest appropriate number, e.g., 44,500.

Exercise 7.2 The difference between estimating the M_r of a protein using SEC and SDS-PAGE (see Chapter 8 and Exercise 8.1).

When a sample of haemoglobin and myoglobin are applied to a 10% SDS-PAGE gel both proteins produced a single band with an estimated M_r of 16,000.

When the samples were subjected to SEC, haemoglobin had an M_r of 64,000 and myoglobin an M_r of 16,000.

Explanation:

Size exclusion chromatography (SEC) separates proteins in their native conformation. This means they retain their secondary, tertiary and quaternary structures (see Chapter 2). In SEC the M_r estimation of a protein will be in its native conformation (size and shape).

Electrophoresis of samples using the detergent SDS (SDS-PAGE) will denature the conformation of proteins unravelling the secondary, tertiary and quaternary structures. They assume linear structures and the M_r estimation is of the denatured conformation (polypeptide).

Myoglobin gave an estimated M_r of 16,000 using both SEC and SDS-PAGE shows that its structure is comprised of a single polypeptide. Haemoglobin gave an estimated M_r of 16,000 using SDS-PAGE and 64,000 using SEC indicating that haemoglobin's native conformation has a quaternary structure comprised of 4 proteins each with an M_r of 16,000. When haemoglobin is brought into contact with SDS the 4 proteins in the quaternary structure lose their native conformation to produce polypeptides of equal M_r.

Answers to Exercise 8.1

Calculations to complete a purification table.

Extract volume 10.0 ml

Protein concentration 2.5 mg ml^{-1}

Step 1 Total protein

Volume (ml) multiplied by the protein mg ml^{-1}

$10 \times 2.5 = 25$ mg

Step 2 The rate of reaction

A 100 µl of extract was assayed in a reaction volume of 1.0 ml in a 1.0 ml semi micro cuvette with a 1.0 cm path length at 25°C with BAPNA. This was measured directly in a spectrophotometer to give an absorbance of 1.45 over a 10 min reaction period.

The change in absorbance at 405 nm min^{-1} is $1.45/10 = 0.145$

Step 3 Using the Beer-Lambert law to convert the change in absorbance min^{-1} into an amount of product formed min^{-1} and eventually into International Units of enzyme activity

Absorbance (A) = path length of the cell (cm) (L) × molar absorptivity (M^{-1} cm^{-1}) (ε) × concentration (M)

$$A = L \times \varepsilon \times C$$
$$0.145 = 1 \times 8800 \times \text{concentration (molar)}$$
$$\frac{0.145}{8800} = 0.000016 \text{ M min}^{-1}$$

$= 16 \ \mu M \ min^{-1}$ (remember that a molar (M) concentration is μmol in 1000 ml)

A) Therefore in a 1.0 ml cuvette we have 16 nmol
B) This has all derived from 100 μl of enzyme producing 16 nmol min^{-1} product
C) Therefore 1.0 ml of enzyme would produce 160 nmol min^{-1}

The International Units of enzyme activity are 1 μmol of product produced (or substrate consumed) min^{-1}.

Therefore from C (above), we have 0.16 units of enzyme activity ml^{-1} of extract.

Step 4 Specific activity

Specific activity is defined as units of enzyme activity mg^{-1} of protein

$$= \text{enzyme activity} \quad \frac{\text{units ml-1}}{\text{Protein concentration (mg ml-1)}} \qquad \text{or} \quad \frac{\text{units } \cancel{\text{ml}^{-1}}}{\text{mg } \cancel{\text{ml}^{-1}}} \ \text{to give} \quad \frac{\text{units}}{\text{mg}}$$

$$= \frac{0.16 \ \text{units ml}^{-1}}{2.5 \ \text{mg ml}^{-1}}$$

$= 0.064$ units mg^{-1} of protein.

Step 5 Total activity

The total units of enzyme activity

$$= \text{units mg}^{-1} \ (\text{specific activity}) \times \text{total protein (mg)}$$
$$= 0.064 \times 25$$
$$= 1.6 \ \text{units}$$

Or units ml$^{-1} \times$ vol (ml)

$$0.16 \ \text{units ml}^{-1} \times 10 = 1.6 \ \text{units}$$

Answers to Exercise 8.2: The molecular weight calculations associated with SDS-PAGE.

M_r standard proteins	$Log_{10} \ M_r$ standard proteins	R_f (relative to the dye front)
250,000	5.40	0.11
150,000	5.18	0.18
100,000	5.00	0.26
75,000	4.87	0.36
50,000	4.70	0.44
37,000	4.57	0.64
25,000	4.40	0.80
15,000	4.18	0.97

• Plot $log_{10} \ M_r$ standard proteins v their mobility relative to the dye front (R_f).

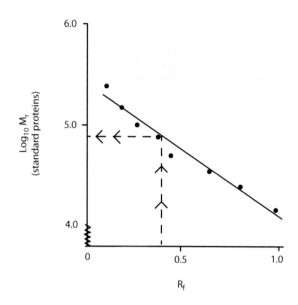

Points to remember when drawing an SDS-PAGE calibration plot:

- Plot a line of "best fit" through the data.
- R_f is a value between 0.0 and 1.0.
- Do not attach the line to either axis. If the line attaches to the y-axis that is an R_f of 0.0 which is the origin. If the line attaches to the x-axis this is a value of 1.0, which is where the dye front has run.
- There are few proteins with an M_r below 10,000 ($\log_{10}$ 4.0) so start the y-axis at $\log_{10}$ 4.0.
- The unknown polypeptide has an R_f of 0.39.
- Using the calibration plot this can be converted into a M_r for the polypeptide of 79,432.8. SDS-PAGE is not that accurate so round the value to the nearest appropriate number, for example, 79,500.

APPENDIX 7: An Alphabetical List of Chromatography (C), Electrophoresis (E), Filtration Equipment (F) and Laboratory Suppliers (LS)

(C) *Agilent Technologies*: Offices throughout the world; access the website for relevant location (http://www.home.agilent.com)

Agilent Technologies LDA UK Limited
Life Sciences & Chemical Analysis Group
Lakeside
Cheadle Royal Business Park
Stockport, Cheshire SK8 3GR
Agrisera, Ltd (Plant protein antibodies. www.agrisera.com)
AB Box 57, SE-911 21 Vännäs, SWEDEN

(C, E and F) *Bio-Rad Laboratories*: Offices throughout the world; access the website for relevant location (http://www.bio-rad.com)

Bio-Rad Laboratories, Inc
Bio-Rad House
Maxted Road
Hemel Hempstead
Hertfordshire HP2 7DX

(C) *CM Scientific* (suppliers of Upchurch, Ltd)
(https://www.cmscientific.com/upchurch.php)

CM Scientific, Ltd
1 Ryefield Court
Ryefield Way
Siliden
BD20 ODL, UK

(C) *Diba Industries* (Omifit columns)

Diba Industries Inc
4 Precision Road
Danbury, CT 06810

(LS) *Fisher Scientific*
(https://www.fishersci.co.uk/gb/en/home.html)

Fisher Scientific UK Ltd
Bishop Meadow Road
Loughborough
LE11 5RG

(C, E) *GE Healthcare*: Offices throughout the world; access the website for relevant location (http://www
.gehealthcare.com)

GE Healthcare UK Ltd
Amersham Place
Little Chalfont
Buckinghamshire HP7 9NA
England

(E) *Engineering & Design Plastics Ltd*
(http://www.electrophoresis.co.uk/)

84 High Street
Cherry Hinton
Cambridge CB1 9HZ, UK

(C) Kinesis Ltd (www.Kinesis.co.uk)
9 Orion Court
Ambuscade Road
Colmworth Business Park
St Neots
Cambridgeshire PE198YX, UK

(C) *Merck KGaA*: Offices throughout the world; access the website for relevant location (http://www.merck
.de/servlet/PB/menu/1001723/index.html). They now also supply Millipore equipment and supplies

Merck House
Seldown Lane
Poole, Dorset
BH15 1TD
United Kingdom

New England Biolaboratories: Offices in the USA; relevant information can be found at (https://www.neb.com/)

New England Biolabs
240 County Road
Ipswich, MA 01938-2723

(F) *Pall Corporation*: Offices throughout the world; access the website for relevant location (http://www
.pall.com/)

Europa House
Havant Street
Portsmouth, Hampshire
PO1 3PD

(C) *Perkin Elmer LAS*: Offices throughout the world; access the website for relevant location (http://las
.perkinelmer.co.uk)

(C) *Phenomenex PLC*: Offices throughout the world; access the website for relevant location (http://www
.phenomenex.com)

Queens Avenue
Hurdsfield Ind. Est.
Macclesfield Cheshire
SK10 2BN, England

Promega: Offices throughout the world; access the website for relevant location and distributors (http://
www.promega.com/)

Qiagen Ltd: Offices in the UK; relevant information can be found at (https://www.qiagen.com
/gb/?akamai-feo=off)

Qiagen House
Fleming Way
Crawley
West Sussex
RH10 9NQ

(F) *Sartorius (Vivascience)*: Offices throughout the world; access the website for relevant location and
distributors (http://www.sartorius.com/)

Sartorius Ltd
Longmead Business Centre
Blenheim Road
Epsom
KT19 9QQ
United Kingdom

(LS) *Scientific Lab Supplies*
(https://www.scientificlabs.co.uk/)

Scientific Laboratory Supplies Ltd
Wilford Industrial Estate
Ruddington Lane
Wilford
Nottingham, NG11 7EP

(E) *SCIE-PLAS*
(http://www.scie-plas.com/)·

Unit 3 Gainsborough Trading Estate
Old Road
Southam
Warwickshire CV47 1HP
United Kingdom

(C) *Shimadzu*: Offices throughout the world; access the website for relevant location (https://www
.shimadzu.co.uk/)

Shimadzu UK Limited
Mill Court
Featherstone Road
Wolverton Mill South
Milton Keynes
Buckinghamshire
MK12 5RD

(C, E, F and LS) *Sigma-Aldrich*: Offices throughout the world; access the website for relevant location
(http://www.sigmaaldrich.com)

Sigma-Aldrich Company Ltd.
The Old Brickyard
New Road
Gillingham
Dorset
SP8 4XT

(C, E, F and LS) *ThermoFisher Scientific Ltd. (includes Perbio Science protein methods)*
(https://www.thermofisher.com/uk/en/home.html#)

Life Technologies Ltd
3 Fountain Drive
Inchinnan Business Park
Paisley PA4 9RF, UK

(LS) *Thistle Scientific Ltd*
(http://www.thistlescientific.co.uk/acatalog/contact-us.html)

DFDS House, Goldie Road
Uddington, Glasgow
G71 6NZ, UK

(C) *Tosoh Bioscience*: Offices throughout the world; access the website for relevant location (http://www
.tosohbiosep.com)

Tosoh Bioscience GmbH
Zettachring 6
70567 Stuttgart, Germany

(C and F) *Waters PLC*: Offices throughout the world; access the website for relevant location (http://www
.waters.com)

Waters Ltd
730-740 Centennial Court
Centennial Park
Elstree
Hertfordshire
WD6 3SZ, UK

(LS) *Web Scientific Ltd* (www.webscientific.co.uk)

Crewe
Cheshire
CW2 5PR, UK

(F) *Whatman*: Offices throughout the world; access the website for relevant location and distributors
(http://www.whatman.com/)

For UK, Ireland, France, Italy, Spain, Belgium, Luxembourg, Portugal, Greece, Cyprus and Malta:

(LS) *VWR International Ltd*
(https://uk.vwr.com/store/)

Hunter Boulevard
Magna Park
Lutterworth
Leicestershire
LE17 4XN

APPENDIX 8: Buffer Tables to Prepare Buffers at a Required pH Value

- To prepare a buffer dissolve the reagent powder in a beaker with lower volume of ultrapure water (18.2 MΩ·cm at 25°C) than the final volume required.
- The use of an ultrasonic bath will aid the dispersion of the solid material.
- When the buffer constituents have completely dissolved, check and adjust the pH then make the solution up to the volume required. The use of a volumetric flask will ensure that the final volume is correct.
- Filter the buffer through a 0.2 mm membrane before transferring to a storage vessel at a suitable temperature.

Remember that for some buffers (e.g., Tris/HCl) the temperature will influence the final pH value.

Always set the buffer pH accounting for the temperature that the buffer will be used in an experiment, e.g., 4°C for a chromatography experiment, which may change to 37°C for the enzyme assay.

Buffers with phosphate ions are not suitable for use with proteins, which require calcium ions because the mixture will form a precipitate at pH 7.0.

McIlvaine's buffer: Valid for pH values between 2.2–8.0.

Prepare a 0.1 M solution of citric acid and a 0.2 M solution of disodium hydrogen phosphate.

Mix the volumes in the table (below) to prepare a 100 ml solution of 0.15 M McIlvaine's buffer

pH	Volume (ml) of 0.2 M Na_2HPO_4	Volume (ml) of 0.1 M citric acid
2.2	2.00	98.00
2.4	6.20	93.80
2.6	10.90	89.10
2.8	15.85	84.15
3.0	20.55	79.45
3.2	24.70	75.30
3.4	28.50	71.50
3.6	32.20	67.80
3.8	35.50	64.50
4.0	38.55	61.45
4.2	41.40	58.60
4.4	44.10	55.90
4.6	46.75	53.25
4.8	49.30	50.70
5.0	51.50	48.50

(Continued)

pH	Volume (ml) of 0.2 M Na₂HPO₄	Volume (ml) of 0.1 M citric acid
5.2	53.60	46.40
5.4	55.75	44.25
5.6	58.00	42.00
5.8	60.45	39.55
6.0	63.15	36.85
6.2	66.10	33.90
6.4	69.25	30.75
6.6	72.75	27.25
6.8	77.25	22.75
7.0	82.35	17.65
7.2	86.95	13.05
7.4	90.85	9.15
7.6	93.65	6.35
7.8	95.75	4.25
8.0	97.25	2.75

REFERENCE

McIlvaine, T.C. (1921) A buffer solution for colorimetric comparison. *J Biol Chem* 49:183-186.

***0.1 M Phosphate buffer*:** Valid for pH values between 5.8 and 7.8:

Prepare 0.1 M sodium di hydrogen phosphate (NaH_2PO_4) and 0.1 M disodium hydrogen phosphate (Na_2HPO_4) (if available use the hydrated salts, which will dissolve without too much difficulty). The use of an ultrasonic bath will aid the dispersion of the solid salt particles.

The dihydrogen salt is the acidic salt with two replaceable H^+ ions.

Mix the volumes in the table (below) to prepare a 100 ml solution of 0.1 M phosphate buffer.

pH	Volume (ml) NaH₂PO₄	Volume (ml) Na₂HPO₄
5.8	92.0	8.0
6.0	87.7	12.3
6.2	81.5	19.5
6.4	73.5	26.5
6.6	62.5	37.5
6.8	51.0	49.0
7.0	39.0	61.0
7.2	28.0	72.0

(Continued)

pH	Volume (ml) NaH$_2$PO$_4$	Volume (ml) Na$_2$HPO$_4$
7.4	19.0	81.0
7.6	13.0	87.0
7.8	8.5	91.5

Source: Adapted from http://www.sciencegateway.org
/protocols/cellbio/appendix/phosb.htm.

0.1 M Tris/HCl buffer: Valid for pH values between 7.2–9.0 (25°C).

These buffers can be prepared by mixing the powders of Tris base with Trizma/HCl and making the volume up to 1000 ml.

pH 5°C	pH 25°C	pH 37°C	Tris base g/litre	Trizma/HCl g/litre
7.76	7.2	6.91	14.04	1.34
7.89	7.30	7.02	13.70	1.60
7.97	7.40	7.12	13.22	1.94
8.07	7.50	7.22	12.70	2.36
8.18	7.60	7.30	12.12	2.78
8.26	7.70	7.40	11.44	3.32
8.37	7.80	7.52	10.64	3.94
8.48	7.90	7.62	9.76	4.60
8.58	8.00	7.71	8.88	5.30
8.68	8.10	7.80	8.04	5.94
8.78	8.20	7.91	7.08	6.68
8.88	8.30	8.01	6.14	7.40
8.98	8.40	8.10	5.28	8.06
9.09	8.50	8.22	4.42	8.72
9.18	8.60	8.31	3.66	9.30
9.28	8.70	8.42	3.00	9.80
9.36	8.80	8.51	2.46	10.26

Source: Adapted from Sigma Aldrich (Supelco data sheet): https://www.sigmaaldrich
.com/Graphics/Supelco/objects/4800/4709.pdf.

Alternatively, 1000 ml of a 0.1M Tris/HCl buffer can be prepared by dissolving 12.11 g of Tris base in 700 ml of ultrapure water (18.2 MΩ·cm at 25°C). The pH should be adjusted with HCl until the required pH value has been reached before the volume is made up to 1000 ml (use a volumetric flask). The solution should be filtered through 0.2 μm filter before storage.

For Tris buffers, the final pH value should reflect the temperature at which the experiment (chromatography buffer or enzyme assay buffer) will be conducted.

Glossary of Terms

ΔG: The change in the Gibbs free energy derived from the Gibbs free energy equation $\Delta G = \Delta H - T\Delta S$.

Absorbance (of light): The $\log_{10}(1/T)$. The values range between 0 and infinity (∞) (spectrophotometers typically measure linear absorbance values between 0 and 3.0).

Agarose: A polysaccharide with many hydroxyl groups. The material can be used to construct biocompatible resins to be used in protein purification.

Agonist: A substance that binds to a receptor and triggers a response in the cell.

Aliquot: A portion of the total amount of solution.

Ampholytes: A mixture of polyamino and polycarboxylic acids.

Ångström (Å): A unit of measurement equivalent to 10^{-10} m (0.1 nm).

Anion: A molecule with a negative charge, which will travel towards a positive electrode (anode).

Antibody: A protein released by B cells in response to a foreign compound (antigen). There are different classes of antibodies collectively known as immunoglobulins.

Antigen: A foreign compound that, when it enters the body, is recognised as foreign and elicits the production of an antibody.

Ascites: Fluid that collects in the peritoneum (which is the membrane that forms the lining of the abdominal cavity).

Aspiration: Removal of liquid using a pipette, syringe or a syphon.

Assay: A process where the concentration of a component (e.g., target protein) as part of a mixture is measured. There are many different types of assay depending on the target protein's biological function, including enzyme assay, bioassay (the effect of a substance on a living organism), immunoassay, antigen capture assay, receptor assay, radioimmunoassay, etc.

Asymmetric: Not the same on both sides of a central line.

Attenuance (of light): Measurement of light scattering as is the case when a spectrophotometer is used to estimate bacterial cell numbers (incorrectly referred to as optical density). When light scattering is low, attenuance reduces to absorbance.

Azocasein: The orange sulphanilamide dye is covalently bonded to the milk protein casein to provide a substrate for proteolytic enzymes.

Bactericide: A reagent which destroys bacteria.

Ballotini beads: Glass beads (0.2–1.0 mm diameter) used to puncture the walls of prokaryotic and eukaryotic cells.

Beer-Lambert law: The absorbance (A) of a solution at a given wavelength (nm) is equal to the path length of the cuvette (l) in the spectrophotometer (1 cm) × (ε) the molar absorptivity coefficient ($M^{-1}\,cm^{-1}$) × (C) the concentration (mol L^{-1}) (also see molar adsorption [absorptivity] coefficient (ε)).

$$\text{Beer-Lambert law} \quad A = l\varepsilon C$$

Example: The absorbance of a solution of NADH is 1.2; calculate the concentration of the solution.

The molar absorptivity coefficient (ε) of NADH at 340 nm is 6.22×10^3.

The path length of the cell is 1.0 cm.

$$\text{Beer-Lambert's law} \quad A = l\varepsilon C$$

$$1.2 = 1 \times 6220 \times C$$

Therefore, C = 0.000193 M (Appendix 2)

Or, C = 0.193 mM or 193 μM

Answer: The concentration of a solution of NADH is with an absorbance of 1.2 is 193 μM.

bis: Occurring twice, as in bis acrylamide or bis Tris propane.

Biogel: A trade name (Bio-Rad) for polyacrylamide gel formed into beads used for protein purification.

Brønsted: Proposed a definition for acid and bases, namely, that an acid is a proton donor and a base is a proton acceptor.

Calmodulin: A small, ubiquitous calcium binding protein which affects the activity of many calcium-dependent enzymes.

Cation: A molecule with a positive charge which will travel towards a negative electrode (cathode).

Chaotropic salts: "Chaos-forming" salts referring to a salt's ability to disrupt the regular hydrogen bond structures in water. They increase the water solubility of non-polar substances and increase the "salting in" of proteins.

Chelating agent: A compound (e.g., EDTA or DIECA) which preferentially binds to metal ions. This reduces or effectively eliminates the metal ions' presence in a solution.

Chromatography: A separation process that distributes analytes (substances) between two immiscible phases: a moving phase and a stationary phase. How they distribute between the two phases is determined by their partition coefficient (K_D).

cis-Configuration: In chemistry this refers to the arrangement of atoms relative to each other. The term "cis" means the atoms in a molecule are arranged on the same side as each other ("this side of").

Concentration: A molar (M) solution is 1 mole of a compound dissolved in 1 litre of water, i.e., the molecular weight in gram dissolved in 1000 ml of water.

Clathrate: A caged/lattice structure formed around a molecule (or structure) trapping and containing that molecule (or structure), e.g., water forms clathrate structures around aromatic rings or aliphatic chains.

Condensation reaction: A chemical reaction between two molecules which results in the elimination of a water molecule from the final structure.

Conformation (of proteins): The three-dimensional shape of the macromolecular chain.

Conjugated (as in secondary antibody): Joined together, e.g., anti-mouse IgG raised in rabbit conjugated to horse radish peroxidase.

Co-ordinate bonds: A covalent bond where both electrons for sharing are provided by one of the atoms.

Co-translational modification (of a protein): The addition to a protein's structure (e.g., a sugar) as the protein is being synthesised on a ribosome. This usually occurs on proteins as they are synthesised into the lumen of the endoplasmic reticulum.

Covalent bond: A chemical bond that involves the sharing of pairs of electrons between atoms.

Critical micelle concentration (CMC): The concentration above which a detergent will start to form micelles (temperature and possibly salt dependent).

Cuvette: A small square tube, sealed at one end, made of plastic glass or quartz (required for UV) designed to hold samples for spectrophotometric analysis.

Dalton (Da): The molecular mass of a compound relative to 1/12 the molecular weight of carbon (i.e., 1).

Dative bonds: See Co-ordinate bonds.

Denatured (conformation of proteins): The native conformation of a protein can be altered by changes in pH, temperature and the presence of detergents. The unravelled native conformation (biologically active) is denatured (biologically inactive).

Dielectric constant: The ability of a medium to reduce the force of attraction between two charged particles. Water has a large dielectric constant (80.4) which is able to weaken the attractive forces between anions and cations (e.g., $Na^+ Cl^-$) resulting in the salt dissolving in the water.

Dipole: A molecular dipole occurs due to the uneven distribution of electrons in an molecule.

DNase: An enzyme which cleaves DNA.

Dounce homogeniser: A homogeniser with a glass mortar and pestle.

E64: An inhibitor of some proteolytic enzymes (sulphydryl).

Electrophoresis: Describes the movement of a molecule under the influence of an electrical field in which the experiment is typically stopped before the sample contacts the electrode.

Empirical: Derived from experimentation, i.e., by trial and error rather than theoretical.

Enantiomer: A pair of chemically identical molecules that are mirror images of each other.

Endoplasmic reticulum: A specialized membranous organelle within eukaryotic cells responsible for the synthesis of many membrane proteins. In addition, the endoplasmic reticulum synthesises proteins exported by the cell as well as proteins to be directed to the lumens of other organelles.

Enzyme: A biological macromolecule (typically a protein but also some ribonucleic acids called ribozymes) that acts as a catalyst increasing the rate of reaction.

Eukaryotes: Organisms that are composed of one or more cells which contain a membrane enclosed nucleus and organelles (e.g., animal, plant, fungi, yeast and most algae).

Fc: The crystallisable portion of an immunoglobulin (the constant region) which is not involved in antigen binding.

Feedstock: The raw material used in an industrial process.

Fines: Chromatography resins can break down as a result of handling and usually float when the resin is resupended. If the fines are not removed, they could block the spaces around and in the resin which would result in high back pressure.

Free radical: A molecule with a reactive unpaired valency electron.

Fungicide: Chemical compounds used to prevent the growth of fungi.

Genome: The whole hereditary information of an organism that is encoded in the DNA including genes and non-coding regions. This can be fractionated to the nuclear genome and mitochondrial genome.

Glycosylation: The addition of saccharide residues to proteins and lipids (see O-linked, N-linked and GPI-linked saccharides).

Gravity: The natural force of attraction that exists between all bodies in the universe ($g = 981 cm s^{-2}$).

GPI-linked saccharides: An amphipathic molecule composed of phosphatidyl inositol, phosphate and sugar residues attached to the N-terminus of some membrane proteins.

Homogenate: Tissue (cell)/buffer mixture resulting from the action of a homogeniser.

Homogeniser: A laboratory machine that disrupts tissue (cells) by cutting, mixing and blending the starting material in a buffer.

Homogenous: When items in a group are similar.

Hydrodynamic volume: The volume of a macromolecule (e.g., protein) in solution. This volume can vary depending on the M_r of the macromolecule, its shape and its interaction with the solvent.

Hydrogen bond: When hydrogen is bonded to a very electronegative atom such as oxygen or nitrogen, the result is a dispersion of charge within the molecule with the oxygen (or nitrogen) side becoming slightly negative and the hydrogen side becoming slightly positive, creating a dipole. Hydrogen bonds exist throughout nature, giving water its unique properties. In a protein's structure, a weak attractive force can be established if these oppositely charged dipole molecules are in close proximity.

Hydronium ion: Water dissociates into a proton and a hydroxyl ion:

$$H_2O \leftrightarrow H^+ + OH^-$$

The proton associates with another water molecule to produce the hydronium ion (a protonated water molecule)

$$H_2O + H^+ \leftrightarrow H_3O^+$$

producing $H_2O \leftrightarrow H_3O^+ + OH^-$

The molar concentration of water is 55.5 and the concentration of H_3O^+ and OH^- at 25°C is 10^{-7} molar. This gives a pH (see definition of pH) of 7 for water and neutral solutions. In practice, because atmospheric CO_2 dissolves in water to produce the acidic bicarbonate ion HCO_3^- the pH of water is usually around pH 5.5.

Hydrophilic (water loving): A molecule or functional group which is hydrophilic will prefer to interact with water or other polar solvents.

Hydrophobic (water hating): A molecule or functional group which is hydrophobic will tend to avoid contact with water or other polar solvents.

Hygroscopic: A substance that readily attracts and retains water.

Hydrostatic pressure: The pressure a fluid exerts or transmits.

Immiscible: Incapable of mixing, e.g., oil and water.

Immunoglobulin (antibody): A protein produced by the lymphocytes which binds to a specific antigen.

Inclusion bodies: Small intracellular insoluble aggregates, usually occurring in bacteria that are used to express recombinant proteins.

Intermolecular: A property or interaction occurring between different molecules or macromolecules.

Intramolecular: A property or interaction occurring within a single molecule or macromolecule.

In situ: Literally means "in place", e.g., exactly where it occurs.

In vitro: Literally means "in glass", e.g., outside a living organism or cell.

In vivo: Literally means "in life", e.g., in a living organism or cell.

Isocratic: A chromatographic mobile phase of constant composition.

Isoelectric point (pI): The pH value when a molecule carries no net charge. The molecule will not move under the influence of an electrical field or bind to an ion exchange resin.

Isoenzymes (isozymes): Two or more forms of an enzyme that catalyse the same reaction but differ from each other in their physical properties, such as amino acid sequence, substrate affinity, V_{max}, tissue expression or regulatory properties.

I.U.: International Units of enzyme activity defined as 1μmol of product formed (or substrate consumed) min^{-1} at a given temperature (usually 25°C).

K_a: The equilibrium constant (association/dissociation constant).

Katal: S.I. unit of enzyme activity defined as 1 mol of product formed (or substrate consumed) sec^{-1} at a given temperature (usually 25°C).

K_{av}: The effective dissociation constant (K_D) in size exclusion chromatography.

K_D: The partition coefficient is a measure of the distribution of a compound between two immiscible phases.

K_m: The Michaelis–Menten constant, which is the substrate concentration which produces half the maximum rate in an enzyme catalysed reaction.

Lectins: Naturally produced proteins or glycoproteins (mainly from plants) that can bind with carbohydrates or sugars to form stable complexes.

Leupeptin: An inhibitor of some peptidase enzymes (serine like and some sulphydryl peptidases). See Chapter 2.

Ligand: A molecule that binds to a specific site on a protein.

Lipopolysaccharide (LPS): A molecule comprising both lipid and sugar residues.

Lysosomes: Organelles containing many digestive hydrolases present in animal cells.

Lysozyme: An enzyme which catalyses the hydrolysis of the β -1,4-glycosidic bonds. It can be used to break down the peptidoglycan complex surrounding Gram-positive bacteria.

Lyotropic salts: The opposite of chaotropic salts, in that they increase the structure of water and increase the "salting out" of proteins.

Microfuge: A bench top centrifuge used to centrifuge small volumes of samples contained in microfuge tubes.

Microfuge tube (Eppendorf tube): Small, cylindrical plastic containers with a conical bottom and a "snap shut" lid. Different size tubes are available for use in a microfuge.

Mitochondria: Organelles present in most eukaryotic cells; their primary function is to convert organic materials into energy in the form of ATP via the process of oxidative phosphorylation.

Mole: 1 mole of any compound is the molecular weight in gram and this contains 6.023×10^{23} molecules (Avogadro's number).

Molar: 1 mole of a compound dissolved in one litre (1000 ml) of water.

Molar absorption (absorptivity) coefficient (ε): Also known as the molar absorbance coefficient or incorrectly as the molar extinction coefficient. The absorbance of a molar solution of a compound in a 1cm path length of light at a given wavelength. The units are $(M^{-1}\,cm^{-1})$ of a compound at a given wavelength. The molar absorptivity coefficient for many compounds can be found in reference books.

For proteins, molar concentrations are not always appropriate and in this case, a 1% (w/v) percent absorptivity at a given wavelength is quoted (e.g., $\varepsilon^{1\%}$ at 280nm for bovine serum albumin = 6.67).

Molecular sieving: Polyacrylamide gels used for the electrophoresis of proteins are polymerised with a fixed pore size (e.g., 5% or 10% polyacrylamide gels). This pore size will allow molecules smaller than the pore to enter but will prevent larger molecules from entering the gel. A 10% polyacrylamide gel used in SDS-PAGE will fractionate polypeptides in the mass range 200,000 to 10,000. If a crude liver cell extract is applied to the gel, only the polypeptides in the 200,000 to 10,000 mass range will be visible on the gel after electrophoresis. Polypeptides with a mass larger than 200,000 will remain at the interface between the stacking gel and the resolving gel.

Monoclonal antibody: The antibodies produced by monoclonal cell cultures. The cell line is derived from one parent cell and the antibodies produced all target one epitope of the antigen.

M_r: The molecular mass of a compound relative to the molecular weight of hydrogen (i.e., 1).

Mutually exclusive: Two or more events that cannot occur simultaneously.

N-linked saccharides: Sugar's residues attached to the amino acid asparagine in a glycoprotein.

Native (conformation of proteins): Proteins are polymers of amino acids which eventually fold to form a compact three-dimensional structure. The shape of the protein may alter depending on the pH, but at the protein's normal resident pH value, the shape can be assumed to be its native conformation.

Nitrocellulose membrane: A form of cellulose membrane which effectively irreversibly binds proteins used in Western blotting.

Nomogram: A two-dimensional graphical calculating device which usually has three scales: two scales represent known values and the final scale is where the answer is read from.

Nucleus: A eukaryotic membrane-bound organelle which contains the majority of the cell's genetic material.

O-linked saccharide: Sugar's residues attached to the amino acids serine or threonine in a glycoprotein.

Orthogonal (chromatography): Separations based upon two or more different properties of molecules using chromatographic methods to resolve a complex mixture (e.g., ion exchange chromatography followed by reversed-phase chromatography).

Particulate: Small insoluble material which can block the pores (and spaces around the pores) of chromatographic resins, resulting in an increase in back pressure. They can be removed using a 0.2 μm membrane filter or by centrifugation at 13,000g for 20 minutes.

Pepstatin: An inhibitor of some proteolytic enzymes (acidic peptidases).

Peptidase: Enzymes which degrade proteins by cleaving the peptide bond, either from internal peptide bonds or the N- or the C-terminus of a protein. They are characterised by key amino acids or other properties required for catalysis, e.g., serine, threonine, cysteine, aspartate, glutamate or metal ions.

Peptidoglycan: A carbohydrate polymer cross-linked by proteins. Crystal-violet stains the peptidoglycan of the cell wall of Gram-positive bacteria.

Peroxisomes: Present in all eukaryotic cells whose role is to remove toxic substances from the cell.

pH: The negative $\log_{10}$ of the activity of hydrogen ions in solution, i.e., pH = $-\log_{10}(a_{H+})$ which is a measure of acidity. In dilute solutions, the activity of hydrogen ions approximates to the molar concentration (moles per litre) of hydrogen ions in solution, i.e., pH = $-\log_{10}[H^+]$.

$$[H^+] = 10^{-3} M (pH 3.0)$$
$$[H^+] = 10^{-7} M (pH 7.0)$$

Note: The logarithmic changes in acidity ($[H^+]$) are converted into a linear pH scale.

Phosphorylation: The addition of a phosphate monoester to a macromolecule, catalysed by a specific enzyme (kinase). Proteins can be phosphorylated on the amino acid side chains of serine, threonine and tyrosine (in addition, histidine may also be phosphorylated in both eukaryotic and prokaryotic cells). Phosphorylation can alter the conformation of a protein resulting in modulation of the protein's activity.

pKa: The negative $\log_{10}$ of the equilibrium constant (K_a), i.e., pKa = $-\log_{10} K_a$. It is a value where the acid and basic forms are in equal concentration.

Planar: This means that all the molecules are in one plane.

Plasma membrane: A phospholipid and protein bilayer approximately 6 nm thick which surrounds the cell. Separating the cellular components from the extracellular environment.

Polar: An uneven distribution of electrons resulting in a charge difference across the molecule.

Polyclonal antibodies: Antibodies raised to a protein in an animal which results in many different IgG molecules being produced against different parts of the protein.

Polysaccharide: A chain of many saccharide units covalently linked together to form a polymer.

Posttranslational modification (of a protein): An alteration of a protein's structure after the protein has been synthesised on a ribosome. The modification can be an addition (e.g., phosphate or sugar) or the removal peptide fragment from the protein's structure. These modifications can activate or moderate a protein's biological role.

Potable: Water that is safe to drink or use for cooking.

Potter–Elvehjem homogeniser: A homogeniser with a glass mortar and a Teflon pestle which can be rotated by hand or machine.

Prokaryotes: Unicellular organisms which do not have a membrane-enclosed nucleus or organelles (e.g., bacteria).

Protein A: A protein (M_r 42,000) found naturally in the cell wall of *Staphylococcus aureus* which binds to the Fc domain of immunoglobulins. The interaction is species and immunoglobulin dependent.

Protein G: A protein (M_r 30–35,000) found naturally in the cell wall of β -haemolytic *Streptococci* C or G strains which binds to the Fc region of immunoglobulins. Antibodies from different species which do not bind well to protein A may bind to protein G.

Proteome: The complete set of proteins encoded by the genome.

Racemate: An equal mixture of enantiomeric isomers.

Radian: 1 radian is the angle subtended at the centre of a circle by an arc with an equal length to the radius of the circle. One revolution of a centrifuge rotor is equivalent to $360^\circ = 2\pi$ radians.

Reducing agents: A substance that chemically reduces other substances, especially by donating an electron or electrons.

R_f (retention factor): The mobility of the standards/samples relative to the dye front (a value between 0 and 1.0).

Resolving gel: A polyacrylamide gel (typically 7.5%, 10% or 12% acrylamide) used to separate complex protein mixture.

Ribosomes: A large complex of proteins and nucleic acids that function to manufacture proteins from mRNA.

Saccharide: A carbohydrate molecule.

Salt bridge (salt bond, ionic bond): Forms as a result of the attractive force between two oppositely charged side chains in a protein's structure. Although relatively weak, they contribute to the stability of a protein's tertiary structure.

Salting out (of proteins): A method of separating proteins of differential solubility in high salt (ionic) concentrations. The salt concentration needed for a protein to precipitate out of the solution differs from protein to protein.

Salting in (of proteins): Most proteins show increased solubility at low salt (ionic) concentrations.

Sephacryl: A trade name (GE Healthcare) for covalently cross-linked allyl dextrose gel formed into beads used for protein purification.

Sephadex: A trade name (GE Healthcare) for cross-linked dextran gel formed into beads used in protein purification.

Sepharose: A trade name (GE Healthcare) for agarose beads (charged polysaccharides removed) used in protein purification.

Silanising: Conversion of active silanol (SiOH) groups on the surface of glass into the less polar silyl ethers (SiOR) groups. This makes the glass surface less adhesive to proteins.

Slurry: A liquid and resin mixture which flows freely.

Solute: A reagent (e.g., sodium chloride) dissolved in a solvent (e.g., water). This applies equally to hydrophobic reagents where the reagent (e.g., flavonoid) is dissolved in an appropriate solvent (e.g., methanol).

Sonication: A method of disrupting biological material by the energy in sound waves.

Stacking gel: A polyacrylamide gel (typically 3–5% acrylamide) which is layered over the resolving gel. In combination with discontinuous buffers, the stacking gel concentrates the sample before it enters the resolving gel.

Stereoisomer: Two molecules with the same atoms arranged differently in space.

Stereospecific: (As in enzymes active site.) The three-dimensional arrangement of atoms in an enzymes active site can accommodate the structure of only one stereoisomer of the enzyme's substrate (e.g. L-amino acids).

Sublimation (of an element or substance): The conversion from the solid phase to the gas phase without entering the liquid phase. This forms the basis of freeze drying.

Substrate: A molecule that an enzyme binds and acts upon.

Superdex: A trade name (GE Healthcare) for size exclusion media to be used in protein purification with high resolving power.

Tetramer: A polymer consisting of four monomers e.g. haemoglobin tetramer alpha2beta2.

Thiol: A compound containing a functional group composed of a sulphur atom and a hydrogen atom (-SH).

Theoretical plates (in chromatography): The height of the theoretical plate is the length in a chromatography column which is the equivalent of a single equilibrium taking place in the immiscible phases (mobile and stationary phases) of the column. The separating power of a chromatography column can be given by the number of theoretical plates.

van der Waals: A weak intermolecular force arising from the polarisation of molecules into dipoles.

Viscosity: A measure of the resistance of a fluid to deform under stress. It can be thought of as a measure of how easy it is to pour a liquid, i.e., water possesses a lower viscosity than vegetable oil.

V_{max}: The maximum rate of an enzyme catalysed reaction.

Zwitterionic: A molecule with both acidic and basic residues, e.g., amino acids.

Index

Page numbers followed by f and t indicate figures and tables, respectively.

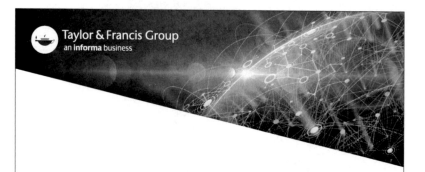

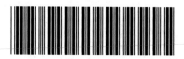